N. Brill

Cash's Textbook of Chest, Heart and Vascular Disorders for Physiotherapists

other books in the series edited by Joan E. Cash

A TEXTBOOK OF MEDICAL CONDITIONS FOR
PHYSIOTHERAPISTS

PHYSIOTHERAPY IN SOME SURGICAL CONDITIONS

NEUROLOGY FOR PHYSIOTHERAPISTS

by Patricia A. Downie

CANCER REHABILITATION
An Introduction for Physiotherapists and
the Allied Professions

CASH'S TEXTBOOK OF CHEST, HEART AND VASCULAR DISORDERS FOR PHYSIOTHERAPISTS

edited by
PATRICIA A. DOWNIE F.C.S.P.

FABER & FABER · London and Boston

First published in 1975
by Faber and Faber Limited
3 Queen Square London WC1
Reprinted 1975 and 1977
Second edition 1979
Printed in Great Britain by
Cox & Wyman Ltd,
London, Fakenham and Reading
All rights reserved

British Library Cataloguing in Publication Data

Cash's textbook of chest, heart and vascular
    disorders for physiotherapists. – 2nd ed.
    1. Cardiovascular system – Diseases
    2. Respiratory organs – Diseases 3. Physical therapy
    I. Cash, Joan Elizabeth II. Downie, Patricia A
    III. Chest, heart and vascular disorders for
    physiotherapists IV. Textbook of chest, heart
    and vascular disorders for physiotherapists
    616.1'062   RC669

ISBN 0–571–04979–6

Contents

Illustrations

PLATES

FIGURES

List of Contributors

C. R. BANNISTER ESQ., M.C.S.P.
Assistant Superintendent Physiotherapist
St. Mary's Hospital, Harrow Road, London W9 3RL

MISS E. A. BEAZLEY, M.C.S.P., DIP.T.P.
Assistant Principal, School of Physiotherapy
St. Mary's Hospital, London W2 1NY

R. BOURNE ESQ., F.R.C.S.
Senior Surgical Registrar
Queen Mary's Hospital, Roehampton, London SW15

MRS. S. E. BROWN, M.C.S.P.
Assistant Superintendent Physiotherapist
Manchester Royal Infirmary, Manchester M13 9WL

DR. L. H. CAPEL, M.D., F.R.C.P.
Physician
The London Chest Hospital, London E2 9JX

MISS D. V. GASKELL, M.C.S.P.
Group Superintendent Physiotherapist
The National Heart and Chest Hospitals
The Brompton Hospital, Fulham Road, London SW3 6HP

MISS D. M. INNOCENTI, M.C.S.P.
Superintendent Physiotherapist
Guy's Hospital, London SE1 9RT

MRS. P. McCOY, M.C.S.P.
Senior Physiotherapist
Coronary Care Unit, Ulster Hospital
Dundonald, Belfast BT16 0RH

J. R. PEPPER ESQ., M.A., F.R.C.S.
Senior Registrar, Thoracic Unit
Guy's Hospital, London SE1 9RT

MISS J. PICKERING, M.C.S.P.
Senior Physiotherapist
Charing Cross Hospital, Fulham Palace Road, London W6 8RF

MISS P. J. WADDINGTON, M.C.S.P., H.T., DIP.T.P.
Principal, School of Physiotherapy
The United Manchester Hospitals
Manchester Royal Infirmary, Manchester M13 9WL

Preface to the Second Edition

In this new edition, I have used the foundations of Joan Cash's first edition upon which to build and develop. A textbook can never lay down an infallible method, technique or approach, nor can it ever cover, even partially, such a large subject as this title. It is built upon principles; where treatments are described the reader must remember that they are only one among various methods, but are included in order to demonstrate the principles. This is particularly so with intensive care, where it is necessary for the physiotherapist to work closely with nurses and doctors; the role of the physiotherapist will vary from unit to unit, and she must be very certain what she can or cannot do. The chapter on Auscultation was requested by many physiotherapists both in the United Kingdom and overseas; I hope it will fulfil a need. The final chapter, on the practical understanding of Lung Function Tests, has been included so that physiotherapists may be given a clinical introduction to lung function in health and illness. For both these chapters I am indebted to Dr. L. H. Capel of the London Chest Hospital.

References and bibliography have been kept to those journals and books which are most easily available; I hope that you will use them and in so doing will be stimulated to look for more. Knowledge is never wasted if it is properly applied. For the physiotherapist, this means in a practical manner to a sick person. Physiotherapy for patients suffering from any of the diseases particularly mentioned in this book must be practical and coupled with understanding. You will need to learn to adapt your treatments to every situation, remembering always that each patient is a unique person who will react and respond differently.

I offer my grateful thanks to all the contributors. I am particularly grateful to the three doctors who accepted my invitation to contribute with enthusiasm. The physiotherapist should work in partnership with the doctor and nurse, and these three medical contributors have adequately demonstrated their belief in this.

Finally, I thank Audrey Besterman for her skill in turning rough, and sometimes odd, diagrams into superb line drawings.

As editor, I would welcome suggestions and constructive criticisms from both student and staff physiotherapists. These books are meant for YOU; unless you write to me, I cannot divine what other aspects you would like covered!

P.A.D.
London 1979

Chapter 1

Basic Anatomy of the Cardio-Thoracic and Vascular Systems

by P. J. WADDINGTON, M.C.S.P., H.T., DIP.T.P.

THE THORACIC CAVITY

The thoracic cage is formed by a bony framework consisting of the twelve thoracic vertebrae, twelve pairs of ribs and their costal cartilages and the sternum.

The thorax is kidney-shaped in cross-section because the ribs extend backwards beyond the plane of the vertebral column before arching forwards. The most posterior part of each rib, the angle, can be identified by an oblique ridge on the external surface. From the angle the rib is directed obliquely downwards and forwards. The degree of this obliquity increases progressively from the first to the ninth rib inclusive, after which the tendency is reversed. The seventh rib is the longest.

Posteriorly the head of a typical rib articulates with demi-facets on the bodies of its numerically equal thoracic vertebra and the one above, as well as with the intervening intervertebral disc, to form a synovial plane joint. The first, tenth, eleventh and twelfth ribs are atypical in articulating with the body of only one vertebra. The tubercles of the upper ten ribs also articulate with the transverse processes of their numerically equal vertebrae forming synovial plane joints.

Anteriorly, of the twelve pairs of ribs the first seven articulate with the sternum and are called vertebrosternal or true ribs. The costal cartilage of the first rib is joined directly to the sternum, forming a synchondrosis, whereas the costal cartilages of the other true ribs form synovial joints with the sternum. The eighth, ninth and tenth ribs articulate with the costal cartilage of the rib above and are called vertebrochondral ribs; the last two pairs are free and are tipped with costal cartilage. They are called vertebral or floating ribs. The lower five pairs together as a group are called false ribs.

The sternum has three parts, from above downwards, the manubrium sterni, the corpus sterni or body and the small xiphoid process. The first costal cartilage articulates with the manubrium. The second articulates at the sternal angle or manubriosternal junction which is easily palpable through the skin as a ridge and is the most reliable point from which to identify the ribs and their costal cartilages. The remaining true ribs articulate with the body of the sternum, the last two (sixth and seventh) with its inferior border.

The gaps between adjacent ribs, or the intercostal spaces, are filled by the intercostal muscles. These are arranged in three layers like the flat muscles of the abdominal wall and their fibres follow a similar direction. Contraction of these muscles effects rib movement and prevents indrawing and bulging of the intercostal spaces due to changes of intrathoracic pressure during inspiration and expiration. The thoracic vessels and nerves are segmental in distribution and follow the line of each rib, lying between the middle and innermost layers of the intercostal muscles and membranes.

The thoracic inlet or upper opening of the thorax is formed by the body of the first thoracic vertebra, the first pair of ribs and their costal cartilages and the upper part of the manubrium sterni. It measures approximately 5cm in an anteroposterior direction and 10cm transversely.

The thoracic outlet or lower boundary of the thorax is formed by the body of the twelfth thoracic vertebra, the last pair of ribs, the lower six costal cartilages and the xiphoid process.

The thoracic cavity is divided from the abdominal cavity by a dome-shaped sheet of muscle and fibrous tissue, the diaphragm. The muscle fibres of this take origin from the perimeter of the thoracic outlet and converge to be inserted into a thin trefoil-shaped aponeurosis, the central tendon, which lies just below the pericardium and blends with it. When relaxed the diaphragm at its highest point rises to the level of the fifth and sixth ribs, being slightly higher on the right than on the left. It will be seen that as well as protecting the contents of the thorax itself, the thoracic cage protects the upper abdominal viscera, i.e. the liver, the stomach and the spleen.

The thoracic cavity is divided into three parts, the right and left pleural cavities and the region in between which is called the mediastinum (see p. 32).

THE RESPIRATORY SYSTEM

The Pleura

Each pleura consists of two layers which are continuous with each other. The lung is surrounded by it rather as if a clenched fist were pressed into a partially inflated balloon. The wrist represents the root of the lung which is formed by structures entering or leaving the lung at the hilum (the area on the mediastinal surface of the lung through which structures enter and leave the lung), that is the bronchus, the pulmonary artery and the two pulmonary veins, the bronchial arteries and veins and the pulmonary plexus of nerves and lymph vessels.

The outer layer or parietal pleura lines the thoracic cavity and is attached to it. The inner visceral layer or pulmonary pleura covers the entire surface of the lungs entering into the fissures and covering the inter-lobar surfaces. The two layers lie one against the other and are lubricated by a thin layer of pleural fluid.

During inspiration the thoracic cage lined by the parietal pleura is enlarged, the lungs covered by the pulmonary pleura expand and air enters. Therefore as inspiration is followed by expiration and so on, there is a continuous sliding of the pulmonary pleura on the parietal pleura.

The parietal pleura is named according to the structures which it covers, thus, the costal pleura covers the ribs, the diaphragmatic pleura the diaphragm, and the mediastinal pleura the mediastinum, starting at the root of the lung. The part of the pleura from the root of the lung extending almost to the diaphragm is called the pulmonary ligament. The cervical pleura extends into the neck through the thoracic inlet.

The Lungs

The lungs occupying the pleural cavities are not identical in size and shape. The left lung is slightly smaller because the heart and pericardium lie more to the left of mid-line than to the right: this modification in the shape of the left lung which accommodates the heart is called the cardiac notch. The right lung, although it is the larger, is slightly shorter because the dome of the diaphragm is slightly raised on that side.

Each lung is divided into two by an oblique fissure which extends into the lung almost as far as the hilum. A line drawn from the third thoracic vertebra posteriorly to the sixth costochondral junction, at which level it reaches the lower border of the lungs, represents the surface marking of the oblique fissure. The part of the lung below this fissure is called the lower lobe. Above the oblique fissure the right lung is divided again by a horizontal fissure extending forwards from the oblique fissure in the axillary line to the fourth costal cartilage (see Fig. 1/1). Thus an upper lobe is formed above the horizontal fissure and a middle lobe is formed below. The left lung is not sub-divided in this way and the whole section is called the upper lobe. The antero-inferior part of the left upper lobe (equivalent to the middle lobe on the right) is called the lingula.

Thus each lower lobe forms the base and the posterior portion of the entire lung and each upper or upper and middle lobes comprise the apex and anterior portion.

The lungs are of a spongy consistency and would be pink in colour were it not for atmospheric pollution.

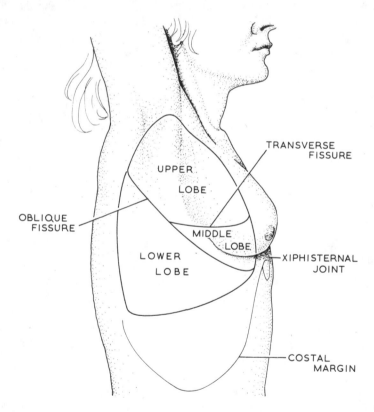

Fig. 1/1   Surface projection of the fissures and lobes of the right lung

THE RESPIRATORY PASSAGES

The respiratory passages, which carry air from the atmosphere to the alveoli, consist of the nose and mouth, the pharynx, the larynx, the trachea and the two main bronchi and their branches within the lungs. It is essential that these should remain open; they are therefore supported by either bone or cartilage as far as the bronchioles (see Fig. 1/2).

The Nose

The nose is divided into two cavities by the nasal septum, formed of thin bone (vomer and ethmoid) and cartilage. The base is provided by the hard palate and the roof mainly by the cribriform plate of the ethmoid bone. The lateral walls are undulating, being crossed in a horizontal direction by three pieces of bone, like the crests of waves, the superior, middle and inferior conchae, which are separated from each other by troughs, the superior, middle and inferior meatuses. The paranasal sinuses, the frontal, maxillary, ethmoidal and sphenoidal, lie within the bones of the skull and open into the lateral wall of each nasal cavity. The nasal cavities and the air sinuses are lined with columnar ciliated epithelium. Anteriorly, where the nasal cavities are open to the atmosphere, lie the nostrils protected by bristle-like hairs. Posteriorly each nasal cavity opens into the pharynx. The opening is called the posterior naris and measures approximately 2·5cm (vertically) by 1·25cm (horizontally).

The Pharynx

The pharynx is a fibromuscular funnel-shaped cavity about 15cm long. It is divided into three parts.

THE NASOPHARYNX

This lies behind the nasal cavities. The roof is formed by bones of the skull. It lies above the soft palate which divides it from the other parts of the pharynx during swallowing. The auditory or Eustachian tubes open one into each side of the nasopharynx, connecting it with the tympanic cavities. This regulates the air pressure on the two sides of the tympanic membranes.

THE OROPHARYNX

This lies behind the mouth, below the soft palate and extends as far down as the larynx.

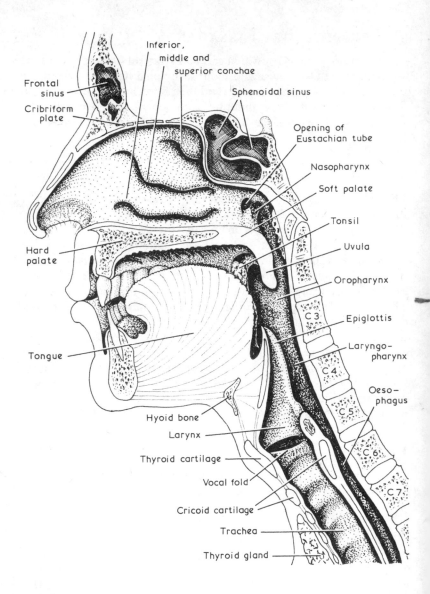

Fig. 1/2   A sagittal section through the nasal and oral cavities, pharynx and larynx

The tonsils are two masses of lymphoid tissue lying in the lateral walls of the oropharynx. They form part of a circular band of lymphoid tissue which acts as a filter, protecting the respiratory tract against infection.

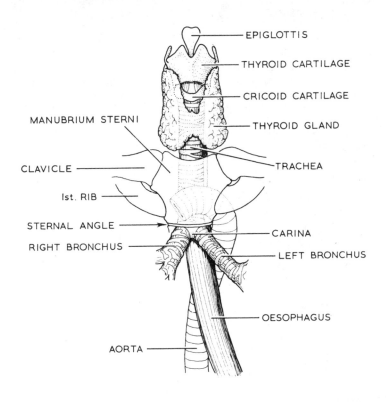

Fig. 1/3   The trachea showing its main relations

THE LARYNGOPHARYNX

This lies behind the larynx.

Air enters the nose, passes into the nasopharynx and from there through the oropharynx and finally into the upper part of the larynx and trachea. These upper respiratory pathways have three important functions: filtering and humidifying the inspired air and, if necessary, raising its temperature to body temperature.

This region has a very rich blood supply.

	Right Lung		*Left Lung*
Upper Lobe {	1. Apical	Upper Lobe {	1. } Apico-posterior
	2. Posterior		2.
	3. Anterior		3. Anterior
Middle Lobe {	4. Lateral		4. Superior } Lingular
	5. Medial		5. Inferior

	Right Lung		*Left Lung*
Lower Lobe {	6. Apical	Lower Lobe {	6. Apical
	7. Medial basal		7. —
	8. Anterior basal		8. Anterior basal
	9. Lateral basal		9. Lateral basal
	10. Posterior basal		10. Posterior basal

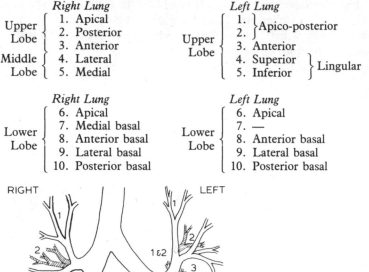

Fig. 1/4 Diagrams to illustrate the bronchial tree and to show the bronchopulmonary nomenclature as approved by the Thoracic Society

The Larynx

The larynx extends from the level of the third cervical vertebra to the lower border of the sixth cervical vertebra and lies between the pharynx above and the trachea below. The shape of the larynx is maintained by two hyaline and elastic cartilages, the thyroid and the cricoid. The thyroid cartilage or Adam's apple consists of two laminae which are fused together anteriorly in mid-line. The cricoid cartilage forms the only complete ring of cartilage, being wider posteriorly than anteriorly. It lies below the thyroid cartilage which fits over it to form two synovial joints. The arytenoid cartilages are two small pyramidal structures which lie interiorly and articulate with the upper posterior border of the cricoid cartilage. The paired vocal cords extend between them and the angle of the thyroid cartilage.

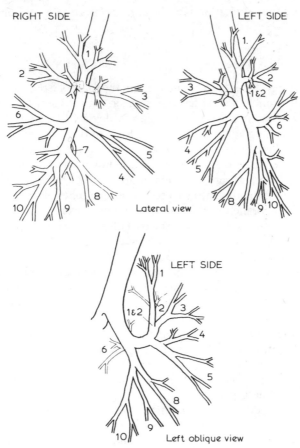

RIGHT SIDE / LEFT SIDE

Lateral view

LEFT SIDE

Left oblique view

The epiglottis lies just above the vocal cords and is shaped like a leaf. It may serve to direct food and liquids into the oesophagus.

The Trachea

The trachea is a tube about 12cm long extending from the cricoid cartilage of the larynx (C.6) to the sternal angle (T.5) where it bifurcates to form the right and left main bronchi. It passes down in an oblique direction, its upper end in the neck being just below the skin and its lower end being adjacent to the vertebral column in the thorax. The framework of the trachea is provided by sixteen to twenty C-shaped pieces of cartilage. The circle is completed posteriorly by smooth involuntary muscle and the cartilages are joined together by fibro-elastic tissue. The cartilage at the bifurcation is shaped to support it and the bifurcation is frequently referred to as the carina (see Fig. 1/3).

The Bronchial Tree

The cartilages of the main bronchi are in the form of irregular plaques. The right bronchus is wider and shorter than the left and is nearly vertical in direction, being only slightly deviated to the right. After entering the lung at the hilum it divides into three branches, one for each of the three lobes. The left main bronchus is longer than the right and is directed more obliquely, passing below the arch of the aorta and in front of the oesophagus and descending aorta. On entering the lung at the hilum it divides into two to supply the lobes of the left lung.

Each lobar branch divides into segmental bronchi and each segmental bronchus together with the part of the lung it supplies is called a bronchopulmonary segment. The segments have both names and numbers (see Figs. 1/4 and 1/5).

These segments can be identified on the surface of the lung and the direction of each segmental bronchus is known although there are variations from the norm. This knowledge is the basis for postural drainage of the lungs (see Chapter 11).

It will be noted that the segments are named according to their position but it should always be borne in mind that the lung is divided by an oblique fissure. Thus the apex of the lower lobe reaches as high as T.3 and lies posterior to be on a level with the posterior and anterior segments of the upper lobe.

Branching of the bronchial tree continues and the diameter of the lumen decreases until at about 0·2mm the tube is known as a bronchiole. Still further branching takes place until the terminal bronchioles are reached. The bronchial tree down to this level has relatively thick walls containing irregular plates of hyaline cartilage. It is lined by ciliated epithelium. The main control of the airway diameter is exerted by circular muscle fibres in the smaller and terminal bronchioles. The bronchioles are prevented from collapsing by the radial traction of the adjacent lung tissue.

The terminal bronchiole is followed by a thin-walled tube, the respiratory bronchiole (see Fig. 1/6).

Alveoli

Leading from the respiratory bronchiole are the alveolar ducts. Each one opens into a large central area, the alveolar sac, around the periphery of which lie the alveoli or air saccules. The cavities are lined

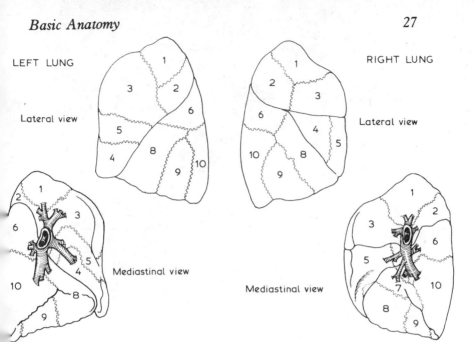

Fig. 1/5(a) Left bronchopulmonary segments

Fig. 1/5(b) Right bronchopulmonary segments

with simple flat epithelium which is in contact with the pulmonary capillary network. At this level gaseous exchange takes place.

COLLATERAL AIR DRIFT

Air can pass between adjacent alveoli through the pores of Kohn unless they are separated by septa, and Lambert has described accessory communications between some bronchioles and adjacent alveoli. This passage of air is called collateral ventilation or collateral air drift.

Blood Supply and Nerve Supply

The bronchial arteries which are branches of the aorta supply the bronchial tree itself and the visceral pleura. The bronchial veins drain into the azygos system.

The pulmonary arteries convey deoxygenated blood to the lungs from the right ventricle and the pulmonary veins (two for each lung) convey oxygenated blood from the capillary network to the left atrium of the heart.

The nerve supply is provided by the autonomic system.

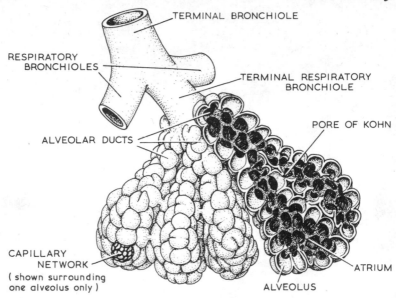

Fig. 1/6   A bronchiole showing the conducting and respiratory parts of the lungs

MECHANISM OF RESPIRATION

Inspiration

IN QUIET INSPIRATION

1. The thoracic inlet remains at rest.
2. The second to seventh true ribs rotate in two directions:

a) About the sternovertebral axis. This is called the 'bucket handle' action. Thus the transverse diameter of the thorax is increased and the subcostal angle widened.

b) About the costovertebral joint in a 'pump handle' fashion so that the anterior end moves upwards increasing the anteroposterior thoracic diameter.

3. The muscle fibres of the diaphragm contract. The upper abdominal viscera are compressed and the abdominal muscles relax to accommodate them. Thus the vertical diameter of the thorax is increased.

On slightly deeper inspiration the diaphragm cannot compress the viscera further and the central tendon becomes the fixed point at the level of T.9. Further contraction of the diaphragmatic muscle fibres causes the lower ribs to rise and the body of the sternum to move forwards. Some authorities doubt this and think that this is probably an integrated activity no matter what degree of diaphragmatic contraction occurs.

As can be seen in Fig. 1/7, when the diaphragm contracts A tends to move up because of rib anatomy. This widens the thorax. Simultaneously B moves down and increases the vertical diameter.

IN DEEP INSPIRATION

The scalene muscles and the sternal head of sternomastoid come into action to raise the first and second ribs, and all the intercostal muscles which aid inspiration are brought into action.

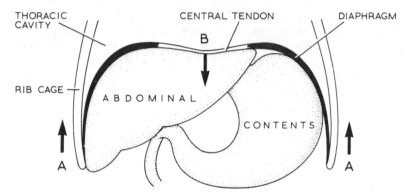

Fig. 1/7   Diagram to show diaphragmatic contraction

FORCED INSPIRATION

This occurs during periods of respiratory distress. Inspiration is increased by the use of pectoralis minor and perhaps pectoralis major and serratus anterior which can be brought into action by fixing the scapula. This is usually done by fixing the whole of the upper limb by gripping something suitably stable, for example a table.

Trapezius, levator scapulae and the rhomboids may also take part if the head and neck are fixed by the necessary muscles.

The scaleni and the sternal head of sternomastoid together with the muscles mentioned under forced inspiration are referred to as accessory muscles of respiration.

Expiration

Normal quiet expiration is due to the elastic recoil of the tissues. Forced expiration is brought about by contraction of the abdominal muscles and latissimus dorsi and in extreme cases by pressure of the arms upon the chest wall.

Coughing

This is a reflex action brought about by stimulation of the sensory nerves present in the larynx or trachea. It may also be caused by stimulation of the afferent nerve endings in the lungs or pleura. All these afferent nerve endings are supplied by the vagus nerve. A short but deep inspiration is followed by closure of the vocal cords. There is a forced expiratory effort which, because of the closed larynx, results in a build-up of high pressure within the lungs and bronchial tree. Suddenly, the vocal cords open and the air thus released escapes with an explosive force carrying with it anything lying in the respiratory passages. Sometimes the air flows at a rate of 70 miles per hour.

Sneezing is a similar mechanism and is caused by irritation of the membranes of the nose. Variations in the position of the soft palate allow the rapid flow of air through the nose and mouth, clearing the nasal pathways.

SURFACE MARKING

Larynx

Third cervical vertebra to lower border of sixth cervical vertebra.

Trachea

Sixth cervical vertebra to sternal angle or fourth to fifth thoracic vertebra. (The sternum articulates with the second costal cartilage at the sternal angle.)

Pleura

Apex 3cm (approx.) above the clavicle beneath the clavicular head of sternomastoid.

A line joining the following points gives the outline.

1. Sternoclavicular joint.
2. Right and left converge to the sternal angle and meet just to the left of mid-line.
3. Vertically down to the level of the fourth chondrosternal junction.
4. Right continues obliquely to the sixth or seventh chondrosternal junction.

Left passes outwards and downwards behind the costal cartilages of fifth, sixth, seventh and eighth ribs.

5. Both right and left pass laterally
    a) eighth costal cartilage – lateral vertical line.
    b) tenth rib   – mid-axillary line.
    c) eleventh rib   – in line with inferior angle of scapula.
    d) twelfth vertebrocostal joint.
6. Otherwise the pleura follows the walls of the thoracic cavity.

Lungs

1. Root – Posterior aspect of the thorax at the level of the fifth and sixth ribs halfway between the medial border of the scapula and the spinous processes.
2. Apex – Above the clavicle beneath the clavicular head of sternomastoid.
3. Sternal angle.
4. Right lung. A line joining the following points:
    a) passes vertically down to the sixth or seventh chondrosternal junction.
    b) sixth costal cartilage – lateral vertical line.
    c) eighth rib   – mid-axillary line.

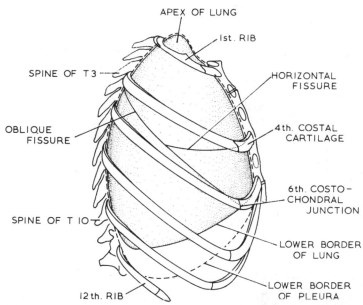

APEX OF LUNG

1st. RIB

SPINE OF T3

HORIZONTAL FISSURE

OBLIQUE FISSURE

4th. COSTAL CARTILAGE

6th. COSTO–CHONDRAL JUNCTION

SPINE OF T 10

LOWER BORDER OF LUNG

12th. RIB

LOWER BORDER OF PLEURA

Fig. 1/8   Diagram to show the lobes and fissures of the lungs and pleura related to the thoracic cage

    d) tenth rib   – line of inferior angle of scapula.
    e) tenth thoracic spine.
5. Left lung. A line joining the following points:
    a) lies behind the left border of the sternum to the fourth chondrosternal junction.
    b) passes outwards along the fourth costal cartilage.
    c) curves down to the sixth costal cartilage.
    d) follows line described for the right lung.
6. Fissures – Oblique fissure on the right and left from the spine of the third thoracic vertebra posteriorly to the sixth costochondral junction anteriorly.

         – Horizontal fissure on the right from the oblique fissure in the mid-axillary line to the fourth costal cartilage anteriorly (see Fig. 1/8).

Diaphragm

Levels vary with the position of the body. The diaphragm takes origin from the margins of the thoracic outlet and rises to the central tendon on each side of which it has a rounded cupola below the lungs and is depressed slightly in the middle.

	Anterior	*Posterior*
Median Portion	Xiphisternal joint	Body T.9. Spine T.8
Right Cupola	fifth rib 1–2cm below right nipple	1–2cm below inferior angle of scapula

	Anterior	*Posterior*
Left Cupola	fifth interspace or sixth rib 2·5cm below left nipple	2·5cm below the inferior angle of scapula

Chest Measurement Levels

1. Fourth costal cartilage.
2. Xiphoid process.
3. Ninth costal cartilage (anterior extremity).

THE MEDIASTINUM

The space in the centre of the thoracic cavity between the pleural sacs is called the mediastinum. On either side, it is balanced by the mediastinal pleura and extends from the thoracic inlet above to the diaphragm below and from the sternum anteriorly to the bodies of the thoracic vertebrae posteriorly. For ease of description, the mediastinum is divided into two parts by a horizontal plane joining the sternal angle (second costal cartilage) to the lower border of the body of the fourth thoracic vertebra. The superior mediastinum lies above and the inferior mediastinum below this imaginary plane (see Fig. 1/9).

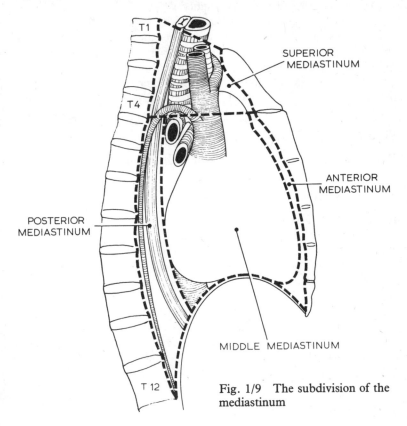

Fig. 1/9   The subdivision of the mediastinum

The main structures contained in the superior mediastinum are, the aortic arch and its three branches, the brachiocephalic, the left common carotid and left subclavian arteries; the brachiocephalic veins, the upper half of the superior vena cava; the phrenic, vagus and left recurrent laryngeal nerves; the trachea, the oesophagus, the thoracic duct and some lymph nodes.

The inferior mediastinum is subdivided into anterior, middle and posterior parts.

The anterior mediastinum lies between the pericardium posteriorly and the body of the sternum anteriorly. It contains fatty tissue and two or three lymph nodes.

The posterior mediastinum is bounded anteriorly by the pericardium and the diaphragm, and posteriorly by the lower eight thoracic vertebrae. It contains the descending thoracic aorta, the azygos and hemiazygos veins, sympathetic and vagus nerves, the thoracic duct and lymph nodes and the oesophagus.

The middle mediastinum is bounded by the other three divisions and contains the heart and pericardium, the ascending aorta, the lower half of the superior vena cava and part of the azygos vein, the bifurcation of the trachea and the two bronchi, the pulmonary arteries, the pulmonary veins, the phrenic nerves and some lymph nodes.

THE CARDIOVASCULAR SYSTEM

The cardiovascular system consists of the heart and the blood vessels.

The Pericardium

The heart and the roots of the great vessels lie in the middle mediastinum enclosed within a fibroserous sac, the pericardium. The outer fibrous layer of the pericardium is cone shaped, the apex blending with the external coat of the great vessels close to the heart and the inferior surface or base fusing with the central tendon of the diaphragm.

The inner serous pericardium is a double layered sac which lines the fibrous sac and covers the heart. The visceral surface, which covers the heart, is separated from the parietal layer, which lines the fibrous sac, by a thin layer of fluid. This allows the heart to move freely within the pericardium.

THE HEART

The heart is a hollow muscular organ the function of which is to act as a pump. It is cone shaped and lies obliquely in the middle mediastinum of the thorax, one-third to the right and two-thirds to the left of the median plane. The base faces backwards and to the right and the apex downwards, forwards and to the left. On average the heart is approximately the size of a clenched fist.

There are four chambers in the heart, the right and left atria and the right and left ventricles. The right atrium lies in front of the left and to the right of the right ventricle, which itself lies in front of the left

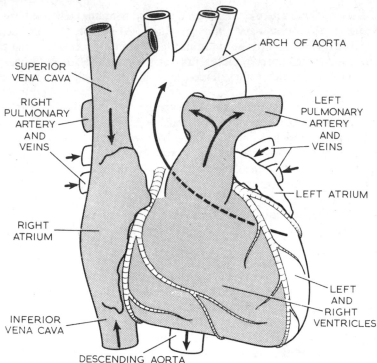

SUPERIOR
VENA CAVA

RIGHT
PULMONARY
ARTERY
AND
VEINS

RIGHT
ATRIUM

INFERIOR
VENA CAVA

DESCENDING AORTA

ARCH OF AORTA

LEFT
PULMONARY
ARTERY
AND
VEINS

LEFT ATRIUM

LEFT
AND
RIGHT
VENTRICLES

Fig. 1/10   The heart and great vessels – a diagram of the anterior view

ventricle, the most muscular chamber (see Fig. 1/10). The apex of the heart is formed by the left ventricle.

The right and left atria are separated from each other by the interatrial or atrial septum and the right ventricle is separated from the left ventricle by the interventricular or ventricular septum. The atria and ventricles are separated from each other by a fibrous septum.

The superior vena cava opens into the upper part of the right atrium. It carries blood from the upper half of the body; beginning at the level of the first right costal cartilage adjacent to the sternum, the superior vena cava ends opposite to the third right costal cartilage. It is formed by the junction of the two brachiocephalic veins. The inferior vena cava, which carries blood from below the diaphragm, is formed by the junction of the common iliac veins. It ascends on the right of the vertebral bodies and enters the mediastinum by passing through the diaphragm level with the lower border of the eighth thoracic vertebra. The inferior vena cava continues upwards and after piercing the pericardium enters the lower part of the right atrium.

The pulmonary trunk, which carries blood from the right ventricle, begins at the pulmonary valve. At the level of the fifth thoracic vertebra it divides into the right and left pulmonary arteries each of which enters the corresponding lung at the hilum. Four pulmonary veins, two from each lung, pierce the pericardium and open into the left atrium.

The blood leaves the left ventricle via the aorta which begins at the aortic valve. The aorta ascends towards the manubrium and passes over the left bronchus before arching backwards towards the body of the fourth thoracic vertebra. The arch of the aorta connects the ascending aorta with the descending aorta which begins at the lower border of the fourth thoracic vertebra. Branches from the aorta supply the heart (coronary arteries), the lungs (bronchial arteries) and the whole of the systemic circulation.

The Valves

Each ventricle has two valves, an inlet and an outlet valve, which control the direction of the flow of blood through the heart. These valves lie on the same oblique plane, in the fibrous septum between the atria and the ventricles (see Fig. 1/11). The atrioventricular valves allow the blood to flow from the atria into the ventricles; the valve on the right side of the heart is called the tricuspid valve and that on the left the mitral or bicuspid valve. The outlet or semilunar valves are the pulmonary valve for the right ventricle and the aortic valve for the left. All the valves have three cusps except the mitral which has two. They are formed by duplication of the endocardium strengthened by fibrous tissue and a few muscle fibres (see Fig. 1/12).

Although the valve mechanism is complex the principle is simple. The valve cusps, which are passive structures, respond to variations in the pressure gradients of the blood flow by floating together and separating again. When the blood is flowing forwards the cusps drift apart so that the flow is unimpeded; the flow gradually slows and then stops and the pressure gradient is reversed. The blood would then flow backwards but for the valves which float together. When the semilunar valves are open the atrioventricular valves are closed and vice versa. When closed during ventricular relaxation, the semilunar valves support the blood which has been pumped into the arteries. When the atrioventricular valves are closed during contraction of the ventricles they have to withstand considerable pressure to prevent backflow. To enable them to do this they are given additional strength in the form of the chordae tendinae. These are delicate tendinous cords which are attached to the margins of the cusps and to the

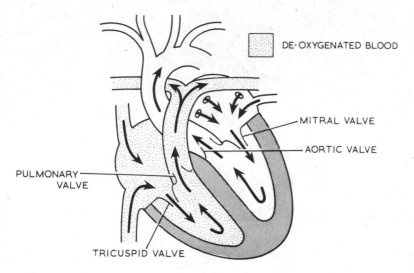

DE-OXYGENATED BLOOD

MITRAL VALVE

AORTIC VALVE

PULMONARY VALVE

TRICUSPID VALVE

Fig. 1/11   Diagram showing the blood circulating through the valves

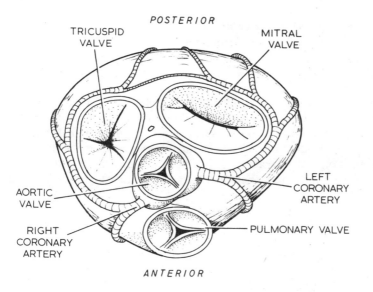

POSTERIOR

TRICUSPID VALVE

MITRAL VALVE

LEFT CORONARY ARTERY

AORTIC VALVE

RIGHT CORONARY ARTERY

PULMONARY VALVE

ANTERIOR

Fig. 1/12   Diagram to show that the four heart valves lie in the same plane

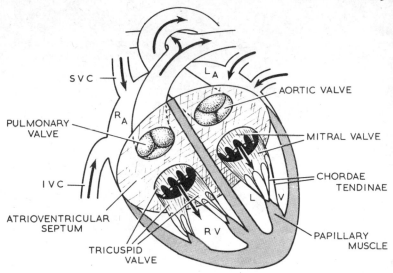

Fig. 1/13   Diagram of the heart to show the valves, chordae tendinae and papillary muscles

papillary muscles of the ventricular walls which contract at the beginning of ventricular contraction (see Fig. 1/13).

The Myocardium

Cardiac muscle is structurally and physiologically unique. The cells are irregular, branched and show striations. At the ends of the cells where adjacent cells join, transverse lines, the intercalated discs, can be identified. Each muscle cell has an inherent property of rhythmical contraction and relaxation. It has been demonstrated that there are electrical connections between adjacent cells which result in the

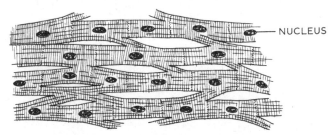

Fig. 1/14   Diagram illustrating the syncytial formation of cardiac muscle

spread of excitation over the intercalated disc. In this way synchronisation of muscle cell contraction occurs. The cell with the most rapid rhythm affects the other cells. Thus the heart functions as a syncytium (see Fig. 1/14), as if there were no membranes separating individual cells.

The cardiac wall is formed of muscle fibres and fibrous rings, surrounding the four valves, to which some of the muscle fibres are attached. Other muscle fibres are in a circular form and attached to each other. The thin walled atria have two layers of fibres, the superficial which enclose both atria and the deep fibres which are looped and arranged at right angles to the superficial. The deep fibres are independent for each atrium.

The walls of the ventricles contain many more muscle fibres than the atria, the wall of the left ventricle being thicker than the right. The arrangement of these muscle fibres is very complex but the basic functional arrangement is of spiral muscle fibres attached to the fibrous rings. When the ventricles contract they shorten both in length and diameter. The contraction wave enters near to the apex and spreads upwards towards the base, causing the blood to move upwards towards the exit valves.

The Endocardium

The endocardium is the inner lining of the chambers of the heart. It is continuous with the lining membrane of the great vessels entering and leaving the heart and is formed by a layer of endothelial cells supported by a layer of connective tissue and elastic fibres. It is thin, smooth and glistening in appearance.

The Conducting System of the Heart

The cardiac muscle, of which the heart is formed, has an inherent property of rhythmical contraction and relaxation. The part of the muscle which has the highest rate of spontaneous discharge is called the sinuatrial (S.A.) node (see Fig. 1/15). This small group of specialised muscle fibres is situated in the right atrium close to the junction of the great veins and is known as the pacemaker. It is embedded in connective tissue and surrounded by autonomic nerve endings. Although the atria are separate chambers the muscle fibres of both are connected. The contraction originated in the S.A. node rapidly spreads causing both atria to contract simultaneously causing the blood to flow into the ventricles.

The atrioventricular (A.V.) node, which is smaller than the S.A.

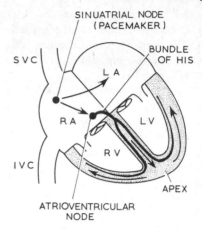

Fig. 1/15 Diagram
illustrating the
conducting system of
the heart

node, lies in the myocardial fibres of the distal part of the right atrium near to the coronary sinus and the tricuspid valve. From this point the atrioventricular bundle (Bundle of His) passes across the atrio-ventricular septum into the upper part of the interventricular septum where it divides into right and left branches. This is the only muscular connection between the atria and the ventricles. These branches pass down into the ventricular muscle lying on either side of the septum. On reaching the apex they turn towards the papillary muscles. The branches spread throughout the ventricular myocardium and are known as Purkinje fibres. The A.V. node, its bundle and proximal part of the limbs are insulated from the rest of the myocardium by a connective tissue sheath.

The Blood Supply to the Heart

Blood is supplied to the heart by the right and left coronary arteries (see Fig. 1/16). These vessels arise from the ascending aorta just beyond the aortic valve. The left coronary artery, which is larger than the right, passes forwards and turns left passing backwards round the left margin of the heart, eventually anastomosing with the right coronary artery. A large branch, the (anterior) interventricular branch, is given off at the point where the artery turns left. This branch anastomoses with the interventricular branch of the right coronary artery. The left coronary artery supplies the left atrium and both ventricles.

The right coronary artery passes forwards and then turns down-wards and to the right giving off a marginal branch. Near its termination it gives off the (posterior) interventricular branch. The sinuatrial and the atrioventricular nodes are usually supplied by branches of the right coronary artery. It also supplies the right atrium and the anterior and posterior surfaces of the right ventricle.

The anastomoses between the two coronary arteries are not usually adequate to give a good collateral circulation should a large branch of a coronary artery be occluded.

The majority of the veins of the heart drain into the coronary sinus which lies between the left atrium and the left ventricle. It ends by opening into the right atrium. The remaining veins open directly into the atria; a few drain into the ventricles.

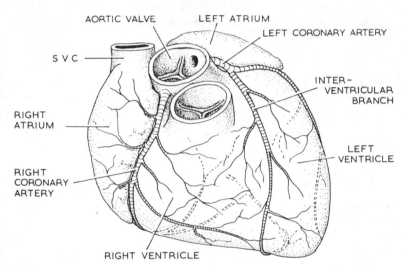

Fig. 1/16 Diagram to show the anterior aspect of the heart showing the coronary vessels

The Nerve Supply to the Heart

The autonomic nervous system supplies the heart with sympathetic and parasympathetic nerves. It is thought that these interact under normal conditions, so that if there is decreased vagal (para-sympathetic) activity leading to an increased heart rate, there will be an increase in sympathetic activity at the same time.

Sympathetic and vagal tone are controlled by nerve cell nuclei which form part of the reticular formation in the medulla oblongata. These nuclei are commonly referred to as the 'cardiac centre' and are themselves subject to control from higher centres (the cortex and hypothalamus).

THE SYMPATHETIC SUPPLY

Nerve cells lie in the upper five thoracic segments of the lateral horns of the spinal cord. Axons pass from these segments to the superior, middle and inferior ganglia, synapse and pass to the heart via the superior, middle and inferior cardiac sympathetic nerves. These nerves supply the sinuatrial node, atrioventricular node and the atrial and ventricular muscle. The chemical transmitter at these post-ganglionic nerve endings is noradrenaline.

The sympathetic system is stimulated at times of stress, e.g. fright, emotion, or during haemorrhage. This leads to an increased heart rate and speed of conduction of the heartbeat and an increased contraction force of the atrial and ventricular muscle so that there is a maximal increase in the cardiac pumping action.

THE PARASYMPATHETIC SUPPLY

The vagal nerve cell bodies lie in the dorsal motor nucleus of the vagus in the medulla. Preganglionic fibres travel in the vagi (tenth cranial) synapsing with ganglion cells near the sinuatrial node, atrio-ventricular node and in the wall of the atria. Post ganglionic fibres supply these structures. The chemical transmitter at these nerve endings is acetyl-choline.

The ventricles have no vagal supply.

The vagi monitor the sinuatrial node, the natural rhythmicity of the node being higher than the normal heart rate. Vagal tone (activity) slows this rate to the normal (about 70 beats per minute). If vagal tone increases, the heart rate becomes slower, e.g. during sleep; on waking the vagal tone decreases and the heartbeat quickens.

SURFACE MARKING

Heart

The apex of the heart lies in the fifth intercostal space about 9cm from midline, a little below and medial to the left nipple where the apex beat can be palpated. The sternocostal surface of the heart can be outlined on the chest wall. The left border of the heart corresponds to a line, convex to the left, drawn upwards and medially from the apex beat to the lower border of the left second costal cartilage 1–2cm from the sternal margin. The right border is denoted by a line, slightly convex to the right, drawn from the upper border of the right third costal cartilage 1–2cm from the sternal margin to the right sixth costal cartilage. This line is at its greatest distance from mid line (3–4cm) in the fourth intercostal space. A line joining the right sixth costal

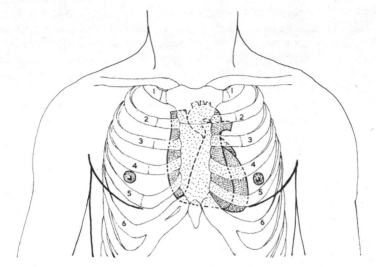

Fig. 1/17   Diagram to show the surface projection of the heart

cartilage to the apex beat shows the position of the lower border of the heart (see Fig. 1/17).

THE BLOOD VESSELS

The systemic blood vessels provide a series of branching tubes taking blood from the left ventricle to distribute it throughout the systemic circulation to the tissues and back to the right atrium. The pulmonary vessels similarly conduct blood from the right ventricle to the lungs for gaseous exchange and return it to the left atrium. The structure and function of these vessels differ in different parts of the system but they all have a smooth lining formed by a single layer of endothelial cells. There are four main types of blood vessel: arteries, arterioles, capillaries and veins.

With the exception of the capillaries the blood vessels are described as having three coats, the outer tunica adventitia, which mainly consists of fibrous tissue organised in a longitudinal manner; the tunica media, or middle coat which consists of smooth muscular and elastic fibres arranged in a circular manner, and the tunica intima, consisting of a smooth layer of flat endothelial cells on a sub-endothelial layer formed of elastin and collagen fibres (see Table 1/1).

The thickness of the vessel walls and their structure vary with their function.

The large arteries leaving the heart convert the intermittent ejection of blood from the ventricles into a continuous though still pulsating stream. To achieve this the large arteries, particularly the aorta, store blood during contraction of the ventricles for distribution when there is no blood leaving the heart. Consequently their walls are thin in comparison to the size of the lumen and contain more elastic than muscular tissue. This elasticity allows them to expand and recoil.

The smaller arteries have fewer elastic fibres and a gradually increasing proportion of smooth muscle fibres. The contraction and relaxation of the muscle fibres allow for the control of blood flow to various parts of the body dependent upon demand.

Table 1/1 To Show Differences in Coats of Arteries and Veins

VESSEL	TUNICA INTIMA	TUNICA MEDIA	TUNICA ADVENTITIA
Large arteries	Endothelial cells. Elastic – collagen fibres with plain muscle.	Elastic membranes separated by fibrous tissue.	Fibrous tissue. Few elastic fibres (thin layer).
Medium arteries	Endothelial cells. Elastic membrane.	Plain muscle cells. Few elastic membranes.	Collagen and elastic fibres. Areolar tissue.
Small veins	Endothelial cells. Connective tissue.	Elastic fibres. White fibrous tissue. Some muscle fibres.	Areolar tissue. Longitudinal elastic fibres.
Medium veins	Endothelial cells. Elastic fibres.	Connective tissue and elastic and muscle fibres.	Areolar tissue and elastic fibres.

The arterioles both large and terminal have muscular walls which control the flow of blood through the microcirculatory units of various tissues (Gray).

In general arterioles open into an intercommunicating capillary network. At this level interchange of gases and substances takes place across the capillary wall which consists of a single layer of flattened endothelial cells on a fine basement membrane.

To serve this function the capillary bed is interposed between the arteries and the veins. However, at various sites in the body there is direct connection between small arteries and veins, these are called arteriovenous anastomoses. If this connecting vessel is patent, blood by-passes the capillary network, and if the vessel is closed blood flows through the capillaries. In this way a local regulation of blood occurs.

Veins carry blood back to the heart and like arteries are described as having a wall composed of three coats. The basic structural difference is in the tunica media which contains only a little muscular or elastic tissue resulting in thinner walled vessels. These are adequate for conveying blood at a much lower pressure.

Since pressure is low and flow is, in many cases, against gravity most veins are equipped with valves. These are formed by part of the inner layer doubled back on itself, strengthened by connective tissue and covered with endothelium. Valves are semilunar in shape and are usually found opposite to each other. The convex edge is attached to the vessel wall and the concave margin is free. They lie close to the vessel wall as long as the blood is flowing towards the heart. If there is any regurgitation, the valves are disturbed and their opposed edges come into contact with each other and prevent back flow. On the cardial side the valve is pouched so that when filled with blood it looks knotted.

The return of blood to the heart is brought about by a number of forces. The deep veins run in the fascial planes between muscle groups where they are subjected to muscle contraction and relaxation. This is particularly important in the lower extremities where the deep veins of the calf lie between soleus and the deep posterior crural muscles, frequently referred to as the leg muscle pump (the soleal pump). The non-elastic, dense fascia of the lower extremities makes the muscle pumps more effective. Blood from the head and neck is assisted back to the heart by the force of gravity. The changes of intrathoracic pressure from atmospheric to subatmospheric (negative) pressure has a suction effect on the blood in the veins near the heart and consequently aids venous return.

The systemic veins are arranged in two groups, superficial and deep. The superficial veins lie in the superficial fascia whereas the deep veins usually accompany the arteries. All venous blood has eventually to pass into the deep veins and there are many communicating veins between the deep and superficial veins. These veins have valves which ensure that the flow of blood is into the deep veins and prevent the reverse flow.

Collateral Circulation

Arteries may end by joining another artery directly, such as occurs in the case of the two vertebral arteries and the radial and ulnar arteries in the hand. Such an anastomosis allows blood to reach the territory of supply in the event of one main artery being blocked. Often it is the smaller branches of the arteries which anastomose, as is seen round joints. This forms the basis of a collateral circulation, so

---

important in arterial injury or disease. If the main artery stem is obstructed, blood can flow from the branches given off proximal to the block into the artery distal through branches given off distally. In the course of time, if the obstruction is not relieved, the branches tend to lengthen and their walls to thicken, so that they become capable of supplying the necessary nutrients and gases to the regions previously supplied by the obstructed vessels.

This collateral circulation tends to develop as the years go by and the needs of the body require it. In disease the state of these collateral vessels will determine the fate of the tissues.

Some arteries, such as those which penetrate the cerebral cortex, do not anastomose other than through the capillary bed. These are known as end-arteries. Obstruction of these arteries will lead to certain cutting off of the blood supply to their territories with consequent death of the tissues.

Nervous Control of Blood Vessels

The smooth muscle in the vessels of the systemic circulation is supplied by nerves from the sympathetic division of the autonomic nervous system. In general these nerves cause the smooth muscle to be in a state of partial contraction due to stimuli continuously sent out from a diffuse network of neurone groups in the reticular formation of the brain stem, frequently referred to as the vasomotor centre.

Research has shown that the pathway of the vasoconstrictor fibres is by the lateral horns of the first thoracic to second lumbar segments inclusive. Preganglionic fibres are the axons of these cells. They leave the cord in the ventral nerve root and emerge in the spinal nerves, to leave these nerves in the white rami communicans to enter the sympathetic trunks. Here they may synapse at once or run up or down to synapse, for the upper limbs in the cervical ganglia and for the lower limbs in the lower lumbar and upper sacral ganglia.

Postganglionic fibres enter the spinal nerves via the grey rami communicans and are carried in both dorsal and ventral rami to be distributed with these nerves. Some fibres pass directly from the ganglia to the larger arteries (see Fig. 1/18).

Most of the fibres for the upper limb pass from the stellate ganglion (inferior cervical ganglion) into the eighth cervical and first thoracic nerves, so entering the lower trunk of the brachial plexus. The majority of the fibres then run in the median and ulnar nerves, fewer are found in the musculocutaneous, radial and axillary nerves. For the lower limb some fibres pass from the lower lumbar ganglia into the lumbar plexus to be distributed with the femoral and obturator nerves. Many pass from the upper sacral ganglia into the sciatic nerve

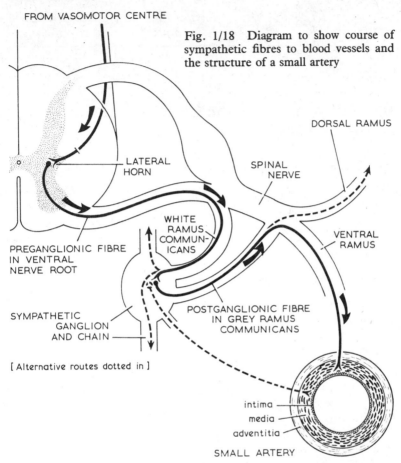

Fig. 1/18 Diagram to show course of sympathetic fibres to blood vessels and the structure of a small artery

to be distributed with the tibial and common peroneal branches (Martin, Lynn, Dible & Aird).

The activity of the vasomotor centre is increased or decreased by nervous and chemical stimuli. Increased activity increases vasoconstriction while decreased activity has the reverse effect.

REFERENCES

Gray's Anatomy. 35th ed. (1973). (Ed. R. Warwick) Longman.
Martin, P., Lynn, B. R., Dible, J. H. and Aird, I. (1956). *Peripheral Vascular Disorders*. Churchill-Livingstone.

BIBLIOGRAPHY

See end of Chapter 2.

Chapter 2

Basic Physiology of the Cardio-Thoracic and Vascular Systems

by P. J. WADDINGTON, M.C.S.P., H.T., DIP.T.P.

RESPIRATION

Purpose of Respiration

Breathing is the first and last act of the respiratory process which is concerned with the intake of oxygen and the elimination of carbon dioxide by the body. Respiration is also concerned with the regulation of the hydrogen ion concentration of the blood.

The process involves:

1. Ventilation – the mass movement of air in and out of the lungs.
2. The exchange of oxygen and carbon dioxide between the alveolar air and the pulmonary capillaries.
3. Blood gas transport to and from the tissues.
4. Gaseous exchange at tissue level.

Act of Breathing

INSPIRATION

This is an active muscular effort designed to enlarge the thoracic cavity, lowering the intrathoracic pressure to a subatmospheric level. As this occurs air flows from a region of higher pressure (atmospheric) to one of lower pressure (subatmospheric).

The inspiratory effort has the following forces to overcome:

1. External forces.
2. Elastic recoil of the lungs and thorax.
3. Frictional resistance to the movement of the tissues.
4. The resistance to airflow by the bronchial tree itself.

EXPIRATION

Normal quiet expiration is caused by the elastic recoil of the tissues. If the resistance given to the moving gases by the non-elastic tissues of the airway is negligible, the return of the lungs to their resting position is quick and easy but where the resistance is above normal, the speed of expiration will be reduced and active contraction of the expiratory muscles may be necessary. The expiratory muscles will be contracted during forced expiratory acts such as blowing and coughing.

Elasticity and Compliance

Both the lungs and the thoracic cage contain tissues which have elastic properties. Elasticity of a body is defined as the property of a body to return to its original shape after it has been distorted by some external force. These structures obey Hook's Law – 'Stress is proportional to strain' or 'Equal increases in a force cause equal increases in length'. The force is provided by the muscles of inspiration. The work in changing the original shape of the body is stored as potential energy which is expended as the body returns to normal. The reciprocal of elasticity is compliance, which is a measure of the distensibility of the lung. In many patients with lung disease compliance is reduced while in some, for example, those with emphysema, it may be increased.

Elastic Forces Acting upon Lungs and Thorax

In the normal subject who is relaxed at the end of quiet expiration the elastic forces of the lungs and thorax balance one another. That is, the tendency of the elasticity of the lungs to empty them is equal to the tendency of the elastic forces of the thorax to expand. If air enters between the pleura of the lung and chest wall, the lung will collapse and the chest wall will move outwards. In conditions such as emphysema where the elasticity of the lung is lost, the unopposed elasticity of the thorax causes it to expand. The elastic forces of the thorax have a limit giving the thorax a fixed capacity which will vary with the individual. Therefore rigidity of the thorax in disease will have an adverse effect on respiration.

Lung elasticity is not solely dependent upon collagenous and elastic fibres but also upon the fact that a surface tension exists between the liquid lining the alveoli and the alveolar gas. This force tends to cause the alveolus to collapse. Therefore the inspiratory muscles must overcome this alveolar surface tension as well as tissue elasticity when they inflate the lungs.

SURFACTANT

It has been shown that passive expiration is not entirely due to the elastic recoil of the tissues and that 'the retractive forces due to surface tension were (are) as important as those due to the elastic tissues of the lung itself' (Crofton & Douglas, 1971).

Surfactant (surface acting agent) is secreted by some of the cells in the alveolar walls. It acts on the mucoid layer controlling surface tension, equalising pressure during inspiration and expiration and between small and large alveoli. Without surfactant the alveoli would collapse.

There is reason to believe the surfactant also 'assists osmotic forces acting across the alveolar capillary membrane and prevents the alveolar lining fluid from drawing further fluid into the alveoli' (Crofton & Douglas).

Frictional Resistance to Respiration

There are two types:

1. The friction caused by the movement of the tissues, that is, the rib-cage, diaphragm, abdominal structures and the lungs themselves during inspiration and expiration.

2. The friction caused during the flow of gases, a) between the molecules of the gases themselves, b) between the gases and the walls of the tubes.

During slow flow in a straight tube the flow is laminar, that is, in straight lines like the laminae of a piece of plywood seen from the side. The air in the centre of the tube flows faster than that at the periphery.

During fast flow in a straight tube the air flowing along becomes turbulent.

Because of the many branching tubes in the bronchial tree, eddy currents are set up which may create turbulence even at moderate flow rates.

The effect of abnormalities in the smooth tubes of the bronchial tree which may be caused by excessive mucus secretions or tumours is to increase the turbulence of the gases passing through.

LUNG VOLUMES

All lung volumes are related to the physique of the subject.

The volume of air that can be expelled from the lungs following the deepest possible inspiration is called the vital capacity (V.C.). The average man will have a V.C. of about 4·5 litres and the average woman 3·2 litres (see Fig. 2/1).

In normal quiet respiration we neither breathe in fully nor out fully. Therefore we have an inspiratory reserve volume (I.R.V.) and an expiratory reserve volume (E.R.V.) in addition to the air passing in and out during quiet respiration which is called tidal volume (T.V.).

$$\left. \begin{array}{l} \text{I.R.V.} = 2\cdot6 \text{ litres} \\ \text{E.R.V.} = 1\cdot5 \text{ litres} \\ \text{T.V.} = 0\cdot4 \text{ litres} \end{array} \right\} = \text{V.C. } 4\cdot5 \text{ litres}$$
(calculated on a total lung capacity of 6 litres)

At the end of quiet expiration, that is, at the resting respiratory level, 3·0 litres of air remains in the lungs. This is called the functional residual capacity (F.R.C.). It is composed of the E.R.V. = 1·5 litres and the residual volume (R.V.) which is 1·5 litres and cannot be forced out of the lungs, remaining in the alveoli.

$$\left. \begin{array}{l} \text{E.R.V.} = 1\cdot5 \text{ litres} \\ \text{R.V.} = 1\cdot5 \text{ litres} \end{array} \right\} = \text{F.R.C. } 3\cdot0 \text{ litres}$$
(calculated on a total lung capacity of 6 litres)

Forced Expiratory Volume

It is usual to measure V.C. with a spirometer, to give an indication of the condition of the patient's lungs. This is most often made using a dry, waterless spirometer, the Vitalograph. If the vital capacity is forced out as rapidly and completely as possible it is called the forced expiratory volume (F.E.V.). A most significant figure in assessing a patient is the F.E.V. which occurs in the first second, the $F.E.V._1$. In a normal person this is usually at least 70% of the total V.C. In patients with diffuse airways obstruction this percentage is considerably reduced. The Vitalograph apparatus produces a permanent record in the form of a graph which may be kept in the patient's notes.

Maximal Ventilation Volume

Another measurement of lung function which is considered to be of clinical value is the maximal ventilation volume or the maximal voluntary ventilation (M.V.V.). The subject is asked to breathe as deeply and rapidly as possible for 15 seconds and the ventilation per minute is then calculated. In normal subjects the volume may be greater than 100 litres per minute.

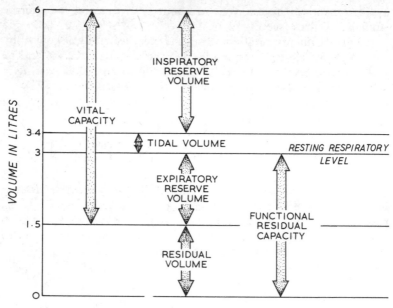

Fig. 2/1   Diagram to show lung volumes

Peak Flow

Peak flow is another lung function test. In this the patient's highest expiratory flow rate during forced expiration is measured. This test is related to F.E.V.$_1$ and M.V.V.

Rate of Respiration

The rate of respiration is about 14 breaths per minute for normal subjects at rest.

Dead Space

The tidal volume passing in and out of the lungs during normal quiet respiration equals about 400ml; of this only 250ml reaches the alveoli. The remaining 150ml is still in the air passages at the end of inspiration and can therefore take no part in gaseous exchange. Therefore the volume of each breath must exceed 150ml. Below this level breathing will not be useful. This 150ml is called anatomical dead space. In patients with a tracheostomy this is decreased.

The air which enters the alveoli is called alveolar air. Of this some may not be used to oxygenate the blood flowing through pulmonary capillaries because too much enters the alveoli in proportion to their blood flow. In some patients a proportion of the alveoli may have no blood flow at all and the air which reaches these cannot be utilised, so that the air passing to and fro serves no respiratory function. The volume of inspired air which enters the alveoli and is of no functional value is also effectively 'dead space' gas. Alveolar dead space plus anatomical dead space is usually called physiological dead space.

Percentage of Gases

	Inspired Air %	Alveolar Air %	Expired Air %
O_2	21	14	16
CO_2	0	6	4
N_2	79	80	80

Air in the alveoli in quiet respiration will be a mixture of the lungs' functional residual capacity and 250ml of the tidal volume. Therefore it will be of a lower oxygen and a higher carbon dioxide content than room air. Expired air will have a higher oxygen and a lower carbon dioxide content than alveolar air because it is a mixture of alveolar air and dead space air which will contain room air percentage of gases.

This larger percentage of oxygen in expired air than in alveolar air is a vital statistic when mouth-to-mouth breathing is being given.

Carriage of Gases–Partial Pressures

The air in the respiratory system is composed of a mixture of three gases and water vapour. The proportions of oxygen and carbon dioxide are variable while that of nitrogen remains the same.

The physical properties of this mixture can be deduced from:

DALTON'S LAWS OF PARTIAL PRESSURES

1. 'The pressure exerted by a mixture of gases is equal to the sum of the pressures which each would exert if it alone occupied the space.'

2. 'The pressure exerted by a saturated vapour depends only upon the temperature and the particular liquid considered.'

BOYLE'S LAW

'The volume of a fixed mass of gas is inversely proportional to the pressure provided the temperature is constant.'

It follows, therefore, that the partial pressure of any gas is proportional to its percentage by volume in the mixture.

Therefore when three gases, oxygen, carbon dioxide and nitrogen occupy the same space, each will contribute to the total pressure in proportion to its concentration. The actual pressure measured in millimetres of mercury will vary with the barometric pressure.

It must be remembered that alveolar air is saturated with water vapour at body temperature. At 37°C water vapour in alveolar air has a pressure of 47mm Hg independent of the gases and not variable with barometric pressure.

PARTIAL PRESSURES IN ALVEOLAR AIR

$$O_2 = 14\% \text{ of } 760—47\text{mm Hg} = 100\text{mm Hg}$$
$$CO_2 = 6\% \text{ of } 760—47\text{mm Hg} = 40\text{mm Hg}$$
That is $P_{O_2} = 100$ and the $P_{CO_2} = 40$

HENRY'S LAW OF SOLUTION

'The quantity of gas going into a simple solution at constant temperature is proportional to the pressure.' Dalton states that

'In a mixture of gases the solubility of each gas varies proportionally with its partial pressure.'

Therefore the movement of gases between a gas and a liquid or between liquids is governed by pressures. The movement is always from one of high pressure to one of low pressure. The movement of gases in the lungs between the alveolar air and the blood, is in a gas to liquid situation, oxygen moving into the blood and carbon dioxide into the air. At tissue level, a liquid to liquid situation, oxygen moves into the tissues and carbon dioxide from the tissues into the blood.

PARTIAL PRESSURES

In alveolar air and arterial blood P_{O_2} is 100mm Hg approx
In alveolar air and arterial blood P_{CO_2} is 40mm Hg approx
In tissues and venous blood P_{O_2} is 40mm Hg approx
In tissues and venous blood P_{CO_2} is 46mm Hg approx

Gases are carried in the blood as a result of:

1. The formation of a solution.
2. Chemical combination.

The amount carried is dependent upon tension or partial pressure.

Carriage of Oxygen

IN SOLUTION – DISSOLVED IN PLASMA

A small volume of oxygen, which can be calculated to be 0·3 vols per cent, is carried in the blood in solution. It is of little significance when oxygen supply to the tissues is being considered.

CHEMICAL COMBINATION – COMBINED WITH HAEMOGLOBIN

The amount of oxygen combined with haemoglobin in a red cell is dependent upon oxygen tension or pressure and can be represented on a graph as an S-shaped curve, the oxygen dissociation curve (see Fig. 2/2). When the Po_2 equals 100 the haemoglobin of the red cells is 97·4% saturated. This is called the arterial point. Because the haemoglobin is nearly 100% saturated at this point the graph is plotted as Po_2 against percentage saturation of haemoglobin. At a Po_2 of 40 the haemoglobin is 70% saturated. This is called the venous point.

The quantity of oxygen which the blood is able to carry is dependent upon:

1. The amount of haemoglobin in the red cells.
2. The number of red cells.
3. The amount of carbon dioxide carried by the blood.

If the Pco_2 is raised less oxygen is carried at a given tension.

The Po_2 of blood as it passes through the lungs is raised from 40mm Hg to 100mm Hg. This represents 5ml of oxygen for every 100ml of blood.

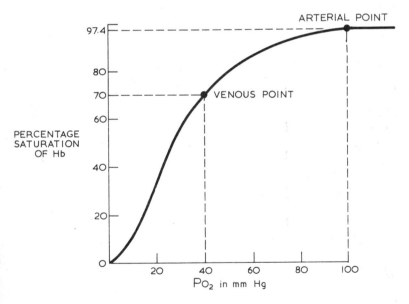

Fig. 2/2   Diagram showing an oxygen dissociation curve

Carriage of Carbon Dioxide

IN SOLUTION

Some carbon dioxide dissolves in the plasma and a small quantity of this reacts with water to form carbonic acid. As carbonic acid is a weak acid very few of its molecules dissociate into H^+ and HCO_3^-

$$H_2O + CO_2 \rightleftharpoons H_2CO_3 \rightleftharpoons H^+ + HCO_3^-$$

In addition, some carbon dioxide dissolves within the erythrocytes.

CHEMICAL COMBINATION

1. Carbon dioxide combines with the amino group of plasma proteins to form carbamino compounds.
2. Carbon dioxide also combines with the amine (NH_2^-) part of the haemoglobin molecule. Oxygen combines with the iron (haem) radical. Saturation of haemoglobin with carbon dioxide occurs at a low partial pressure and the reaction is very speedy, requiring no catalyst.
3. Formation of bicarbonate. Carbon dioxide from the tissues enters the plasma and diffuses quickly across the cell membrane into the erythrocyte. Because of the presence within the red cells of the catalyst carbonic anhydrase, the reaction $H_2O + CO_2 \rightleftharpoons H_2CO_3$ is accelerated.

Reduced haemoglobin which results from the release of oxygen to the tissues acts as a base and mops up the H^+ released from the H_2CO_3 $\rightleftharpoons H^+ + HCO_3^-$. The HCO_3^- thus liberated diffuses out of the red cell and is replaced by Cl^- from the plasma. This maintains the ionic balance across the cell membrane and is called the chloride shift. Within the red cells the Cl^- combines with K^+ forming potassium chloride and in the plasma HCO_3^- combines with Na^+ to form sodium bicarbonate.

In the lungs the haemoglobin becomes oxygenated and the process is reversed.

Carbon dioxide dissociation curves of blood and plasma can be plotted (see Fig. 2/3) but full saturation of the blood by carbon dioxide does not occur. Therefore they are not plotted in the same way as the oxygen dissociation curve, that is, as percentages of saturation. They are plotted as partial pressures against volumes per cent. Over the normal range of Pco_2 there is only a slight curve so that it nearly represents a straight line.

Maintenance of Blood pH

In health the pH of the blood is maintained within very narrow limits, i.e. 7·35–7·45. This is a slightly alkaline solution. The acidity or

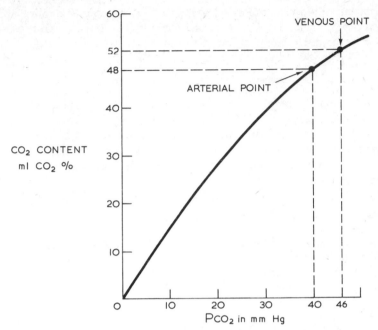

Fig. 2/3   Diagram showing a carbon dioxide dissociation curve

alkalinity of a solution is dependent upon the concentrations of hydrogen ions H^+ and hydroxyl ions OH^-. The use of the pH method is a way of expressing this and is sometimes referred to as the hydrogen ion concentration, to which it is inversely related. pH 7 indicates a neutral solution. Any figure below seven shows acidity, i.e. an increase in hydrogen ion concentration, any figure above seven indicates a decrease in the hydrogen ion concentration and therefore an alkaline solution.

The pH of whole blood or plasma depends upon the ratio of the bicarbonate and carbonic acid present. The blood bicarbonate is an important chemical buffer in the regulation of acid-base balance.

Carbon dioxide from the tissues is constantly entering the blood and combining with water to form carbonic acid. Under normal conditions an equal amount of carbon dioxide is expelled by the lungs and the pH of the blood is not affected. If this elimination of carbon dioxide is reduced the carbonic acid content of the blood will rise. This increase in acid will cause the pH to fall. A reduction in pH is referred to as acidosis.

If there is an increase in the ventilation of the lungs and carbon dioxide is expelled at above the normal rate the CO_2 and H_2CO_3

concentration in the blood will fall, it will become more alkaline and the pH will rise, i.e. a proportionate rise in bicarbonate will cause a rise in the pH. This is called alkalosis.

Control of Respiration

Respiration is an involuntary activity which to a certain extent is under voluntary control. One can stop breathing and control its rate and depth but breathing cannot be stopped for an indefinite period; approximately 45 seconds is the maximum. Breathing is also modified at an involuntary level during such activities as speaking, swallowing and coughing.

Nervous Control of Respiration

Spontaneous respiration is due to a rhythmic electrical discharge from a group of nerve cells in the reticular formation of the brain stem, mainly in the lower part of the floor of the fourth ventricle in the medulla. This area is called the respiratory centre. Some cells form the expiratory centre and are situated more posteriorly than the group of cells forming the inspiratory centre but their territories overlap. Although this area has been designated as the respiratory centre, it is now thought that for normal respiration it is necessary for the whole of the reticular formation to be functioning. Damage to the respiratory centre is in many cases fatal.

From this area impulses are sent to C.3, 4 and 5 for relay to the diaphragm via the phrenic nerve and to the thoracic spinal cord for relay by the intercostal nerves to supply the intercostal muscles, the diaphragm and the abdominal muscles.

The exact way in which the neurones of the reticular formation interrelate has yet to be established but from this area rhythmic inspiratory and expiratory impulses are discharged. These can be influenced by afferent impulses reaching the area.

THE HERING-BREUER REFLEX

Many vagal afferent fibres are present in the walls of the small air passages. They are sensitive to stretch. When the lungs are inflated, impulses are generated which have an inhibitory effect on the inspiratory centre. The greater the stretch the greater the inhibition.

When the lungs are deflated for a prolonged period there is an increase in inspiratory effort. Again it is considered that afferent impulses are conveyed along vagal afferent fibres.

Some authorities consider that both these reflexes form the

Hering-Breuer reflex. In man the Hering-Breuer reflex is very weak.

COUGH REFLEX

The vagus nerve probably carries the afferent impulses initiated by the irritants which stimulate a cough reflex. The upper part of the respiratory tract is sensitive to mechanical irritants while the alveoli are sensitive to chemical substances.

PRESSURE

The carotid sinuses and carotid bodies are affected by pressure and are called baroreceptors. When they are stimulated by a rise in blood pressure this has an inhibitory effect on the respiratory centre. A fall in blood pressure has the opposite effect.

CHEMORECEPTORS

The carotid bodies which lie one on each side of the carotid bifurcation and the aortic bodies which lie near the arch of the aorta are sensitive to oxygen lack. Their afferent impulses pass along the glosso-pharyngeal and vagus nerves respectively and share the same nerve trunk as the afferents of the baroreceptors. They have a stimulating effect on the respiratory centre. N.B. The direct effect of anoxia on the respiratory centre is depressing.

Stimulation of the respiratory centre by oxygen lack is not a very important factor under normal conditions, as haemoglobin is easily saturated with oxygen at normal or even below normal rates of ventilation. However, it is important at high altitudes where the oxygen concentration in the atmosphere is low, resulting in inadequate oxygenation of haemoglobin.

In some respiratory diseases the patients may 'learn' to tolerate high carbon dioxide levels in the blood. Stimulation of the respiratory centre by oxygen lack can then become a vital factor.

In these cases it can be dangerous to give the patient too much oxygen as this stimulation to respiration will thus have been removed.

OTHER INFLUENCES

A change in body temperature, especially a sudden cooling, for example if one were to jump into the sea on Christmas Day, will cause hyperventilation.

It is thought that the proprioceptors present in the muscles of respiration may influence the respiratory centre.

The respiratory rate is influenced by higher centres and changes in rate, depth and rhythm are brought about by emotional factors.

The respiratory centre is depressed during sleep causing an increase in alveolar carbon dioxide.

Chemical Control of Breathing

CARBON DIOXIDE

It is a matter for debate whether the Pco_2 or the hydrogen ion concentration of the blood is the most important single factor to stimulate the respiratory centre producing both an increase in the rate and depth of respiration.

If the air in the alveoli has a high Pco_2 the arterial blood being in equilibrium with it will also have a high Pco_2. This high level of carbon dioxide will increase ventilation by directly affecting the respiratory centre.

An increase of carbon dioxide in the blood is reflected in a rise of carbon dioxide, in the form of carbonic acid, in the cerebrospinal fluid. The rise in the hydrogen ion concentration thus effected has an excitatory influence on the respiratory centre which lies in the floor of the fourth ventricle.

The blood pH is kept constant by the balance of bicarbonate and carbonic acid. The kidneys regulate the bicarbonate concentration of the plasma despite variation in the dietary intake. An increase in the amount of carbonic acid, due to a rise in the carbon dioxide in the blood, will be reflected in an increase in the hydrogen ion concentration. This is represented by a fall in pH. A fall in the pH of the blood has an excitatory effect on the respiratory centre. (Release of acids other than carbonic, e.g. lactic acid from exercising muscle or ketoacids in diabetes will stimulate breathing in a similar way.)

It must be remembered that Pco_2 and pH are interrelated as the amount of carbon dioxide in solution in the blood is dependent upon carbon dioxide tension.

Very high concentrations of carbon dioxide in the blood have a narcotic effect and can lead to unconsciousness and death.

OXYGEN TENSION

Oxygen lack as given above is registered by the chemoreceptors which influence the respiratory centre via afferent nerve impulses. This therefore can be classified as nervous control.

The direct effect (chemical) of oxygen lack on the respiratory centre is depressing.

MULTIPLE FACTOR THEORY

The phrase 'Multiple Factor Theory' (Guyton, 1969) draws attention to the situation that no one factor regulates the respiratory centres although some factors are more important than others.

TABLE OF NORMAL VALUES

Lung Volumes based on a Capacity of 6 litres

Vital Capacity (V.C.)	= 4·5 litres
Residual Volume (R.V.)	= 1·5 litres
Expiratory Reserve Volume (E.R.V.)	= 1·5 litres
Functional Residual Capacity (F.R.C.)	= 3·0 litres
Tidal Volume (T.V.)	= 0·4 litres (400ml)
Inspiratory Reserve Volume (I.R.V.)	= 2·6 litres
Forced Expiratory Volume in the 1st Second (F.E.V.₁)	= 70% V.C.
Maximum Ventilation Volume (M.V.V.)	= 100 litres
Anatomical Dead Space	= 150ml

Partial Pressures

Alveolar Air and Arterial Blood P_{O_2} = 100mm Hg; P_{CO_2} = 40mm Hg
Tissues and Venous Blood P_{O_2} = 40mm Hg; P_{CO_2} = 46mm Hg
Blood pH = 7·4 (slightly alkaline)
Vital capacity of the average male = 4·5 litres approx
female = 3·2 litres approx
Rate of Respiration 14–20 per minute

THE FUNCTIONING OF THE HEART

The Heart as a Pump

The heart acts as a pump to keep the blood circulating round the body. In fact it acts as two separate pumps, the right side of the heart pumping the blood from the systemic circulation to the lungs and the left side of the heart pumping the blood from the lungs to the systemic circulation.

The Cardiac Cycle (see Fig. 2/4)

The *cardiac cycle* begins with the initiation of the heart beat in the sinuatrial node; this is followed by the contraction of the atria. When the electrical impulse has passed through the atria, there is a short pause during which the contraction wave is moving along the atrio-ventricular bundle. The ventricles contract and blood is ejected into the arteries.

Contraction and relaxation of heart muscle are called respectively systole and diastole.

The cycle is 0·8 seconds long and is made up of an atrial part (systole 0·1 seconds and diastole 0·7 seconds) and a ventricular part (systole 0·3 seconds and diastole 0·5 seconds) giving a complete diastole (atrial and ventricular) of 0·4 seconds. Therefore on average, at rest, there are 70 cycles per minute. This is called the resting heart rate.

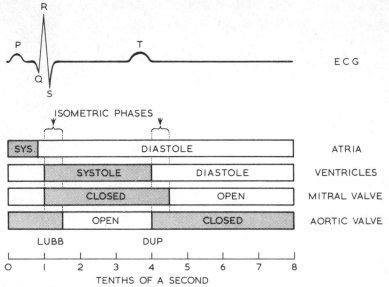

ECG

ISOMETRIC PHASES

SYS.	DIASTOLE	ATRIA
SYSTOLE	DIASTOLE	VENTRICLES
CLOSED	OPEN	MITRAL VALVE
OPEN	CLOSED	AORTIC VALVE

LUBB   DUP

0   1   2   3   4   5   6   7   8
TENTHS OF A SECOND

Fig. 2/4   Diagrammatic representation of the cardiac cycle

Heart Sounds

The heart valves are passive structures which respond to pressure gradients and offer almost no resistance to the forward flow of blood. It is the closure of these valves which causes the basic two heart sounds.

The flow of blood through the heart can be described as beginning while the atria are relaxed and filling with blood from the great veins. Isometric ventricular diastole begins, atrial pressure rises and the atrioventricular valves open, allowing blood to flow rapidly and then more slowly into the ventricles. The ventricles are 70% full of blood before the atria contract. The heart beat is initiated and a wave of contraction spreads over the atria, the great veins are sealed and pressure increases in the atria and ventricles. With the spread of the contraction to the ventricles, the intraventricular pressure rises and the atrioventricular valves float up and close causing the first heart sound 'LUBB'.

The heart muscle continues to contract but the blood is incompressible and therefore there is no change of volume; this is called the isometric contraction phase. The pressure rises in the closed ventricles until it exceeds that in the aorta and pulmonary artery whereupon the semilunar valves open and blood is ejected into the arteries. As the blood leaves the ventricles, pressure increases in the blood vessels and decreases in the ventricles; the valves close causing the second heart sound 'DUP', the ventricles begin to relax and the cycle begins again.

As systole is shorter than diastole there is a shorter interval between the first and second than between the second and first heart sounds.

Cardiac Output

The term *cardiac output* is used to denote the amount of blood pumped out by each ventricle per minute. It depends upon the heart rate and the stroke volume and is expressed in the following equation.

$$\text{Cardiac Output} = \text{Heart Rate} \times \text{Stroke Volume}$$

The average in the adult population is 5 litres per minute.

Heart Rate

The term *heart rate* implies the number of heart beats per minute and depends upon the rate at which the sinuatrial node initiates a contraction of the heart muscle. The sinuatrial node is controlled by a group of nerve cells in the reticular formation of the brain stem. This area situated in the medulla is referred to as the cardiac centre. The two parts of the autonomic nervous system have opposite effects on the sinuatrial node. In a state of rest sympathetic activity is minimal and parasympathetic activity via the vagus nerve (vagal tone) acts to inhibit the node. The greater the vagal activity the slower the heart rate. Sympathetic activity is of particular importance during exercise and emotional experiences. This works in conjunction with the release of the hormones adrenaline and noradrenaline. The heart rate is affected by impulses from higher centres. During emotional excitement the heart accelerates, however, sudden emotional shock may result in a slowing down of the heart rate.

The heart rate is affected by changes in blood pressure, a rise in blood pressure will cause a reduction in heart rate and a fall in blood pressure will cause a rise in heart rate. These changes are effected via the baroreceptors. When the rise in blood pressure is due to an increase in cardiac output such as occurs in exercise, it would obviously be undesirable for the heart rate to be reduced to below resting levels. In this event (exercise) the effect is to reduce the increase in heart rate which otherwise would occur.

It has been shown that an increased return of blood to the heart causes an increase in heart rate but no receptors which could result in reflex activity have been found. This is called the cardio-accelerator reflex (Bainbridge effect). It is therefore considered that this is simply due to an increased filling of the right atrium in which the sinuatrial node is situated.

Stroke Volume

Stroke volume is the output per ventricle per beat. It is determined by the extent of filling of the ventricles and by the force and completeness of ventricular contraction. Thus one of the major factors determining the amount of blood pumped by the heart each minute is the rate of venous return. Consequently the heart must adapt itself to a varying input of blood. This basic relationship between venous return and contractibility is explained in Starling's law of the heart which states: 'Within physiological limits, the heart pumps all the blood that comes to it without allowing excessive damming of blood in the veins' (Guyton, 1974). The law shows that within defined limits, the force of contraction is related to the length of the muscle fibres.

It would appear therefore 'that an increase in heart rate would always give an increase in cardiac output. Starling using his heart–lung preparation on the other hand found that an increase in heart rate had no effect on cardiac output. These two views are diametrically opposite. It now appears that the truth is somewhere between the two' (Green, 1976).

THE SYSTEMIC CIRCULATION

The term systemic circulation refers to the circulating system of blood vessels other than those involved in the pulmonary circulation.

Blood like all fluids flows from a region of high hydrostatic pressure to a region of low hydrostatic pressure. Thus the pressure gradient affecting the blood in the systemic circulation is that between the high pressure resulting from left ventricular contraction and consequently present in the aorta and large arteries and that existing in the great veins and the right atrium. These are called respectively the arterial blood pressure or by tradition, the blood pressure, and the venous blood pressure. The mean value of arterial blood pressure is 100mm Hg whereas venous blood pressure is at atmospheric or 0mm Hg. The pressure is that exerted by the blood on the vessel walls.

Resistance to the flow of blood is given by the blood vessels in inverse proportion to the size of their lumen. The smaller the vessel the greater the resistance.

The resistance of the blood vessels to blood flow is called the peripheral resistance.

It can be seen that the pressure gradient within the systemic circulation (arterial blood pressure 100mm Hg minus venous blood pressure 0mm Hg) and the peripheral resistance oppose each other in effecting the blood flow.

This is expressed in the following equations:

$$\text{Cardiac Output (Blood Flow)} = \frac{\text{Blood Pressure}}{\text{Peripheral Resistance}}$$

or

Blood Pressure = Cardiac Output × Peripheral Resistance

An adequate arterial blood pressure is necessary to ensure the supply of blood to the tissues. Cardiac output has been discussed on p. 63.

Peripheral Resistance

Approximately one half of the resistance to the flow of blood in the systemic circulation is at the level of the arterioles. A small alteration in the diameter of the arterioles in any one area can make a great difference to the blood flow in that area.

The smooth muscle in the walls of the arterioles is supplied by the sympathetic nervous system, stimulation of which, except in a few areas, causes constriction of the arterioles. Under normal circumstances a state of continuous partial constriction exists. This is called sympathetic or vasoconstrictor tone. The sympathetic nervous activity is controlled by a diffuse group of nerve cell nuclei in the reticular formation of the brain stem frequently referred to as the vasomotor centre. An increase in the number of sympathetic impulses will cause vasoconstriction, a decrease in the size of the lumen of the arterioles; a decrease in activity will cause vasodilatation, an increase in the size of the lumen of the arterioles.

Factors Influencing Sympathetic Activity

The *baroreceptor system* is a pressure regulating system and consists of many small nerve receptors situated in the aortic arch and at the bifurcation of the common carotid arteries, the carotid sinus. As arterial blood pressure rises nerve impulses to the medulla increase and inhibit the activity of the vasomotor centre causing a reduction in vasomotor tone. The reverse is true, a fall in arterial blood pressure will cause an increase in vasomotor tone.

The level of carbon dioxide in the blood reaching the vasomotor centre affects its activity. A rise in the level of carbon dioxide above normal causes an increase in arterial blood pressure and consequently an increase in the blood flow and nutrition to the tissues, the rapid metabolic activity of which resulted in the high levels of carbon dioxide which activated the process.

The vasomotor centre is also influenced by oxygen lack both directly by the blood supplying the area and indirectly via the chemoreceptors in the aortic and carotid bodies. When stimulated the result is an increase in vasomotor activity.

Also influencing the vasomotor centre is the cerebral cortex so that emotional stress may result in increased activity.

Sensory receptors, especially those concerned with pain, modify the centre's activity, either increasing it in response to mild pain or reducing it in response to severe pain.

The control of blood vessels by the nervous system is concerned with the overall distribution of blood so that, for example, during exercise blood is diverted from the gastro-intestinal tract and kidneys to the muscles. A rise in body temperature will cause vasodilation of the arteries of the skin, which increases blood flow and consequently heat loss. The reaction to a fall in body temperature has the opposite effect so that heat loss is diminished.

Local Factors Affecting Blood Flow

Local blood flow is also influenced by heat and cold and by metabolites. The latter are released from the active tissues, and are able to overcome the sympathetic tone and dilate arterioles and capillaries, both directly and through the axon reflex. This can be seen in the triple response when the skin is stimulated or a vasodilator such as histamine is introduced. The first stage is the appearance of a red line due to capillary dilatation, and is the result of the released H-substances. The second stage is the appearance of a bright red flare due to the dilatation of the arterioles following stimulation of the axon reflex. Finally a weal appears due to the increased exudate of fluid from the dilated capillaries. This triple response is used therapeutically to produce a very local increased blood flow.

Heat has a direct effect upon the walls of the small blood vessels causing dilatation and also acts indirectly by causing release of metabolites. Temperatures between 10° and 20°C constrict the arterioles, stasis occurs in the capillaries, oxygen is lost to the tissues and the local area becomes cyanosed. If the capillaries constrict, the skin will become white. Green points out that in some people the blood vessels are unduly sensitive to cold, which causes long-lasting vasoconstriction. This is seen in sufferers from Raynaud's disease.

Blood Viscosity

The more viscous a fluid flowing through a vessel, the greater the resistance to the flow. Under normal circumstances the viscosity of the blood remains constant. The concentration of red blood cells, which may be abnormal in disease, is the most important factor in either increasing or decreasing the viscosity of the blood.

Thus peripheral resistance can be altered without a change in the size of the arterioles.

THE PULMONARY CIRCULATION

In contrast with the systemic circulation the pulmonary circulation is a low pressure system. Its function is to transport blood to and from the lungs where gaseous exchange takes place through the capillary membrane and epithelial lining of the alveoli.

Because of the circulatory nature of blood flow the same amount of blood which flows through the systemic circulation must flow through the lungs. To accommodate increases in the amount of blood entering the lungs the blood vessels are expansile so that the resistance to blood flow decreases as the rate of blood flow increases. Vascular distensibility is reduced with age. Another factor allowing for an increase of blood flow is that all available vessels are not in use at rest. The mean pressure in the pulmonary artery is given as approximately 17mm Hg (Kelman) or 13mm Hg (Guyton) which can be compared with a mean systemic arterial pressure of 90mm Hg (Kelman) or 100mm Hg (Guyton). Guyton (1969), writes that the pressure gradient in the systemic circulation is approximately 100mm Hg whereas in the pulmonary circulation it is 9mm Hg (13mm Hg – mean pulmonary artery pressure minus 4mm Hg – mean pulmonary venous pressure) i.e. about one-eleventh of the total resistance in the systemic circulation.

Control of Pulmonary Circulation

According to Crofton and Douglas (1971), the control of pulmonary vascular resistance in the normal lung is based on the pressure of O_2 and CO_2 in the blood. Anoxia increases pulmonary vascular resistance. No effective nervous control of pulmonary vascularisation is known.

Pulmonary Oedema

Under normal conditions the low pressure in the pulmonary capillaries together with a blood plasma colloid osmotic pressure of 28mm Hg tends to draw fluid into the capillaries. However in disease, for example, mitral stenosis and left ventricular failure which results in an increase in the pressure in the pulmonary capillaries, the pressure gradient may be reversed causing fluid to pass through the capillary membrane into the lung i.e. pulmonary oedema.

REFERENCES

Crofton, J. and Douglas, A. (1975). *Respiratory Diseases*, 2nd ed. Blackwell Scientific Press.

Green, J. H. (1976). *An Introduction to Human Physiology*, 4th ed. Oxford University Press.

Guyton, A. C. (1974). *Function of the Human Body*, 4th ed. W. B. Saunders Co.

Kelman, G. R. (1977). *Applied Cardiovascular Physiology*, 2nd ed. Butterworth and Co.

BIBLIOGRAPHY

Best, C. H. and Taylor, N. B. (1959). *The Living Body*, 4th ed. Chapman and Hall Ltd.

Cotes, J. E. (1975). *Lung Function – Assessment and Application in Medicine*, 3rd ed. Blackwell Scientific Publications.

Hamilton, W. J. and Simon, G. (1971). *Surface and Radiological Anatomy*, 5th ed. W. Heffer and Sons Ltd.

Last, R. J. (1972). *Anatomy – Regional and Applied*, 5th ed. Churchill-Livingstone.

Mitchell, G. A. G. and Patterson, E. L. (1970). *Basic Anatomy*, 2nd ed. Churchill-Livingstone.

Passmore, R. and Robson, J. S. (Eds. in Chief, 1971). *A Companion to Medical Studies*, 3rd ed., Vol. 1. Blackwell Scientific Publications.

Rawling's Landmarks and Surface Markings, 9th ed. (1953). (Revised by Robinson, J. O., 1953). H. K. Lewis and Co. Ltd.

ACKNOWLEDGEMENTS

The author acknowledges with thanks the cooperation she has received from Miss E. A. Beazley and Miss J. Pickering, in allowing her to use their material which previously appeared in the First Edition of this book. It has helped her to make the Anatomy and Physiology section a complete and concise entity. She also acknowledges the very real help she has received from Miss J. Nicholas, M.C.S.P., DIP.T.P., of the Manchester Royal Infirmary in the writing of this chapter. Figure 1/4 is reproduced by kind permission of the authors, Dr. A. F. Foster-Carter and Dr. G. Simon, and the Editor of *Thorax*.

Chapter 3

Cardiac Arrest and Resuscitation

by J. R. PEPPER, M.A., F.R.C.S.

CARDIAC ARREST

This may be defined as a sudden cessation of a functional circulation. It is an emergency which demands prompt recognition. The absence of carotid or femoral pulses is sufficient. There is no need to listen for the heart beat or look for dilated pupils.

Aetiology

The heart arrests either in asystole or in ventricular fibrillation. Asystole is due usually to hypoxia, for whatever reason, or complete heart block. Ventricular fibrillation is commonly the result of an electrolyte imbalance e.g. hypokalaemia.

The common causes of cardiac arrest are:

1. Massive pulmonary embolus which obstructs the circulation and produces myocardial hypoxia.

2. Myocardial infarction which can lead to sudden death probably due to ventricular tachycardia and fibrillation.

3. Pericardial tamponade which restricts filling of the heart.

4. Tension pneumothorax which produces an acute shift of the mediastinum compressing the opposite lung and the heart.

5. Increased vagal tone which can occur during induction of general anaesthesia and may lead to a cardiac arrest when associated with hypoxia and acidosis.

Less common causes include anaphylactic reactions to drugs and air embolism.

RESUSCITATION

Unless the circulation can be rapidly restored, irreversible brain damage will occur within three (3) minutes. The priority therefore is to restore the circulation and ventilate the lungs.

If there is no board under the mattress the patient is transferred to the floor so that effective cardiac massage can be given. External cardiac massage in adults is applied by placing one hand over the other at the lower end of the sternum. The arms should be held straight as this is less tiring for the operator who may have to continue massage for several minutes before further help is available. A rate of massage of 60 per minute is the aim in adults, 80–90 per minute in children. In infants and small children the heart lies higher in the thorax so that the massaging hands should be placed over the mid-sternum. Care should be taken to avoid sudden compression of the abdomen as this may cause the liver to rupture.

Initially ventilation is achieved by mouth-to-mouth breathing or a face mask and Ambu bag, taking care to maintain an airway. The patient should be intubated with an endotracheal tube swiftly and skilfully; until such skill is available it is safer to continue ventilation by face mask, keeping a close watch on the airway.

While this is going on, medical help will have arrived and an intravenous line and E.C.G. monitor will be set up. If the heart rhythm is ventricular fibrillation, D.C. counter-shock is given starting at 100 Joules (in adults) to restore sinus rhythm. If asystole is present, 1 in 10 000 adrenaline is injected either directly into the right ventricle through the chest wall or into a central venous line to induce ventricular fibrillation which can then be treated by D.C. shock. Sodium bicarbonate is given to correct the acidosis which invariably develops following a cardiac arrest.

The patient who has recently undergone open heart surgery is in a special situation. If, after giving adrenaline and continuous external massage for one minute, there is no improvement the chest is re-opened via the recent wound. There are many recorded instances of patients surviving this procedure and leaving hospital in good health.

Once a cardiac output has been restored as shown by the return of the carotid or femoral pulses a search is made for the cause of the arrest and appropriate action taken. An anti-inflammatory steroid, dexamethasone, is generally given as prophylaxis against the development of cerebral oedema. However, the patient may slide into a state of low cardiac output which is insufficient to meet the needs of the vital organs; brain, kidneys and heart.

Low Cardiac Output

When such a state exists a vicious cycle develops (see Fig. 3/1).

If this cycle is allowed to continue, cardiac arrest will inevitably recur. On an intensive care unit such a state should be recognised early from the following features:

1. Poor urine output; less than 30ml per hour in an adult.
2. Cool peripheries and if the core and toe temperatures are being measured there will be an increase in the core: toe gradient.
3. Mental confusion deteriorating eventually to unconsciousness.
4. An increasing tendency to acidosis.

Although the causes of low cardiac output are many, the basis of treatment is the same. Initially the filling pressure of the heart is

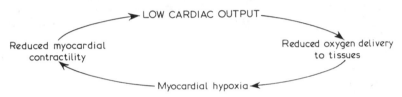

Fig. 3/1   Diagram illustrating the vicious cycle resulting from a low cardiac output

examined by measuring the central venous pressure (right atrial pressure). In some instances it is useful to measure the left atrial pressure as well. Due to the relationship between cardiac output and the filling pressure of the heart as described in Starling's law of the heart, there is a critical range for optimal functioning of the heart. If the right atrial pressure is below this range which is +5 to +15mm Hg, blood, plasma or plasma expanders are given to raise the pressure. By raising the right atrial pressure to the upper limit of this range the heart is placed in the optimal physiological situation. In many instances this simple measure will suffice to restore a normal circulation.

If this is not enough, attention is directed to the state of myocardial contractility. This can be altered by the administration of synthetic catecholamines the commonest of which are isoprenaline and adrenaline. Recently dopamine has come into regular use because of its special beneficial effect on the kidneys. Other drugs in use include salbutamol and noradrenaline. A further drug has appeared recently called dobutamine. All these drugs increase the rate and force of contraction of the myocardium but in practice it is their effect on heart rate which is the limiting factor.

If after applying these measures the patient has not improved an attempt may be made to reduce the peripheral resistance. The aim of this treatment is to reduce the minimum pressure which the left ventricle has to generate in order to open the aortic valve; and thus to reduce the work done by the left ventricle. This is achieved by the administration of peripheral vasodilator drugs which reduce the sympathetic vasoconstrictor drive to arterioles. Hence, whole new vascular beds which were closed are opened up and the capacity of the circulation increases. For this reason the central venous pressure will fall and in order to maintain the heart at its optimal filling pressure, several units of blood or plasma will need to be given. This type of treatment is potentially lethal unless the central venous pressure is maintained. Drugs which are used include chlorpromazine (Largactil), phentolamine (Rogitine), nitroprusside (Nipride).

In addition the patient may be placed on intermittent positive pressure ventilation (I.P.P.V.), to reduce oxygen requirements by taking over the work of the respiratory muscles and to gain better control of the arterial oxygen tension. The acid base balance is also closely maintained and corrected when necessary.

Until recently no other routine measures were available but there are now various forms of cardiac assist devices of which the intra-aortic balloon pump is the only one in regular clinical use.

Intra-Aortic Balloon Counterpulsation

The relationship between the *supply* of oxygen to the myocardium and the *demand* by the energy processes of the myocardium for oxygen becomes critical in low cardiac output states. Drugs which increase the contractility of the myocardium and thus the cardiac output tend to do so at the expense of increased demand by the myocardium for oxygen. Such drugs may increase demand beyond the available supply and thus build up an oxygen debt. Counterpulsation provides a way of improving the ratio between supply and demand.

The concept of counterpulsation is based on the finding that myocardial oxygen consumption is dependent upon the pressure generated by the left ventricle. Counterpulsation does two things: first it increases the diastolic perfusion pressure and second it reduces the systolic pressure against which the left ventricle contracts (a similar effect to that of the peripheral vasodilator drug).

A special balloon catheter is introduced into the descending thoracic aorta via a femoral artery. When the balloon inflates blood is displaced and the diastolic pressure in the aorta is increased. When the balloon deflates the systolic pressure is reduced and the capacity of the aorta for blood increases.

The catheter is attached to an electronically controlled actuator. The R wave of the E.C.G. (see Fig. 2/4) is the trigger which is picked up by the control unit. The effect is delayed so that the balloon is inflated during diastole when the aortic valve is closed. Since the majority of coronary blood flow occurs during diastole and is dependent upon diastolic perfusion, the selective elevation of diastolic pressure by the balloon will increase coronary blood flow. Shortly before the onset of left ventricular systole the balloon is deflated. This reduces the systolic pressure against which the left ventricle ejects its blood and so reduces work and hence myocardial oxygen consumption by the left ventricle.

The counterpulsation pump is used in two clinical situations. First in the operating theatre to enable a struggling heart to take on the load of the circulation and so come off cardiopulmonary bypass. Second to assist a patient in low cardiac output, either following open heart surgery or as a means of holding a severely ill patient with coronary artery disease for a limited period before emergency coronary artery vein bypass surgery is done.

Chapter 4

Auscultation

by L. H. CAPEL, M.D., F.R.C.P.

The art of auscultation was introduced into medicine by Laennec in the early part of the nineteenth century, and it was he who devised the stethoscope. He set out to relate what he could hear to what he found post mortem. That is, to relate what he heard to the structural changes in the lungs. Nowadays we have the chest radiograph for the study of structural changes in the lungs, and use auscultation mainly to try to relate what we hear to functional changes in the lungs. That is, we use the stethoscope to tell us something of how air moves in and out of the different parts of the lungs, and then speculate on what this might tell us about the condition of the lungs. This article presents the modern view of breath sounds as developed by Dr. Paul Forgacs, perhaps the first advance in the subject for a century and a half.

LUNG SOUNDS

Lung sounds are divided into breath sounds and added sounds (Fig. 4/1). *Breath sounds* may be normal or abnormal. *Added sounds* are always abnormal: they are divided into crackles, which are short sharp interrupted sounds, and wheezes, which are prolonged and musical.

Breath Sounds

Breath sounds are sounds of a mixture of intensities and frequencies of about 200 to 2000 Hertz (cycles per second, i.e. just below middle C and four octaves above). These are the sounds heard with a stethoscope placed at the root of the neck. They are generated by turbulent airflow in the pharynx and larger airways. Turbulent airflow, that is airflow disturbed by multitudes of eddies like the swirling seen round the pontoons of a bridge, contrasts with laminar or smooth airflow, which is silent. Airflow in the smaller airways is laminar and silent.

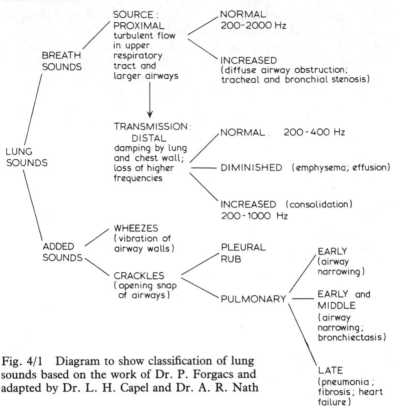

Fig. 4/1 Diagram to show classification of lung sounds based on the work of Dr. P. Forgacs and adapted by Dr. L. H. Capel and Dr. A. R. Nath

The breath sounds generated in the larger airways are transmitted via the alveoli of the lungs to the listening stethoscope on the chest wall. The alveoli damp off the higher frequency sounds, so lower pitched sounds only are heard (about 200 to 400 Hertz). These lower pitched sounds are normal breath sounds heard at the lung bases. Thus the alveoli are filters and not generators of breath sounds.

Breath sounds may be normal or abnormal in their *generation* and normal or abnormal in their *transmission* through the lungs.

1. Abnormal *generation* of breath sounds occurs in bronchitis and asthma when air flows at increased speed through normal airways; this increase in speed increases turbulence and the amount of noise made. This noisy breathing can be heard when the patient coughs or breathes forcibly.

2. Abnormal *transmission* of breath sounds can result from an increase or reduction in the damping off of the higher frequencies. Pneumonia consolidates the lung. Consolidated lung is more solid

than normal lung and transmits the breath sounds better: high frequency sounds are less damped, and so the bronchial breath sounds of the larger airways are then heard over the pneumonic lung, at the lung bases, for instance. Pleural effusion reflects the breath sounds away from the stethoscope listening over the effusion and the intensity of breath sounds is reduced. Emphysema and pneumothorax increase the damping of all the frequencies, and breath sound intensity is reduced. Effusion is easily distinguished from emphysema and pneumothorax as a cause of reduced intensity breath sounds by percussion: the note is dull with an effusion and resonant with emphysema and pneumothorax.

Added sounds

In the past the added sounds were given a variety of names, and no agreement on them was reached. We shall call them crackles and wheezes.

CRACKLES

Crackles are short sharp interrupted sounds. They may be described as fine, medium and coarse according to their loudness, and early, middle and late according to the part of the inspiratory cycle in which they appear. Crackles heard early in inspiration, usually only a few and not loud, are characteristic of patients with severe airway narrowing; crackles heard early and in mid-inspiration are characteristic of patients with bronchiectasis. Crackles heard late in inspiration (late inspiratory crackles), are heard in pulmonary fibrosis, in pneumonia and in heart failure. If crackles are heard in inspiration they will often be heard in expiration.

All crackles tend to repeat from breath to breath, so the same pattern of crackles will be heard from breath to breath as the same pressure and volume conditions of the lungs are repeated. They persist after coughing. Late inspiratory crackles (but not the others) are heard always over dependent parts of the lungs, for example the lung bases, and they will go with a change of posture which brings the dependent part uppermost; for example, if the patient's right base is listened to while he lies on his right, and then turns on to his left side, the stethoscope remaining in position. When he turns once more so that his right side is again dependent, then the crackles return.

It is believed that all this is explained if a crackle is the opening snap of an airway just closed and leading to a partially deflated territory of the lungs. The lung can be partially deflated by the hydrostatic pressure of extra liquid in the lungs in heart failure and by a tendency to retraction of the lungs in fibrosis. In early inspiratory crackles and in early and mid-inspiratory crackles the airways which crackle have been closed by the air trapping mechanism during the previous expiration. In all crackles the sound arises when the lung expands enough to draw the walls of the airway in question apart and air rushes in.

If the chest radiograph shows evidence of pulmonary fibrosis, congestion or bronchiectasis, then crackles will usually, but by no means always, be heard. Further, crackles may be heard though the radiograph is normal.

WHEEZE

A wheeze is a continuous musical sound. It may be of high, medium or low pitch. Wheezes are generated by the vibration of airway walls the faces of which just touch: as air rushes through they vibrate like a reed, or like the sound amusing to children when air from an inflated balloon rushes through the neck if this is held taut. The lung wheezes like a reed instrument and not like an organ pipe. The waxing and waning of wheeze with successful management of asthma may reflect change in congestion of the wall of the airway and change in bronchospasm.

CRACKLE-WHEEZE

A crackle-wheeze may be heard, towards the end of inspiration typically, in patients with resolving asthma. The airway opens with a crackle and the walls then vibrate with a wheeze. This tends to support the suggestions that this is how crackles and wheezes are generated.

Listening to the Lungs

Make sure the stethoscope earpieces are comfortable and fit snugly. A stethoscope with a diaphragm only is convenient – it slips into a pocket, and can be slipped under the chest of an immobile patient. Listen first while the patient makes a deep slow inspiration and expiration. This brings out any crackles. Then listen while the patient makes a deep forceful inspiration and expiration. This brings out any wheezes. Regular practice in those with normal and abnormal lungs brings confidence: critical use of the stethoscope will add to the interest and success of your work.

BIBLIOGRAPHY

Forgacs, Paul (1978). *Lung Sounds*. Baillière Tindall.

Chapter 5

Intensive Care – I

by P. J. WADDINGTON, M.C.S.P., H.T., DIP.T.P.
revised and enlarged by S. E. BROWN, M.C.S.P.

WHAT IS INTENSIVE CARE?

Progressive patient care has always been a feature of hospital life. In the traditional type of ward, patients who require constant care and supervision are placed in beds near to the Sister's office where they are always under the watchful eye of the staff passing to and fro. As the condition of the patient improves he is moved farther down the ward where the supervision based on simple geography will be less.

With the development of more sophisticated equipment and techniques the commissioning of intensive care units became a natural development of the graduated ward method. Such units ensure the best and most economical use of personnel and equipment.

In large hospitals it is usual to have several units where specialised patient care is given, for example a respiratory care unit; cardiac surgery units separate for adults and children; a transplant unit; a coronary care unit and a neonatal unit. Some hospitals have intensive care units which combine two or more of these units. Intensive care and supervision of patients is given on all these units and yet the role of the physiotherapist varies from unit to unit. In the coronary care unit her aim will be progressive rehabilitation and only rarely will she be required to treat the patient's chest. The question therefore may be asked: 'What do we mean by intensive care?' Many patients receive intensive physiotherapy, for example, in a thoracic surgery ward or rehabilitation centre, but this is not usually classified as intensive care.

Intensive care is the term used to describe the high quality of specially trained staff and supervision available to the acutely ill patient in a single unit.

RESPIRATORY CARE UNIT

The majority of patients admitted to this unit will require mechanical aid in some form, even if this is only suction, to maintain adequate ventilation. However, a proportion will need close and continual observation only, for a short period e.g. a patient who has received a stab wound, one who has self-administered a drug overdose or a patient in the immediate postoperative stage.

CARDIAC SURGERY UNITS

The majority of the patients in these units will have undergone open heart surgery. However, a few may have received closed heart surgery and need particularly close observation e.g. a pregnant woman or a patient with poor respiratory function test results.

THE NEO-NATAL UNIT

The majority of the babies in this unit will have been born prematurely and the unit may be partially split into medical and surgical areas.

The transplant and coronary care units usually contain only those patients to whom the titles refer.

The essence of effective intensive care is teamwork and, as in any good team, the members have certain basic skills and knowledge in common but it is the blending of different talents which together make an effective whole. Everyone has one simple objective, the recovery of the patient. The personnel of the unit will include the physician or surgeon, the anaesthetist, nursing staff, the technicians who maintain the equipment and the physiotherapists. The services of the radiographers and the laboratory technicians are regularly required. In some units either the physician or surgeon will be in charge, in others the anaesthetist.

It is obvious that intensive care is a service which must be available 24 hours a day, seven days a week, including Christmas Day and Boxing Day. This is not to say that a physiotherapist has always to be on duty all night. In many cases this is not necessary; usually if the patient has been treated at regular intervals during the day and again in the evening he can be safely left at night. He needs his sleep too. Where practical an 'on call' service should be available.

HISTORY

Modern intensive respiratory care is a development of the work of a Danish doctor, Dr. H. C. A. Lassen and an anaesthetist, Dr. B. Ibsen who, in the poliomyelitis epidemic in 1952, were faced with the problem of treating patients who could not swallow or breathe, which with the equipment available at the time was a fatal combination.

The first coordinated records of attempts to design breathing machines appear to be associated with the founding of the Humane Society (later the Royal Humane Society) in 1774. In relatively modern times (1929) a practical breathing machine was designed by Dr. Phillip Drinker, an engineer of Harvard University. This respirator and its successors, were based on the negative (subatmospheric) pressure principle. It was called the 'iron lung' by the general public; the correct name of this type of respirator is the tank or cabinet respirator.

The tank respirator was an air-tight box designed to take the whole of the patient's body and limbs, leaving the head outside. Ways had to be found to ensure a good seal round the neck. In the original tanks the patient was placed on a drawer on wheels which could be pulled out from inside the cabinet. An improved model, the Smith-Clarke Cabinet Respirator, Alligator Model was produced in 1952. As the name implies, the lid of the respirator was hinged at the foot end and it opened rather like the jaws of an alligator. This was quick and easy to operate when the patient could not be cared for through the portholes which were placed at intervals along each side. It also had a face mask or mouthpiece which the patient could use when the cabinet was open.

In normal respiration a muscular effort produces a gradual increase in the volume of the thorax, pressure is reduced to subatmospheric levels and air enters the lungs via the respiratory passages from the nose and mouth which are at atmospheric pressure. This reduced pressure in the thorax also aids venous return to the heart. Because the surface of the body is at atmospheric pressure there is a favourable pressure gradient between the blood in the peripheral veins and the right atrium.

The cabinet respirator was attached to bellows which created a negative (subatmospheric) pressure within the box. The patient's nose and mouth, outside the box, were at atmospheric pressure. Thus air flowed into the patient's lungs until the difference between the pressure within the tank and the pressure within the lungs was equal to the elasticity of the lungs and the chest wall. This was an effective method of ventilating the lungs but it had an adverse effect on venous return to the heart. The peripheral veins were within the box, thus they were at subatmospheric pressure too and therefore there was no advantageous pressure gradient to aid venous return. To counter this it was usual to introduce a positive pressure phase into the cycle, especially for patients who were in the respirator for a long period.

There is a vital flaw in this method of ventilation when it is used for patients who cannot swallow and maintain a clear airway. Secretions from the mouth which could include vomit may be drawn into the patient's lungs as well as air. The patient then either drowns or his lungs are damaged by the secretions. In some centres especially in the United States of America a cuffed tracheostomy tube (a tube in the trachea which bypasses the upper respiratory tract and is designed to prevent secretions from there from entering the lungs) was used to overcome this problem. The method worked well but the patient in the tank was a very difficult nursing problem at best. A new method of ventilating patients who could not swallow was necessary. Today, except for a few old 'polio patients' who may sleep in the tank, it is unlikely that a negative pressure respirator will be used; the positive pressure ventilator is a much more practical proposition even for the patient who can swallow.

The method instituted by Dr. Lassen was based on two ideas, the maintaining of a clear airway and the use of positive pressure ventilation, that is blowing air into the lungs, which at the beginning was provided by manual pressure on a rubber bag as used in anaesthetics. The manpower was provided by medical students working day and night on a rota basis. It was not long before a mechanical ventilator was designed to undertake this onerous task. Since that time a number of ventilators have been developed in an effort to produce the perfect piece of apparatus.

The main features in maintaining a clear airway, as given by Dr. Lassen, are:

1. High tracheostomy.
2. Well-fitting tracheostomy tube.
3. Humidification.
4. Repeated suction of the trachea and main bronchi.
5. Postural drainage, frequent changes of position and squeezing of the thorax followed by aspiration.

These rules still apply today.

THE ROLE OF THE PHYSIOTHERAPIST

The physiotherapist in the modern intensive care unit, where patients may or may not be receiving artificial ventilation, will be surrounded by a variety of mechanical aids, some of which she will need to use. But her simple basic role is three-fold:

Chest Care

1. To assist in maintaining adequate ventilation by loosening and removing secretions from the lungs.
2. To ensure that the free breathing patient is adequately ventilating all areas of the lungs.

Movement

1. To instruct the patient in free active exercises to maintain mobility and adequate muscle power and aid venous return.
2. To maintain full range joint movement and muscle length by passive movements where the patient is paralysed. This will also aid venous return.
3. To ensure that the positioning of the patient is compatible with the maintenance of good posture.

General Care

1. To have an understanding of the patient, his condition and the medical problems involved.
2. To appreciate the nursing programme and techniques.

THE ROLE OF THE PHYSIOTHERAPIST EXPANDED

The most overwhelming impression when walking into an intensive care unit for the first time is that the room is full of equipment, coupled with a certain amount of mechanical noise. When this is associated with very ill patients and seemingly ultra-efficient staff it can be, for some people, a rather worrying experience. However the equipment is easy to understand, the physiotherapy techniques are basic and there are many people on hand should an emergency arise. It is not long before a physiotherapist working on such a unit becomes a skilled member of the team.

The Equipment and its Uses

Standard pieces of equipment, such as ventilators, humidifiers and suction apparatus, have been developed by a number of engineers and doctors. The design will vary in detail but in basic principles of operation each will follow a common pattern. It is only possible to outline these basic principles. Anyone entering an intensive care unit for the first time should familiarise herself with the equipment in that unit and with the routine to be followed in an emergency such as an electrical failure, the breakdown of an individual ventilator, a cardiac arrest or respirator failure.

ENDOTRACHEAL TUBES, TRACHEOSTOMY TUBES AND AIRWAYS (see Fig. 5/1)

The purpose of these tubes is to maintain a clear airway. They were originally made of red rubber, now it is more usual to find plastic tubes in use.

The endotracheal tube is one which passes either through the mouth (oral) or the nose (nasal), the pharynx, the larynx and into the trachea. They vary in size and design. There are two basic tubes, the plain and the cuffed. The nasal endotracheal tubes are made of much thinner materials than the oral tubes: this allows the lumen to remain almost as large as for the oral tube but the overall diameter is less. The cuffed oral tube is usually the type chosen for adult patients, especially those on ventilators whereas the plain nasal tube is that most commonly used for small children and babies. To maintain the endotracheal tube in place a piece of cotton tape is tied firmly round the tube. For easy release this is tied in a bow at the side of the neck.

The use of endotracheal tubes can only be a temporary measure as prolonged intubation may cause inflammation and ulceration of the larynx. It is usually considered that 3 to 4 days is the time for safe use. However, plastic tubes may be used for a week without adverse effect.

There are two types of tracheostomy tubes in common use, the cuffed plastic tube and the uncuffed silver tube.

Tracheostomy is an operation, usually performed under a general anaesthetic, in which a short horizontal incision is made in the neck and a small window or fenestra fashioned in the trachea. To ensure that the tracheostomy tube will be parallel with the walls of the trachea it is necessary for the surgeon to perform a high tracheostomy at the level of the second and third or third and fourth tracheal rings. If the tracheostomy is too low the tube may extend beyond the carina, enter the right main bronchus and thus prevent air from entering the left lung. It is normal practice for an endotracheal tube to be in place

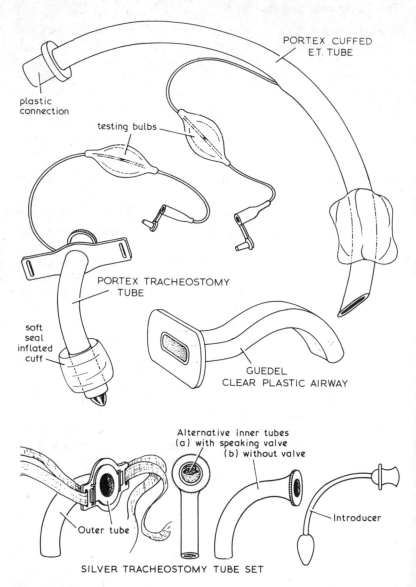

PORTEX CUFFED
E.T. TUBE

plastic
connection

testing bulbs

PORTEX TRACHEOSTOMY
TUBE

soft
seal
inflated
cuff

GUEDEL
CLEAR PLASTIC AIRWAY

Alternative inner tubes
(a) with speaking valve
(b) without valve

Introducer

Outer tube

SILVER TRACHEOSTOMY TUBE SET

Fig. 5/1   Diagram showing endotracheal and tracheostomy tubes and an airway

during this operation. It is withdrawn to just above the operation site to enable the surgeon to test the tracheostomy tube.

The tracheostomy tube should provide a clear airway with a low resistance to the flow, it should be well-fitting to prevent damage to surrounding structures, and the possibility of accidental displacement should be reduced to a minimum. A right-angled cuffed rubber tube with a metal connecting piece for use with a ventilator was designed by Spalding and Smith in 1959. The plastic cuffed tube is now in common use. This tube has a straight arm lying in the trachea, parallel to the walls so that no pressure is exerted on the tissues, and a short section at right angles to this lying in the tracheostome (see Fig. 5/2).

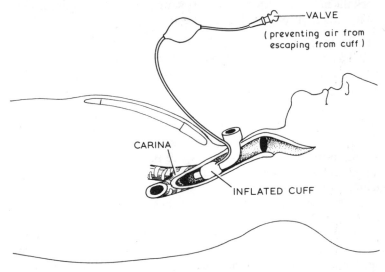

Fig. 5/2   Diagram of cuffed tube in situ

The tube is secured in position by a piece of cotton tape fastened round the patient's neck, again in the form of a bow for easy release.

The cuffed form of endotracheal and tracheostomy tube is designed to ensure a good seal between the tube and the trachea. A cuff is a short band of thin plastic, bonded to the outside of the tube. It can be inflated by a syringe via a small tube which is incorporated into it, one end of which lies outside the patient. Care must be taken not to over-inflate the cuff as pressure on the adjacent structures can cause ulceration by impairing the circulation. Only enough air should be used to create a seal. It is possible, with practice, to judge the correct amount by listening, if necessary with a stethoscope. There should be no audible hissing sound when the patient is receiving artificial ventilation; when the patient is off the ventilator, no air should escape from the mouth or around the tube. A patient with an inflated cuff cannot speak as no air is passing over the vocal cords.

Most tracheostomy tubes now in use have a large volume low pressure cuff which ensures a larger area of contact and reduces the possibility of undue pressure being exerted at any point.

With these soft-seal cuffs, some centres feel that it is necessary to release the cuff at intervals. However there is evidence to suggest (Ching, 1971), that prolonged use of these tubes may lead to tracheal stenosis if the cuffs are reduced at regular intervals due to pro-gressively higher inflationary pressures. It is therefore advisable to check the inflation with the pressure gauge designed for this purpose.

The functions of the cuffed tube are:

1. To facilitate access to pulmonary secretions.
2. To prevent substances from the mouth from entering the lungs.
3. To help maintain positive pressure ventilation by preventing air from escaping round the tube.
4. To bypass an obstruction preventing ventilation.

All endotracheal and tracheostomy tubes reduce the anatomical dead space by about one half but this is usually negligible in com-parison to the physiological dead space present in the free breathing patient. There is therefore some doubt as to whether intubation facilitates ventilation in these patients.

Tracheostomy and endotracheal tubes are sized from 2·5mm in-creasing by 0·5mm to 11·0mm.

The silver tracheostomy tube cannot be used for connection to a ventilator and is used in the intermediate stage before finally closing the tracheostomy. It is sometimes a permanent feature for patients following laryngectomy. It usually has an inner tube which can be removed for cleaning. Some have a valve which allows the patient with a larynx to speak.

The disadvantages of tracheostomy are the increased danger of infection and the loss of humidification. Dry gases entering the trachea can cause crusts to form and a blockage of one of the res-piratory passages may occur.

Opinions differ as to the frequency with which tracheostomy tubes should be changed. Within a few days of operation there is a firm track from the skin to the trachea and after this there is usually no difficulty in changing the tube.

Occasionally it may be necessary to use an airway to facilitate suction through the mouth. All physiotherapists should be familiar with the airway, which is frequently in position when a patient returns from theatre. It is a simple tube, usually made of rigid plastic, flattened vertically, with a flange to prevent it from slipping past the teeth and into the mouth completely. It has a right-angled curve so that the tube fits over the tongue and down into the pharynx. Airways vary in size. An airway facilitates artificial ventilation when used in conjunction with an anaesthetic bag and mask during resuscitation but cannot be used for intermittent positive pressure ventilation. It serves the simple purpose of preventing the tongue falling backwards and suffocating the unconscious patient; it also gives a clear pathway for suction in both the conscious and the unconscious patient. To insert, put the airway into the mouth with the curved end pointing upwards. Once in the mouth it is rotated through 180°. It is then in position to restrain the tongue, protect the suction catheter from being bitten and direct it into the pharynx.

HUMIDIFICATION

Humidification is the moistening of the air or gases we breathe. This is one of the functions of the upper part of the respiratory tract.

Artificial humidification is necessary for patients in the following circumstances:

1. *When breathing through endotracheal or tracheostomy tubes*. The natural humidification and warming function of the upper respiratory tract is bypassed if a patient is breathing either through an endotracheal or tracheostomy tube. Dry air at lower than body temperature passing over secretions in the bronchial tree extracts moisture from them causing crusts to be formed. These crusts may partially block the trachea or main bronchus or occlude one of the smaller airways. They are very difficult to remove. Ciliary action is diminished in the absence of adequate humidification. Artificial humidification is therefore essential for the maintenance of adequate ventilation. The vast majority of ventilators incorporate some form of humidification. Patients who have a permanent silver tracheostomy tube seem to acclimatise themselves to the lack of humidification and provided the inner tube is cleaned regularly suffer no gross ill-effects.

2. *When breathing air to which gases have been added*. These gases are completely dry and will require considerable humidification and it may be considered advantageous to the patient to augment the natural humidification process.

3. *When secretions are abnormally thick*. Humidification will facilitate their removal.

There are several methods of achieving humidification, but the majority have the two same problems to a greater or lesser extent.

Condensation in the tubes is one of these and when using apparatus where this pertains, care must be taken to ensure that the tubes are emptied at regular intervals. It is very distressing for the patient when water enters a tracheostomy tube. The other problem is that humidifiers are liable to become infected by bacteria and introduce this infection into the patient's respiratory system. Careful sterilisation of the apparatus is essential.

HUMIDIFIERS

NEBULISERS

There are two types of nebuliser in common usage today. One is pneumatically powered and the other is ultrasonic.

a). Pneumatically powered nebulisers. Examples of the pneumatically powered nebuliser are the Ohio de-luxe nebuliser, the Bard Inspiron nebuliser, the Bird 500ml nebuliser and the Puritan all-purpose nebuliser (see Fig. 5/3).

In all these nebulisers the fine mist of liquid particles is formed in accordance with Bernoulli's principle. A high pressure jet of gas is blown across the top of a fine tube set in a bath of water. Water is then drawn up the tube and entrained into the stream of gas having been further broken up on an anvil. The large droplets condense in the humidifier so that only a fine mist of small particles is delivered to the patient. The Bard Inspiron, Ohio and Puritan nebulisers may have the addition of an immersion heater which increases the relative humidity of the gas.

The devices named above are all large volume nebulisers and if a drug, e.g. a mucolytic agent or a bronchodilator, is to be administered to the patient a smaller nebuliser is often more suitable. Examples of these are the Bird Micronebuliser and the Hudson and Wright nebuliser.

b). Ultrasonic nebulisers. Examples of the ultrasonic nebuliser are the Mistogen and Monaghan ultrasonic nebulisers (see Fig. 5/4a). Humidification is produced in a nebuliser by water dropping on to a high speed rotating metal plate or vibrating crystal. One drop at a time, the water is shattered into micro-droplets. These droplets can be extremely small and 97% may be up to 1 to 5 microns in diameter (Chamney, 1969).

Because large quantities of droplets are produced, this form of humidification is very effective in loosening sticky secretions. Care must be taken to observe the patient and the degree of humidity as the effect of over-humidification would result in considerable discomfort to the patient and could result in actual drowning.

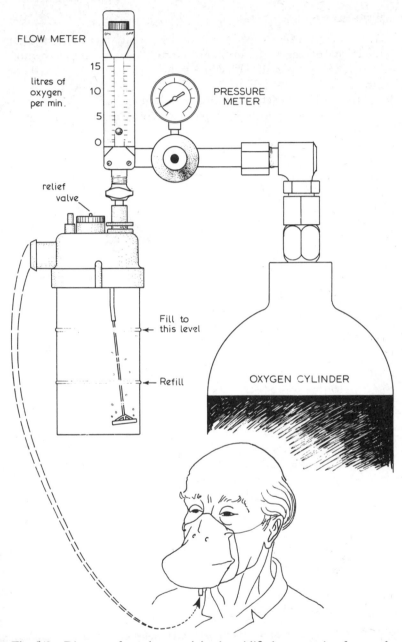

FLOW METER

litres of oxygen per min.

15

10

5

0

relief valve

PRESSURE METER

Fill to this level

Refill

OXYGEN CYLINDER

Fig. 5/3   Diagram of a patient receiving humidified oxygen via a face mask

WATER BATH HUMIDIFIERS

a). *Steam kettle*. This type of humidifier usually incorporates a fan which blows air across the surface of a water bath containing a heating element, the temperature of which can be regulated and the water maintained at between 37 to 60°C. The air or gases which leave the humidifier are fully saturated at the set temperature.

The main problem with this type is that considerable condensation

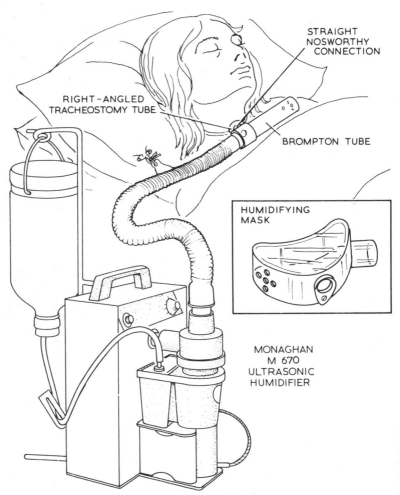

Fig. 5/4(a)   Diagram of a patient with a tracheostomy receiving humidification via an ultrasonic humidifier. The inset shows the polythene box which can be used instead of the Brompton tube

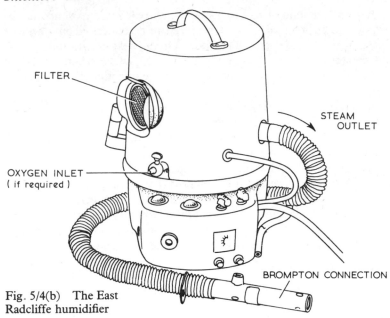

FILTER

STEAM
OUTLET

OXYGEN INLET
(if required)

BROMPTON CONNECTION

Fig. 5/4(b)   The East
Radcliffe humidifier

occurs and that, although the temperature of the humidified air
leaving the kettle is known, the temperature after it has passed
through the delivery tube is difficult to control. The best temperature
to be achieved is 33°C in the trachea.

The hot water has the effect of killing bacteria. All the
humidification produced with the steam kettle method is in the form
of a vapour which is not effective in loosening thick secretions.
Droplets are required for this. The East Radcliffe humidifier (see Fig.
5/4b) and the Cape humidifier are examples of the steam kettle type of
humidifier.

b). Bubble-through humidifiers. The Bennett Cascade is an example
of a heated bubble-through humidifier producing a vapour, often
attached to a ventilator.

Devices which 'humidify' gases by bubbling them through cold
water are *not* effective.

CONDENSERS

These humidifiers can only be used by patients with either an endotracheal or tracheostomy tube. They are usually used during the
process of weaning the patient from the ventilator and although
probably only suitable for short periods, enable the patient to be
mobile and independent of machinery.

No water is added to the gases which reach the patient but the vapour which is contained in the expired air is condensed out on a wire mesh, usually made of stainless steel. On the next inspiration some of the condensed water is picked up as droplets. This method is aimed at preventing loss of moisture and will only be effective if the patient is well hydrated.

In some centres during chest clearance when the secretions are very thick and difficult to remove, the physiotherapist will introduce normal saline i.e. 0·9% sodium chloride into the endotracheal or tracheostomy tube using a syringe. The maximum quantity is 2ml.

Distilled water and a solution of bicarbonate of soda have also been used for this purpose but it is believed that distilled water can cause pulmonary oedema and a strong solution of bicarbonate of soda has been shown to damage mucous membrane and depress ciliary activity. However, a very weak solution of bicarbonate of soda at pH 7·4 may be safe to use. Normal saline is a physiological solution.

PRECAUTION

All forms of humidification that require a container of water should be checked at frequent intervals to ensure that the level of water in the container has not fallen below the minimum mark. This applies particularly to heated models as heated dry air will soon dry out secretions and cause the formation of crusts which could lead to complete blockage of an airway.

Methods by which Humidified Air can be Introduced into the Respiratory System

Humidification is effectively delivered to the patient only by wide-bore tubing, because too much condensation will occur in narrow-bore tubing.

A FREE BREATHING PATIENT WHO IS NOT INTUBATED

a) A face mask (see Fig. 5/3).

b) A mouthpiece which the patient has to hold. This method is frequently used with a nebuliser as a method of giving a short period of humidification prior to chest clearance.

A FREE BREATHING PATIENT WITH A TRACHEOSTOMY TUBE

a) A tracheostomy humidifying tube (Brompton tube). This is made of plastic and it fits directly onto the wide-bore tubing and the tracheostomy. This method of delivery is also suitable for patients with an endotracheal tube.

b) Tracheostomy mask. These are now usually disposable and made from flexible plastic though some rigid plastic boxes are still in use.

A PATIENT ON INTERMITTENT POSITIVE PRESSURE VENTILATION (I.P.P.V.)

It is essential that patients receiving I.P.P.V. receive humidification. A humidifier is usually incorporated into the ventilator. The majority of humidifiers used for this purpose are heated. The ideal temperature at the entrance to the endotracheal or tracheostomy tube is thought to be 34°C±2°C.

Vapour or Droplets for Humidification?

Vapour is a humidified gas containing particles of liquid of less than one micron in diameter i.e. invisible.

Droplets are particles of liquid exceeding one micron and so visible.

Vapour is ineffective in loosening thick secretions but is adequate for compensating for the loss of upper respiratory tract humidification.

SUCTION

The frequent removal of secretions from the respiratory passages is an essential part of the treatment of the patient requiring intensive respiratory care.

Some patients will be able to cough at either a voluntary or reflex level, others will not. It is unusual for the very ill patient who is able to cough and co-operate in the treatment, to be able to do so effectively enough to maintain a clear airway at all times. Secretions may remain in the pharynx. Suction will then be necessary to remove them. If it is necessary to induce the patient to cough at a reflex level, suction will again be required to remove the secretions. Other patients who are unable to cough either because they are so deeply unconscious that the reflex cannot be stimulated or because of the paralysis of the expiratory muscles, will require suction to clear the secretions which have been moved from the lungs by postural drainage and manual techniques.

Suction should be given:

1. Whenever secretions can be heard.
2. Before and after a change of position.
3. Before and during the release of the cuff.
4. If the patient looks distressed and changes colour.
5. If the minute volume (M.V.) drops. (Minute volume is the

amount of air either inspired or expired in one minute. It is usual to measure the M.V. of expired air as this is considered to be a more reliable guide.) It is usually taken and recorded hourly by the nursing staff using a volume meter. The level of the M.V. should be noted by the physiotherapist before and after the treatment as it is an indication as to the state of the patient.

SUCTION APPARATUS

Suction Pumps (see Fig. 5/5). Nature abhors a vacuum and does its best to fill it. This is the principle upon which suction apparatus is

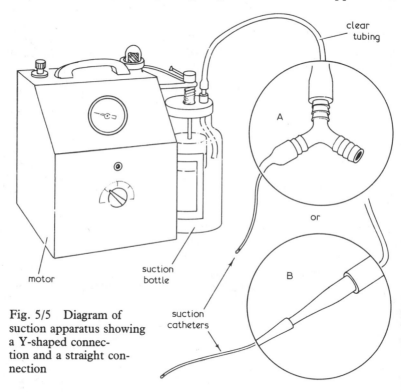

clear
tubing

A

or

B

motor

suction
bottle

Fig. 5/5   Diagram of
suction apparatus showing
a Y-shaped connec-
tion and a straight con-
nection

suction
catheters

built. There are four basic types of apparatus which may be classified according to the power used to create the vacuum or suction force. This vacuum is filled simultaneously with its production, by substances (air, water, sputum, blood) passing down the suction tube.

1. Electrical suction apparatus which is powered from the mains. This type has its own small motor with an on/off switch.

2. Suction apparatus designed to work from a vacuum point

adjacent to the patient's bed; again there is an on/off switch. The power in this instance is provided by a large motor situated at some convenient site within the hospital grounds.

3. Foot pump: here as the name suggests, the power is provided by the individual operator. This type of pump was the only one available in the period when intensive care was developing. Today a foot pump is rarely used but one should be available in case of a power failure.

4. Battery operated, portable suction apparatus. This type, like the electrical apparatus, works from its own small motor and has an on/off switch. The machine should be tested at frequent intervals to check the batteries.

Each suction pump has either one or two suction bottles, depending upon the design, partially filled with some antiseptic solution. The connecting tubes enter through the lid which is secured in such a way as to prevent leakage. Usually the lid is maintained in position by two metal clamps controlled by screws.

If the apparatus has not been used for some time or if it has only just been cleaned, it is advisable to test it with water before use. If suction is not adequate it is wise to check the lids of the bottles to see that they are well screwed down and to check that the sealing washers are in position. Inspect all the tube connections and it is even possible that the on/off switch could be in the wrong position!

Suction tubing. This leads from the bottle on the suction machine to the connection for the suction catheter. Nowadays the tubing is usually made from clear plastic for easy viewing of secretions, and is disposable, though rubber tubing is still found in some centres.

Connections. These are usually plastic and either clear or semi-transparent. A clear connection must be used with rubber tubing in order to take note of the type of secretions passing through the tube. Most connections have three holes, one at each end and one at the side or in the case of the Y – connection three arms. The catheter and tubing fit onto the opposite ends leaving the open aperture for the operator to use. This opening offers less resistance to the suction force than does the catheter and so the suction takes the line of least resistance and air is taken in through the hole. To apply suction to the tip of the catheter the operator places a finger over the opening.

Catheters. Soft, clear, plastic, disposable catheters sizes 4 to 16 French Gauge are commonly used. It is important to select the correct sized catheter for suction; the catheter should not exceed half of the diameter of the endotracheal or tracheostomy tube. If the catheter fits the tube closely, when suction is applied the alveoli will tend to collapse as insufficient air will enter the lungs to neutralise the negative pressure being applied through suction.

Some hospitals still use the soft rubber catheters which are particularly useful for nasal suction as they are softer and more flexible than the plastic catheters. These are not disposable and need to be returned to the Central Sterilising Supply Department (C.S.S.D.) for sterilisation after use.

The catheter must have two holes close together on opposite sides of the suction end. If one hole becomes adherent to the mucous membrane of the respiratory tract, the resistance at that point will be greater than at the unobstructed hole. Therefore, air will pass through this hole and the suction force exerted on the membrane will be contained.

Bronchoscopy or Pinkerton's catheters should also be available for use in an intensive care unit. These are extra long catheters with a curved end of reinforced rubber. Normally when using a straight catheter if one penetrates farther than the carina, the catheter will enter the right main bronchus which is almost a direct continuation of the trachea. Using a Pinkerton's catheter with the head side flexed to the right there is a greater chance of the catheter entering the left main bronchus.

'Airflow' catheters are available in some intensive care units. These are costly but are invaluable for the suction of patients who have had tracheal or laryngeal surgery and are undergoing anti-coagulation therapy. At the tip of this catheter as well as the usual two holes is an outward spreading flange. By the action of movement in the trachea the air which the catheter meets is buffered around the flange and so prevents the tip from having any contact with the trachea either during its insertion or removal.

All catheters must only be used once then thrown away or if rubber placed with other unsterile catheters in a separate bowl.

Suction Trolley. All the equipment needed should be set out suitably on a trolley:

Plastic gloves
Suction catheters
Lubricating jelly
Bowl of sodium bicarbonate (this solution is passed through the
    catheter after suction to clear secretions and act as a solvent)
Bowl of gauze swabs, for transferring the jelly to the end of the
    catheter
Forceps (if used)
Bowl of antiseptic solution for unsterile catheters, if rubber catheters
    used
Bags for discarding disposable objects.

Suction Technique

Some centres use forceps for introducing catheters and others use only gloves, but in both cases a clean technique must be used as the risk of introducing infection into the respiratory tract is high.

Techniques will vary slightly from unit to unit and the physiotherapist should adopt the method advocated by the medical personnel in charge of the unit in which she is working.

Way of Entry for a Suction Catheter. There are three possible routes by which a suction catheter may be introduced into the respiratory tract: the nose, the mouth and via a tube. Passing a catheter, particularly via the nose and mouth is a very uncomfortable procedure for the conscious patient. It must be done with the correct combination of gentleness and firmness and is the direct product of the attitude of mind of the operator. Fear or distaste for the job in hand will result in either ineffective or over-vigorous use of the catheter. If possible, it is advisable to make one's first attempts at suction in this way on an unconscious patient. He will not be distressed and the operator can gain that confidence which is necessary to use any form of apparatus efficiently.

1. When using the nose as a mode of entry the patient's neck is extended so that the head is tilted backwards resting on a pillow. A lubricated catheter is held between the fingers and thumb of a gloved hand and introduced into the nose. It is directed slightly upwards and backwards until the tip reaches the posterior naris where a little resistance may be felt. A way through can usually be found by carefully rolling the catheter between the index finger and thumb. If the patient has a Ryle's tube in position it has been found in practice easier to use the same nostril. The catheter seems to slide along the first tube and through the posterior naris easily.

The catheter then enters the pharynx. The position of the catheter beyond this point cannot be determined accurately. It may curl up in the mouth but this is a rare occurrence and it can be seen. Some authorities doubt if the catheter reaches beyond the pharynx and into the upper part of the bronchial tree but the fact remains that on some occasions a cough reflex can be elicited and on others the patient begins to retch. It is certain that if the patient is conscious and able to co-operate by taking deep breaths with the mouth open and the catheter is only advanced during inspiration, a cough reflex can be stimulated in the majority of cases. By using this method of advancing the catheter during inspiration even in the unconscious patient success is achieved in a high percentage of attempts.

The nose is a very successful way of entering a suction catheter into the respiratory tract. Unfortunately for the patients it is very uncomfortable but if they are well prepared and able to co-operate the majority tolerate it extremely well.

2. The mouth is a relatively unsatisfactory mode of entry unless the patient is extremely co-operative and even then it may be necessary to use a lubricated airway. The mouth is such a large cavity that it is easy to misdirect the catheter and it is not unusual to see the suction end re-appear between the teeth. The patient may bite the catheter unless an airway is used.

3. Most commonly the catheter is introduced into an endotracheal or tracheostomy tube, which presents no difficulties. However, it must be remembered that if a patient is dependent upon a ventilator the time available for suction is strictly limited. To get some idea of the patient's tolerance one should exhale as far as possible and note how long one can remain comfortable without taking a breath.

Suction. The catheter is advanced as far as possible, care being taken to ensure that suction does not take place during the entry phase. Considerable damage has been shown to be done to the mucous membrane even by the most skilful operator and suction on the way in is considered to be especially traumatic. The modern connector is designed to prevent this. If a three-hole connector is not available the catheter itself can be pinched to prevent suction from taking place. Suction is started by occluding the open hole of the connection with the thumb of the other hand. The catheter is then slowly and gently withdrawn using intermittent suction. As it is removed it is rotated first one way and then the other between the finger and thumb. If a pool of secretions is reached, there is a pause until it is clear, always remembering the time factor for the patient dependent upon a ventilator. Under no circumstances should the 'tromboning' method be used, i.e. a vigorous up and down movement.

If the catheter appears to be blocked it is occasionally possible to clear it by moving the thumb off and on the open hole of the connection.

After suction the ventilator patient is re-attached immediately.

The suction end of the catheter is then placed into the bowl containing a solution of bicarbonate of soda and cleared. It is then discarded and the connection returned to its holder, the suction tube secured, the bowls re-covered and the glove removed.

If a specimen of sputum is required for bacteriological study a special sputum trap can be fitted in between the connection and the suction catheter.

INTERMITTENT POSITIVE PRESSURE VENTILATION (I.P.P.V.)

In patients who are receiving I.P.P.V., inspiration occurs when air under positive pressure (above atmospheric pressure) enters the lungs. Air continues to flow until the pre-set inspiratory cycle of the ventilator is reached and then expiration will take place either passively or with the aid of a negative expiratory phase. As the intrathoracic pressure is raised above atmospheric pressure the pressure gradient between the periphery and the right atrium hinders venous return. This may lead to a reduction in cardiac output and hypotension.

Following the development of the original method of I.P.P.V. many machines have been produced. It is usual to classify them as time cycled, volume cycled and pressure cycled. This classification refers to the inspiratory phase.

In a time-cycled ventilator the rate and duration of inspiration and expiration are pre-set. The volume of gases delivered to the patient depends on the flow rate of the gases to the patient. The higher the rate, the more gas is received by the patient in the set time.

Most time-cycled ventilators have spirometers and pressure gauges built into the machine so that both the tidal volume and/or minute volume as well as airway pressure can be readily observed. These ventilators are often the type selected for long-term ventilation cases. Examples of these ventilators are the Phillips AV1 ventilator, the Servo 900 ventilator (see Fig. 5/6), the East Radcliffe ventilator and the Cavitron paediatric ventilator.

A volume-cycled ventilator is one in which inspiration ends when a

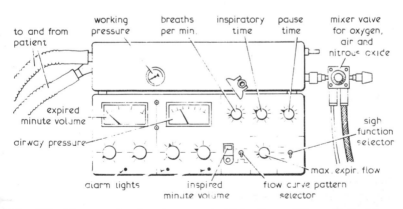

Fig. 5/6   Diagram showing the controls of the Servo 900 ventilator (time-cycled)

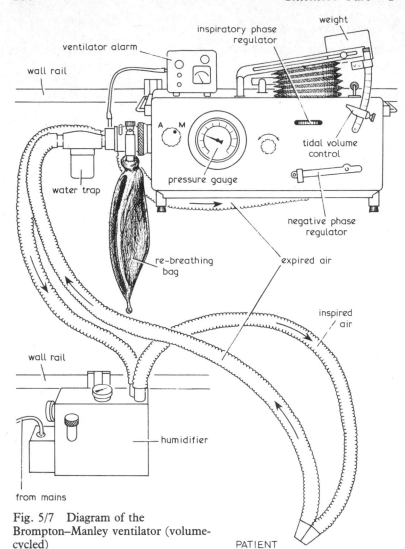

Fig. 5/7   Diagram of the
Brompton–Manley ventilator (volume-
cycled)   PATIENT

pre-set volume has been delivered to the patient. A pressure gauge will
depict any sudden alteration of pressure in the circuit which might be
due to a plug of sputum in one of the main bronchi or to a degree of
resistance on the part of the patient. Some volume-cycled ventilators
run off electricity, for example the Monaghan 250 and Cape ventilators and some are pneumatically powered. An example of the latter
is the Brompton-Manley, (see Fig. 5/7) one of the most commonly

used ventilators and which operates as soon as the gas flows into the ventilator.

Examples of pressure-cycled ventilators are the Bird (see Fig. 5/8a), the Bennett and the Harlow ventilators. These ventilators operate to a pre-determined pressure and when this pressure of gas is reached in the patient's lungs and the tubes leading to him, the flow of gas is cut off and expiration occurs. Of these the Bird is probably the most popular (see Fig. 5/8b). The Bird Mark 7 or 8 is powered by gas under pressure. It can be connected either to a cylinder or to a piped system of oxygen or compressed air. When air is used as the driving force oxygen may be added, or if oxygen is used as the driving force 100% oxygen or a mixture of oxygen and entrained atmospheric air can be given. This mixture is reputedly 40% oxygen though it may prove to be considerably higher. The ventilator can be cycled automatically or be set to be triggered by the free breathing patient who requires assistance. The sensitivity control can be finely adjusted so that the slightest inspiratory effort by the patient producing a small negative pressure within the ventilator will trigger the inspiratory phase. If required the ventilator can be operated manually.

Oxygen can be fed into all ventilators and a humidifier is either built into the original design or it can be incorporated into the circuit.

The physiotherapist will not be required to adjust the ventilator and set the controls. This is usually done by the anaesthetist or physician in charge but she should be able to identify the controls and read the dials, although the records will be kept by the nursing staff. The only exception to this is when the Bird is being used as part of the chest clearance programme.

The patient with an endotracheal or tracheostomy tube will be attached to the ventilator by tubes with plastic swivel connections. These connecting tubes can be quite heavy and if not carefully adjusted can pull uncomfortably on the tracheostomy tube. Some modern ventilators have an adjustable jointed metal arm which will take the weight of these tubes. Another method which is not quite as effective, is to attach the tubes to the sheet or pillow, if used, by cotton tape and a safety-pin or artery forceps.

The Bird ventilator is not always used in conjunction with an endotracheal or tracheostomy tube. It can be used with a mouthpiece or a face mask.

INTERMITTENT POSITIVE PRESSURE BREATHING

Intermittent positive pressure breathing, commonly known as I.P.P.B., is a form of assisted breathing which can be a valuable

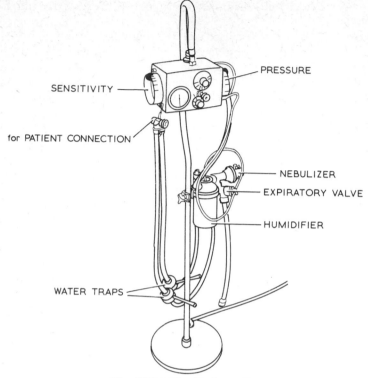

Fig. 5/8(a) The Bird ventilator

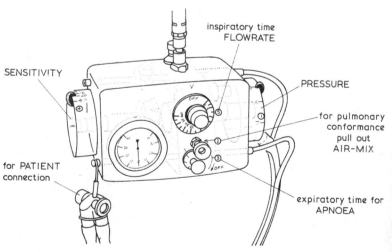

Fig. 5/8(b) Diagram showing the controls of the Bird ventilator

adjunct to physiotherapy, particularly in the treatment of respiratory disease. It is thought to provide more effective aeration of the alveoli and will aid the removal of retained secretions, and it is also a means of administering drugs directly to the airways.

Pressure-cycled machines with a patient-triggering mechanism are employed. The Bird and the Bennett ventilators are most commonly used for this type of treatment and various models are available. They are mainly driven by compressed gas (oxygen or air), but electrically powered ventilators are also obtainable, the latter being more suitable for use in the home.

In hospital, each machine should have several breathing head assemblies which will consist of tubing, nebuliser, exhalation valve and mouthpiece or mask; thus one ventilator can be used to treat several patients each day. There is no risk of cross-infection providing each patient has his own breathing head assembly, although precautions should be taken if a patient is infected with a resistant strain of bacteria. In this case the machine being used should not be moved to other patients, and should be sterilised with ethylene oxide gas when the patient concerned no longer needs I.P.P.B. The breathing head assemblies may be cold sterilised in a suitable disinfectant; Quats or Cidex, being two brands which are frequently used. Your pharmacist will advise on suitable products for this type of sterilising.

Controls

The controls will vary slightly according to the make of ventilator, but basically are as follows:

THE INSPIRATORY PRESSURE LIMIT

This determines the maximum pressure generated by the ventilator. The pressure received by the patient is indicated by a gauge on the machine and should equal the setting; this will not be reached if there is any leak in the circuit, e.g. around the mouthpiece or mask, or if the patient breathes through his nose; under these circumstances the ventilator will not cycle into expiration. When patients exhale before the ventilator has reached the pre-set pressure, the needle on the gauge will swing round to a very high pressure.

THE AIR-MIX SELECTOR

When the ventilator is driven by oxygen this will entrain atmospheric air. The exact percentage will vary with the make of ventilator; some manufacturers state that the mixture is 40% oxygen and 60% atmospheric air, but this can vary.

THE EXPIRATORY TIMER

This will automatically cycle the ventilator but is not usually necessary for I.P.P.B.

THE SENSITIVITY CONTROL

This is used when the machine is to be patient-triggered and can vary the amount of inspiratory effort needed to cycle the machine. It prevents the flow of gas during expiration until the generation of a small negative pressure by the patient causes the machine to cycle into inspiration. The sensitivity control can usually be adjusted so that the slightest effort to breathe in on the part of the patient is sufficient to trigger the machine into the inspiratory phase.

THE MANUAL CONTROL

Most ventilators have some means of manual control.

THE FLOW-RATE CONTROL

In the Bird, this control acts as an on/off switch and also controls the rate at which gas is delivered to the patient. At higher settings the flow-rate is increased so that the cycling pressure is reached sooner. This will reduce the tidal volume but as the overall respiratory rate per minute is increased the minute volume may be greater. To increase the tidal volume and allow deeper inspiration, the flow-rate control should be turned down. When the flow-rate is reduced and the machine is run off oxygen, the percentage of inspired oxygen will increase. The Bennett has a flow-sensitive valve and the flow of inspired gas adapts to the resistance in the individual patient's airway.

Preparation for Treatment

1. Fill the nebuliser with the prescribed solution. This solution should always be prescribed by the physician or surgeon in charge of the patient. Most nebulisers hold at least 5ml of solution which will last about 15 minutes. Normal saline is frequently used but a bronchodilator may be ordered. For example, a 2·5mg dose of salbutamol will consist of 0·5ml of 0·5% salbutamol diluted with 4·5ml normal saline. Glycerols are not usually suitable for use in I.P.P.B. nebulisers.

2. Connect breathing head assembly to the ventilator and connect the ventilator to the driving gas.

3. Set the controls of the ventilator. An average setting for the Bird Mark 7 is Pressure 15, Flow-rate 7, Sensitivity 7, although these may

have to be varied according to the requirements of individual patients.

4. Turn on the ventilator to check that the nebuliser is functioning correctly and that there are no leaks in the breathing head assembly.

Indications for Intermittent Positive Pressure Breathing

In some countries I.P.P.B. is used instead of physiotherapy, but it should only be used as an adjunct to physiotherapy when other measures have not been effective. Indications are as follows:

1. Sputum retention in medical and surgical conditions.
2. Hypercapnia, as in acute exacerbations of chronic bronchitis.
3. Severe bronchospasm as in status asthmaticus.
4. The re-education of paralysed respiratory muscles and as an aid to expectoration when this type of patient has a respiratory infection.

Treatment of the Patient

I.P.P.B. can be used to assist the removal of bronchial secretions, during postural drainage, but if bronchospasm is the dominant factor as in asthma, it is better to give a bronchodilator via the ventilator about 15 minutes before attempting to make the patient cough. These drugs may be given 4-hourly.

Physiotherapists are often asked to treat patients in respiratory failure at the stage of impending coma. The patient is confused, drowsy and unable to cough effectively; in this situation the ventilator can be invaluable and intubation may often be avoided.

With this type of patient it may be necessary to use a mask and it is helpful to have another physiotherapist or nurse to assist with the treatment. If possible the patient should be turned onto his side, one physiotherapist or the nurse should hold the mask over the patient's face ensuring that there is an airtight fit and that the jaw is in the correct position, while the second physiotherapist vibrates the chest on expiration. It is important to observe the chest movement during the treatment as patients with poor rib excursion could get a build up of CO_2 in the mask during treatment. Correct adjustment of the inspiratory pressure and flow-rate should overcome this problem. During treatment the patient frequently becomes more rational and is able to cough effectively after about 10 minutes, but it may be necessary to continue the procedure for longer. The patient should be observed for signs of increased drowsiness and if it occurs, it should be reported to the doctor. If no results have been achieved after 15 minutes, naso-pharyngeal suction should be considered. Treatment should be repeated for 15 to 20 minutes at 2, 3, or 4-hourly intervals, except during the night when the frequency of treatments can generally be reduced. As the patient's condition improves the number of treatments can be cut down and eventually discontinued.

I.P.P.B. can also be used in the re-education of paralysed respiratory muscles. Here the sensitivity should initially be set so that the effort required to initiate inspiration is minimal; by decreasing the sensitivity the patient will have to make more effort. In this way the machine may be used to wean patients from non-triggered positive pressure devices or from tank respirators.

Contra-Indications to I.P.P.B.

1. History of pneumothorax.
2. Large bullae or cavities in the lung.
3. Haemoptysis.
4. Active tuberculosis.

Maintenance of Equipment

It is advisable to have a supply of spare parts for the breathing head assembly as washers and springs will occasionally need to be replaced. It is also necessary to have the ventilators overhauled and cleaned every three months.

EQUIPMENT, DRUGS AND MONITORING USED IN INTENSIVE CARE UNITS

Anaesthetic Bag

In most intensive care units an anaesthetic bag is used for manual hyperventilation, however some centres use a self-inflating bag such as the Ambu-bag (see Fig. 5/9).

An anaesthetic bag is a thin rubber bag usually sealed at one end. To the open end may be attached a Waters canister containing soda lime which absorbs carbon dioxide to prevent rebreathing. An adjustable metal expiratory valve will be next in the circuit, this will have a side-arm for the attachment of the hose supplying the gas. This circuit is attached to the endotracheal or tracheostomy tube by a catheter mount, a length of flexible tubing and a plastic swivel connector (see Fig. 5/10).

Some centres do not use Waters canisters. Some units use plastic Rubens valves which prevent rebreathing. As these do not have a

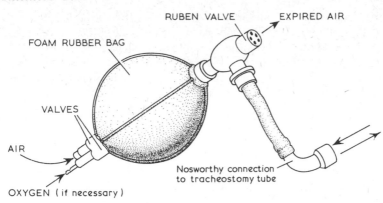

RUBEN VALVE   EXPIRED AIR

FOAM RUBBER BAG

VALVES

AIR

OXYGEN (if necessary)

Nosworthy connection to tracheostomy tube

Fig. 5/9   Diagram of the Ambu self-inflating bag

side-arm the gas is supplied to the other end of a double open-ended anaesthetic bag.

AMBU-BAG (see Fig. 5/9)

This is a self-inflating rubber bag lined with foam rubber which returns to its original shape and size following compression. It is usual to have a Rubens valve in circuit.

Both bags are used in the same way during manual hyper-ventilation.

Administration of Oxygen

The majority of patients in an intensive care unit will require oxygen-enriched air. The amount required will be assessed by the anaesthetist or physician and his judgement will be made firstly by the clinical appearance of the patient and secondly by laboratory analysis of a blood sample which will give the P_{CO_2}, P_{O_2} and the pH.

Patients receiving I.P.P.V. will receive oxygen through the ventilator. Free breathing patients with endotracheal or tracheostomy

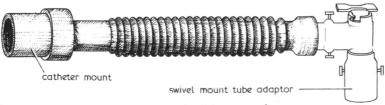

catheter mount

swivel mount tube adaptor

Fig. 5/10   A flexible connection

tubes will receive humidified oxygen and air either through a box type tracheostomy mask or through a tracheostomy humidifying tube (see Fig. 5/4a). With this tube the patient can receive approximately 70% oxygen with the hole opposite to the tracheostomy tube closed and a flow of 8 litres per minute of oxygen, or approximately 50% oxygen with the hole open.

Oxygen is administered to patients without a tracheostomy or endotracheal tube via a face mask (see Fig. 5/3) or nasal spectacles.

There is a large selection of masks available for the administration of oxygen. Some masks are able to give different concentrations of oxygen dependent on the oxygen flow supplied to the mask. Other masks are supplied with a selection of venturi collars enabling a single mask to give a variety of concentrations, for example, the Med-Econ mask and the Mix-o-Mask.

There has been some discussion concerning the provision of humidification with controlled oxygen therapy (Webber, 1976). Vickers Medical Company have provided a cuff, the Humivent, which fits onto the barrel of the Ventimask. Providing at least 10 litres per minute of air is passing through the Humivent from the humidifier, the oxygen concentration to the patient from the mask receiving the stipulated flow of oxygen via the usual narrow-bore tubing, will not be affected.

Analgesia

The use of analgesia to facilitate chest clearance must not be overlooked. Physiotherapy treatments should take place after the patient has received his analgesia whether it be given intravenously, orally or intramuscularly.

INTRAVENOUS ANALGESIA

When a patient requires artificial ventilation it may be necessary to sedate him heavily to prevent the inevitable anxiety and resulting tension of a frightened, conscious patient. Sometimes these patients are given doses of pancuronium bromide (Pavulon), a muscle relaxant, to partially or completely paralyse them and so eliminate any muscular tension or effort which might prevent adequate ventilation.

These patients although unable to move can feel, think and hear so that it is important to give them either analgesia or tranquillisers in conjunction with pancuronium bromide so that they are neither in pain nor distressed mentally.

Intravenous analgesia should only be given when a patient is receiving artificial ventilation as the action of the respiratory centre will be

depressed and respiration may cease if unaided. Drugs given intravenously take effect within a few seconds. Piritramide, morphine,
papaveretum and pethidine are examples of the analgesics that can be
given intravenously.

INTRAMUSCULAR ANALGESICS

The same drugs listed above may also be given intramuscularly and
when given this way do not act so readily on the respiratory centre.
Analgesics are usually given in this way for the immediate postoperative period following surgery or for acute pain and take about 10
to 20 minutes to take effect.

ORAL ANALGESICS

These are seldom used in the intensive care unit and are neither so
effective nor as quick acting as the former two means. Examples of
oral analgesics are paracetamol, Distalgesic and Fortral which may
also be given intramuscularly and intravenously.

EPIDURAL ANALGESIA

If the surgeon knows that because of the surgical procedure to be
undergone, the patient will suffer a large degree of pain postoperatively, he may ask the anaesthetist to insert at the relevant
vertebral level a catheter into the epidural space. This catheter will be
attached to a bacterial filter which is kept strapped to the patient and
through which local anaesthetic such as lignocaine is administered
when necessary by an anaesthetist. This is a most effective short-term
means of giving analgesia.

ENTONOX

This analgesic gas consists of 50% oxygen and 50% nitrous oxide and
can be delivered to the patient either via a face mask if the patient is
breathing spontaneously or by means of the ventilator or anaesthetic
bag for an intubated patient.

a) Face mask. In the circuit is a patient-triggered demand valve and
care must be taken to ensure that, when holding the mask to the face,
the patient achieves a good seal and that he inspires deeply enough to
trigger the valve. This can be heard in action. The gas is contained in a
cylinder for easy transportation or there may be a wall nitrous oxide
point, delivering the gas from a central source. The patient is asked to
breathe deeply for two or three minutes, the mask is then removed and
the patient assisted to cough. The analgesic effects last up to five
minutes. For some patients Entonox may take up to ten minutes to
take effect.

b) The ventilated patient may receive a mixture of nitrous oxide and oxygen, though not necessarily in the fifty–fifty proportions of Entonox to keep him sedated while ventilated. The advantage of this means of analgesia over intravenous analgesics is that once the nitrous oxide is turned off the patient regains awareness within a few minutes whereas injected analgesia may take several hours to wear off.

c) Anaesthetic bag. If the technique of manual hyperventilation is to be used during physiotherapy treatment of a ventilated patient, the patient may be gently 'bagged' with Entonox for a few minutes before treatment begins to help sedate the patient.

Records and Patient Monitoring

The purpose of the intensive care unit is to ensure that the patient receives the best care, treatment and supervision. Records must be kept so that a clear picture of the patient's condition can easily be appreciated by all the staff.

Methods and charts will vary from unit to unit but it is usual to record the following: minute volume, respiratory rate, pressure readings from the ventilator, size of tracheostomy tube, blood pressure, pulse, temperature and level of consciousness of the patient. Space will also be allocated on which drugs and treatments including physiotherapy and times of X-ray, etc. may be recorded. A fluid chart may be necessary and the diet indicated.

There are many items of monitoring equipment in the intensive care unit which, though not concerning the physiotherapist directly, contribute a large part in the overall care of the patient.

A brief description of some of the equipment to be found is given below.

ELECTROCARDIOGRAPH

Most patients in the respiratory intensive care unit, cardiac surgery unit and coronary care unit will be attached to one of these machines. The electrical activity of the heart is continuously displayed on a screen, relayed from three or four electrodes positioned on the patient's body.

CENTRAL VENOUS PRESSURE (C.V.P.) LINE

The C.V.P. line is a very thin flexible catheter. It is often inserted into one of the internal jugular veins or subclavian veins reaching into the superior vena cava or right atrium. It is used for measuring the pressure of blood in the right side of the heart in kilopascals.

ARTERIAL LINE

This line is frequently inserted into one of the radial arteries and is used to measure the radial blood pressure. It is also used for obtaining arterial samples of blood for blood gas analysis. It is necessary to know if the patient is being adequately ventilated and this is reflected in the oxygen and carbon dioxide tension in the arterial blood, Pa,O_2 and Pa,CO_2.

The process of blood gas analysis and the assessment of the acid-base balance used to be a long and complicated process. A much speedier method has been developed by Dr. P. Astrup, a Danish biochemist, and his colleagues. The apparatus, the Micro-Astrup apparatus, which is named after its inventor, can produce the necessary information from a small sample of blood. Capillary blood can also be analysed in this way.

MASS SPECTROMETER

Some intensive care units now have the use of these monitors which are capable of reliable continuous and immediate gas analysis. The samples for analysis may either be obtained by a probe inserted into the expiratory tube of a ventilator or from an arterial blood sample.

X-rays, which in many cases will be taken routinely, may be displayed on a viewing box and should be studied prior to treatment.

Positive End Expiratory Pressure (P.E.E.P.)

P.E.E.P. is a term used more and more in intensive care units and refers to the fact that the patient's lungs are receiving a positive pressure throughout the whole respiratory cycle. Instead of the normal ventilatory cycle during which the pressure returns to zero during expiration, the pressure will only fall to a pre-determined pressure usually between 1 to 10cm H_2O (0·098–0·98 kPa). If for example P.E.E.P. is set at 3cm H_2O (0·294 kPa) the patient is given his pre-set amount of gas which might read a pressure of 20cm H_2O (1·96 kPa). At the end of inspiration the pressure falls to 3cm H_2O (0·294 kPa) and so the patient expires passively but not completely. The effect of P.E.E.P. is to hold alveoli open continuously even during expiration and it is used when gaseous exchange is inadequate even with high oxygen percentages as measured by blood gas results and the clinical presentation of the patient.

The conditions for which P.E.E.P. may be used include persistent pulmonary oedema, fibrosing alveolitis and respiratory distress syndrome.

Sighing

Into modern ventilators is built a sighing device. A patient on a ventilator normally receives a fairly constant volume of ventilation for the period he is attached to the ventilator. Some anaesthetists believe that over a period of time this constant volume will reduce lung compliance and so they use the sighing circuit in the ventilator. This circuit introduces a deep breath every so often into the respiratory cycle. The sigh may be introduced every so many breaths e.g. per 100 or every so many minutes, according to the type of ventilator used, as set by the anaesthetist.

Emergency Procedure – Failure of the Power Supply

It is necessary for all the staff of an intensive care unit to be familiar with the means by which the ventilators in that unit, using electrical power, can be changed from mains to battery or operated by hand. In case the power failure occurs in the hours of darkness there should be emergency lighting available. Most hospitals have an alternative power supply.

REFERENCES

Chamney, A. R. (1969). 'Humidification requirements and techniques'. *Anaesthesia*, **24**, 4.
Ching, N. P. et al (1971). 'The contribution of cuff volume and pressure in tracheostomy tube damage.' *Journal of Thoracic and Cardiovascular Surgery*, **62**, 402.
Webber, B. A. (1976). 'Humidification with controlled oxygen therapy'. *Physiotherapy*, **62**, 192.

BIBLIOGRAPHY

See end of Chapter 7.

Chapter 6

Intensive Care – II

by P. J. WADDINGTON, M.C.S.P., H.T., DIP.T.P.
revised by S. E. BROWN, M.C.S.P.

TECHNIQUES OF CHEST CLEARANCE

Positioning

The positioning of a patient so that gravity contributes to chest clearance is a standard procedure. A knowledge of the basic postural drainage positions (see Chapter 11) is essential to any physiotherapist doing chest work. However, in the intensive care unit to be able to position the patient accurately for all the bronchopulmonary segments is the exception rather than the rule, for either the patient's condition or the mere fact that he is on a ventilator will prevent it.

The patient with a head injury may or may not be put into a head down position because of the possibility of raising intracranial pressure. This will be decided by the neurosurgeon. Another factor here is that the patient may have a bone flap removed, in which case it may not be desirable to turn him onto that side. A compromise may be reached whereby his body is turned as far as possible while his head remains in the supine position. The patient who has had a cerebrovascular accident may have high blood pressure, in which case the head down position will again be contra-indicated.

It may not be possible to put a patient with a flail chest, due to fractured ribs, into side lying and a compromise may again have to be made. Patients having peritoneal dialysis may have to remain in one position for the duration of the treatment.

If one considers a patient receiving I.P.P.V. through a tracheostomy tube but with no contra-indications preventing accurate postural drainage, the presence of the tubes will not allow it. Therefore it is very important that collapse of the dorsal segments should be prevented by not allowing the patient to lie on his back at all, at least during the early stages of his illness. He should be nursed in side lying.

A respiratory care unit should be equipped with tipping beds which work from a central fulcrum. It should be possible for one person to operate such a bed. The bed should be able to tilt from side to side as well as from end to end. This enables patients who are unable to be positioned in side lying to be tilted on the bed therefore altering the line of gravity.

The normal two-hourly turning programme which is the rule for the average patient, may be modified to a two and one regime, if indicated by the condition of the chest.

Bearing all the factors of the patient's condition in mind, it must always be the physiotherapist's aim to place him in the most advantageous position to aid chest clearance. The simple fact of moving the patient may have the effect of loosening secretions. If one is not being successful one should make some adjustment to the patient's position.

Coughing

Effective coughing is the most efficient method of removing secretions from the respiratory system. Under normal conditions these secretions are moved along by the cilia of the epithelial lining of the bronchial tree, until they reach a point where a cough reflex is stimulated. Coughing is also under voluntary control. It is axiomatic therefore that coughing followed by expectoration is the method of choice for chest clearance.

Many patients requiring intensive respiratory care can cough voluntarily, for example, following cardiac surgery or with diffuse airways obstruction. It will be necessary to support the rib-cage and aid the movement of secretions by positioning and assisted expiration. On occasions supportive pressure over the abdomen will help the patient to cough effectively.

In the majority of conscious patients requiring intensive care voluntary coughing will not be completely successful. The patient will either tire or because of inhibition, due to pain and fear, be unable to clear the chest completely. A suction catheter may be employed either to aspirate secretions from the pharynx or to stimulate a cough reflex which will be followed by aspiration.

Suction catheters may also be used to stimulate a cough reflex in an unconscious patient. If the patient is deeply unconscious it may not be possible to elicit the reflex.

Manual Techniques

COARSE CHEST SHAKING

This is the technique most commonly used in the intensive care unit for a ventilated patient. The physiotherapist places her hands suitably on the chest wall with her elbows slightly bent but with her body well positioned over the patient, if necessary kneeling up on the bed. If the patient is in supine lying the physiotherapist can either place both her hands on the anterior aspect of the chest wall, or one hand anteriorly and the other posteriorly. For large patients it is usually more effective to place both hands anteriorly. When the patient is in side lying the hands may be placed either together on the lateral wall of the chest or anteriorly and posteriorly.

As the patient pauses at maximum inspiration the physiotherapist should vigorously shake the chest using her body weight and continue to shake through expiration. On inspiration the physiotherapist should relax and repeat the technique through each expiration.

The degree of vigour applied should vary according to the pathology of the patient. The surgical patient will probably experience more pain than the medical patient and treatment should be moderated accordingly. Normally if the patient has been sedated prior to treatment little pain should be experienced by the patient. A patient with osteoporotic or cracked ribs would require vibrations, *not* coarse shaking.

VIBRATIONS

This technique is not as effective as coarse shakings in loosening secretions but in the conscious, spontaneously breathing surgical patient are all that may be tolerated. For a patient with fractured ribs vibrations are the only suitable technique.

In the intensive care unit vibrations are applied in the whole expiratory phase as are coarse shakings with the hands placed as above. However, instead of the whole body weight being transmitted to the patient as in shaking, the movement is brought about by contraction of the pectoral muscles and biceps. As the muscles contract to bring the hands towards each other vibration should take place; it is *not* a smooth compression of the chest wall.

CLAPPING

For some medical patients this technique is most effective. The hands should be slightly cupped and applied alternately to the chest wall with a quick flexion and extension of the wrist. This percussive technique should be applied either over clothes or a towel so as not to inflame the skin.

Manual Hyperventilation

Manual hyperventilation or 'bag squeezing' as it is often called plays an important part in the physiotherapy treatment of a ventilated patient. Such patients often have few secretions but many will have large quantities of sputum which must be removed.

During the treatment of a patient with copious secretions but who is breathing spontaneously, the physiotherapist would normally ask the patient to take deep breaths prior to coughing. A ventilated patient cannot do this, and so is given deep breaths manually to fully expand the lungs and loosen secretions. The actual compression of the anaesthetic bag is often performed by an anaesthetist though in some centres the physiotherapist will receive instruction in its use.

Prior to use the bag should be connected to the gas source, whether it be piped oxygen, air or a mixture of gases e.g. Entonox, or alternatively to a gas cylinder. In both gases the flow rate of gas should be at least 10 litres per minute (l/min). Seldom is 100% oxygen needed.

The bag is connected to the endotracheal or tracheostomy tube, taken in both hands and compressed; the aim is to fully dilate the bronchi and completely aerate the alveoli. Inflation should be at a steady rate until maximum expansion of the lungs is achieved, this is held for a split second before a quick release of the bag to allow for maximal elastic recoil of the lungs so forcing the secretions upwards towards the carina. Maximal effect of this technique is achieved if a physiotherapist with hands suitably positioned on the chest wall, commences coarse shakings at the point of maximum inspiration, a fraction of a second before the bag is released and continues to shake until inflation is restarted. Accurate co-ordination between the two parties is essential for effective treatment.

After five or six breaths of this nature the patient should be aspirated. Shaking should continue during suction to facilitate the removal of the secretions. This may have been indicated earlier by a spontaneous cough of a conscious patient, or wet sounds produced on inflation indicating the presence of secretions high in the bronchial tree.

This treatment should be continued until the chest is clear, which may include a change of the patient's position midway through treatment. However the frequency and length of treatment is entirely dependent upon the state of the patient's chest and his general condition. It may need to be performed hourly as in the case of a collapsed

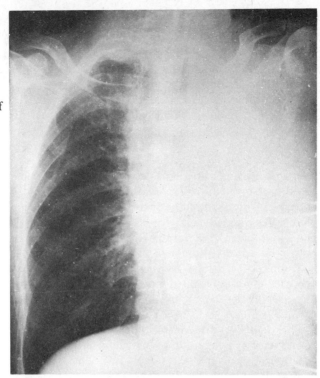

Plate 6/1
Radiograph of
a collapsed
left lung

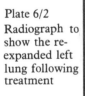

Plate 6/2
Radiograph to
show the re-
expanded left
lung following
treatment

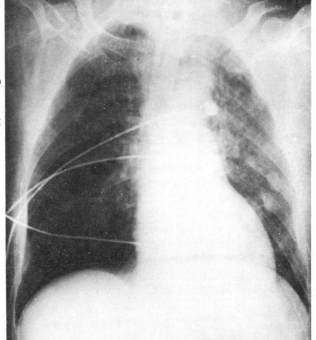

lung (see Plate 6/1), in order to re-expand the lung (see Plate 6/2), or as infrequently as once or twice daily. Even in a ventilated patient with minimal secretions, one such treatment a day is often advocated to maintain lung compliance.

In the adult a 2 litre bag is adequate for treatment, for a child a 1 litre bag will suffice and a 500ml bag should be sufficient for babies.

Precautions

As stated previously patients receiving I.P.P.V. tend to have a lower blood pressure than when breathing spontaneously. During manual hyperventilation the positive pressure in the chest is increased and the blood pressure will tend to fall further. Therefore if the patient's blood pressure is low prior to treatment, manual hyperventilation may be contra-indicated.

The effect of manual hyperventilation tends to be negated in the presence of an unclamped chest drain draining a pneumothorax, as the gas will take the line of least resistance and come out of the chest drain.

This treatment is contra-indicated in the presence of surgical emphysema or a pneumothorax with no chest drain in situ, as the high inflationary pressures may result in further leakage of gas into the pleural space leading to lung collapse.

Some ventilators may be operated manually and have an anaesthetic bag in circuit available for manual hyperventilation e.g. Brompton – Manley (see Fig. 5/7).

MOVEMENT

Some form of movement will be a part of the treatment of a patient requiring intensive care. Occasionally a fully conscious patient will be able to co-operate by doing routine maintenance exercises, others, for example following cardiac surgery, will be able to take part in active assisted movements of their limbs. A percentage of patients in the intensive care unit will either be unconscious or paralysed and therefore will require passive movements. It is not the purpose of this chapter to give detailed instruction in the techniques of passive movements but here are a few points to note.

Particular care should be taken to ensure that full extension of the hips is maintained, by doing this movement in side lying when possible. Some authorities feel that a full range abduction of the hip is undesirable in the paraplegic or tetraplegic patient, as this degree of mobility at the hip joints may be a disadvantage to a patient in calipers.

Special attention should be paid to the maintenance of full mobility in the shoulder girdle and glenohumeral joints. These joints seem particularly vulnerable to the development of progressive limitation of movement when the patient is nursed in side lying.

It is possible while maintaining full range joint movement to neglect to produce the full range extensibility in muscles which act over more than one joint. This is particularly so in the long flexors and extensors of the fingers. By passively moving the limbs in the patterns used in facilitation techniques this difficulty can be quickly and easily overcome.

Other points to note, are the importance of maintaining full range passive and accessory movements in the foot and in the hand, particularly the range between the metacarpals. The distance between the thumb and the index finger is another point to consider. The value of the hand as a functioning unit is dramatically diminished if the thumb is fixed in adduction.

In many cases passive movements will be given in side lying as the supine position can be detrimental to the state of the chest.

Problems of spasticity should be treated using one of the many methods available.

For some patients movement may extend beyond the level of maintenance. A progressive exercise programme may be instituted before the patient is able to breathe adequately without a ventilator. Although this situation will not occur often, this aspect of movement should not be overlooked or neglected.

As an adjunct to the maintenance of full range movement, accurate positioning is of great importance for the unconscious or paralysed patient. The positioning of every patient must be considered, but in some cases the patient's general condition will not allow him to be placed in the ideal position from the locomotor point of view. The vast majority of conscious patients with voluntary movement will recover in a relatively short time and there will be little likelihood of contractures developing.

The unconscious or paralysed patient, who will possibly require prolonged care, will be nursed in side lying and turned two-hourly. It is very important that the patient should remain in the lateral position and not subside into a position 45° to the horizontal. As well as the considerations of chest and pressure areas, the true side-lying position will allow the limbs to be placed accurately. Pillows and sandbags will have the desired effect. One pillow is placed between the patient's back and the mattress and another between the mattress and the frame of the bed. With two pillows so placed the patient cannot roll onto his back. The lower leg is extended and the upper leg is placed on two pillows with the hip and knee flexed about 70°. Both feet are kept at right angles by sandbags or by a combination of pillows and sandbags. The lower shoulder should be adjusted to a comfortable position, usually with the scapula pulled through a little so that the patient is not actually lying on the point of the shoulder. The upper hand and forearm usually rest on the patient's thigh and the lower one on a pillow, the fingers and wrists are kept in a good position, i.e. fingers semiflexed, thumb abducted and wrist extended, by a roll of gamgee tissue. As the patient is turned two-hourly throughout the 24 hours the positioning of the limbs will be reversed at regular intervals.

Spasticity is always a problem and will have to be accommodated in the best way possible.

The positioning of the patient in bed is the joint responsibility of the nursing and physiotherapy staff. Nurses trained in intensive care and neurosurgical work will be aware of the importance of positioning. It is also advisable to seek the assistance of the nursing staff in giving simple passive movements, which should be done at every turn and for the conscious paralysed patient whenever he becomes uncomfortable.

Precaution

Most patients will have several intravenous lines and possibly an arterial line in situ and care should be taken during movements whether they be active or passive to ensure that these lines are not dislodged.

GENERAL NURSING CARE IN WHICH THE PHYSIO-THERAPIST MAY BE INVOLVED

In most intensive care units there will be room to manoeuvre around all four sides of the bed. The patient will be without clothes, which only hinder nursing procedures and may cause pressure sores. The temperature of the room will be sufficient to enable him to be nursed covered only by a sheet. Some patients will dribble from the mouth, in which case the head should be placed either on a rubber sheet covered by paper tissue or on a piece of a paper incontinent sheet which will protect the bed and in either case can easily be changed. Suction of the mouth may be necessary.

The staff must be aware of the dangers of facial palsy, which will prevent the patient from closing the eyes completely or there could be sensory loss affecting the cornea. Irritation, from foreign bodies present in the atmosphere or pressure from the bed linen, may cause corneal ulceration. Micropore or some equivalent adhesive tape with or without the use of a gauze pad may also be used as a protective measure.

Although the general care of the patient is primarily the responsibility of the nursing staff, everyone working in an intensive care unit must be willing to give assistance when necessary and also be very observant of both the patient and the equipment, from the ventilator to the monitor and the intravenous drip.

Turning the patient is a part of physiotherapy treatment and should coincide with the regular turning routine. Speed and efficiency are necessary, especially when turning a patient who is dependent upon a ventilator. Where possible the patient should not be allowed to be supine. It is desirable to have three but essential to have two people to complete the turn of a patient unable to help himself. Having removed as much equipment as possible to the other side of the bed, the operators stand at the side of the bed towards which the patient is facing. The most experienced person takes charge and controls the patient's head and tubes; the second operator stands at hip level and if a third is available she stands opposite to the legs. The pillows are removed and the side-lying position maintained. The operators place their arms as far as possible under the patient's body, pressing down into the mattress to avoid hurting the patient. He is then detached from the ventilator and simultaneously lifted clear of the bed, drawn towards the near side and turned. The patient is immediately re-attached to the ventilator and a pillow placed in his back. Shortly afterwards the patient's chest should be aspirated because of the change of position. The patient's position is adjusted and the pillows replaced. It may be necessary to change the sheets at this time.

Good nursing will prevent the development of pressure sores and such routines as regular turning and lifting the patient clear of the bed during turning, should be adhered to. In some units the patients are nursed on sheepskins which are very effective.

Many patients will be tube fed, and again physiotherapy treatment involving tipping will need to be timed accordingly, as it is not advisable to tip a patient head down following a feed.

The physiotherapist should be aware of basic nursing techniques and this knowledge should be constantly applied to the general care of the patient and co-operation with the nurses.

TREATMENT

Full details of treatment, for the varied conditions which will require intensive respiratory care, will be covered in the appropriate chapters.

The aim at this point is to indicate the way in which the equipment and techniques available to the physiotherapist are utilised in certain basic situations.

As a general rule patients will be treated four-hourly, three times daily with as many treatments in between as necessary or as few as once or twice daily entirely depending on the general condition of the patient and his chest condition. Occasionally a patient will require treatment at intervals throughout the night.

In a few centres the nursing sisters will have been taught the basic physiotherapy techniques during a postgraduate intensive care course and can therefore carry out routine treatments during the night. Anything more than routine, for example a patient requiring I.P.P.B. or the treatment of a collapsed lobe of a lung probably require the skills of the physiotherapist on call.

The Free Breathing Unconscious Patient

This may occur in cerebrovascular accident, head injury or following neurosurgery. It may or may not be possible to stimulate a cough reflex. In the simple situation the patients will have normal lungs.

As these patients have disease-free lungs the problems of ensuring good ventilation will not be increased by the presence of excessive secretions. However, it is unlikely that the patient will be breathing deeply ensuring good air entry to all segments of the lungs. Patients may or may not have a tracheostomy.

It is unlikely that the patient will be tipped during treatment, as this may either cause a rise in blood pressure or an increase in intracranial pressure and the state of the chest will not present any serious problems which would make tipping a necessary procedure. He will be nursed in alternate side lying.

If the patient has a cough reflex the most effective method of moving secretions will be to stimulate a cough. This can be done in two ways, either by shaking and vibrations or by using a suction catheter, which will then be in a position to aspirate. A combination of these methods is very effective. As well as assisting in chest clearance, shaking during expiration will increase the depth of respiration and improve the ventilation of the lungs.

The patient will first be treated on one side and then turned to the opposite side to complete chest clearance. If the physiotherapist detects the presence of secretions which are not responding to simple side lying and coughing, the positioning of the patient should be adapted as far as possible to the standard postural drainage position for the area.

If the patient is so deeply unconscious that a cough reflex cannot be stimulated, the physiotherapist will have to rely on the squeezing effect of shaking. In this case, aspiration without an endotracheal or tracheostomy tube will be relatively ineffective, as the secretions will remain in the trachea and the possibility of the suction catheter reaching this level via the nose or mouth is debatable. Such a patient is liable to develop a chest infection and/or segmental or lung collapse.

Patients who have either an endotracheal or a tracheostomy tube in situ will need humidification.

Full range passive movements will be given.

The Free Breathing Conscious Patient who is Able to Co-operate

He will usually require a percentage of oxygen and therefore he will be wearing a face mask or nasal spectacles.

There are essentially two types of patient in this group: the first is in the early postoperative period, some following cardiac surgery, and the second has diffuse airways obstruction. Both types of patient will require humidification because they are breathing a percentage of dry gas but the patient with chronic lung disease is likely to have copious sticky sputum, the removal of which will be assisted by humidification incorporating a mucolytic agent, or bronchial spasm which may respond to a bronchodilatory drug.

All these patients will be able to co-operate by coughing but it is unlikely that their efforts will be effective enough to ensure adequate chest clearance.

Following cardiac surgery, patients will be in some pain, with a large incision, chest drains and a drip as well as being wired for monitoring. The first method of chest clearance is breathing followed by assisted coughing. The physiotherapist will assist the patient by using gentle pressure with vibrations during expiration, either over the ribs or sternum. At a suitable point the physiotherapist will stabilise the chest while the patient coughs. After some time the patient may tire and may not be able to get sputum beyond the pharynx. At this point nasal suction is indicated. Following good pre-operative preparation the vast majority of patients are remarkably co-operative.

At times, either due to fatigue or inhibited by fear, the patient will not be able to cough. It will then be necessary to use the catheter as a means of stimulating a cough reflex as well as for aspiration.

Many patients at this stage have few secretions; however some will have copious secretions and should be suitably positioned for drainage as far as the presence of tubes etc. will allow. For the first few days patients should not be tipped but otherwise positioned as required.

The chest X-rays will always be available and should be studied prior to treatment.

Assisted active exercises will follow chest clearance. The free breathing patient with chronic lung disease may be reluctant to take up a position to aid chest clearance but with explanation and persuasion he will usually co-operate.

Treatment is frequently preceded by a short period on the ultrasonic nebuliser; occasionally a patient will be on a nebuliser for a prolonged period. As the patient has an intact chest wall, vibrations and shakings will be used to move secretions. The patient's efforts may be ineffective and suction will be necessary to assist him.

I.P.P.B. is used in some centres and is found to be of benefit to all patients in this group as a means of gaining adequate lung expansion and as a means of assisted coughing.

A very small percentage of conscious patients with varying conditions will be found to be unable or unwilling to cough effectively and therefore reflex coughing and suction will be necessary.

A Patient with a Damaged Chest Wall, some Ability to Breathe but Requiring I.P.P.V. to Ensure Adequate Respiration

FLAIL CHEST

In severe chest injury where there are multiple fractures, especially if both sides of the rib-cage are involved, the anterior part of the chest wall will be flail. Paradoxical breathing will occur, i.e. in inspiration the relatively damaged part of the chest wall will be drawn in. The reverse will happen on expiration. There is also a shunting to and fro of air in adjacent bronchi, which results in the loss of a larger area of effective lung than that directly affected by the injury.

The ventilation of the lungs is seriously impaired by this situation, added to which the airway may be obstructed by blood, and blood and air will have entered the pleural cavity. The patient will probably have an underwater seal chest drain in situ (see p. 138).

To ensure a clear airway and adequate ventilation the patient will have been given a tracheostomy and placed on I.P.P.V. The I.P.P.V. also acts as a form of internal splintage and prevents paradoxical breathing. It is probable that the patient will be placed on a self-triggering ventilator. Ventilation will be continued for 10 to 14 days or until the ribs stabilise. It is possible that the patient may have sustained other injuries and therefore if conscious he will be in great pain.

Positioning to aid drainage of the lungs will be very restricted if at all possible and may simply consist of tipping the mattress from side to side, by means of pillows placed between the mattress and bed frame.

It is obvious that direct pressure on the damaged part of the thorax in this situation cannot be contemplated. Manual hyperventilation can be helpful in loosening secretions.

Suction will be necessary to remove the blood and secretions from the trachea. Many of these patients are conscious and the vast majority have a cough reflex which will be stimulated by the suction catheter. Coughing will be extremely painful and the physiotherapist should use her hands to stabilise the rib-cage while the nurse aspirates.

FRACTURED RIBS

Fractures of the ribs usually occur near to the angle and in the majority of cases are caused by direct violence.

The fracture of one or two ribs will be very painful and the patient will be unwilling either to breathe deeply or cough effectively. Breathing exercises and assisted coughing will be all that the patient requires.

Patients with moderate chest injuries cannot cough adequately and maintain a clear airway. It may be necessary to insert a tracheostomy tube and aspirate. If the cuff is inflated inhalation of foreign matter will be prevented. This is of particular importance if the patient is unconscious. If the majority of ribs on one side are fractured, the tendency will be for the patient to rely solely on the unaffected side and in a few days, the lung on the painful side could collapse if adequate treatment is not given.

Active assisted movements will be given where and when indicated.

Patients with Diseased Lungs and Difficulty in Maintaining a Clear Airway and Adequate Ventilation but with an Undamaged Chest Wall and Some Ability to Breathe Spontaneously

This type of patient usually has an acute exacerbation of his diffuse airways obstruction.

As the patient will attempt to breathe he may be nursed on a self-triggering ventilator. A mixture of air and 40% oxygen is frequently given and drugs such as bronchodilators or mucolytic agents, may be added to the humidifying system.

If artificial ventilation is expected to be of short duration an endotracheal tube may be used; for prolonged ventilation the patient will need a tracheostomy.

All the usual methods of chest clearance may be used to remove the copious quantities of sputum. There is unlikely to be any contra-indication to tipping and the intact chest wall allows shaking to be used, although this may be difficult in patients with overinflated chests. Vibrations may be easier and more effective. Suction will be given at frequent intervals and reflex coughing may be stimulated.

The number of treatments given in the 24 hours will be dictated by the condition of the patient but it must not be forgotten that he will need some rest.

The patient will be encouraged to do simple maintenance exercises.

The Patient who has Paralysis of the Muscles of Respiration with Complete or Partial Incompetence of Swallowing and Gross or Complete General Paralysis

This state may occur in polyneuropathies, myasthenia gravis, a drug overdose or tetanus.

Tetanus is rare in England, but it is seen in the Third World particularly among children. The use of the paralysing drug curare to control the spasm in conjunction with I.P.P.V. has proved to be a most successful form of treatment.

With the exception of the patient suffering from a drug overdose, the patients suffering from the diseases listed above are completely conscious. This is sometimes difficult to remember with any patient who is totally paralysed as he will appear to be unconscious. It is very easy to talk over such a patient, entirely forgetting that he will be able to hear what is being said. Even patients whom we believe to be unconscious may not be totally unaware when staff are speaking near by, even if they are unable to respond. It is obvious that great care should be exercised when talking to a colleague close to such patients and one should make a point of talking to the patient and explaining what is happening, if there is any possibility that he might understand.

Treatment of these patients is time consuming and it is important that the patient is left long enough in each position for drainage to take effect.

A well tried treatment routine starts with the patient in the side-lying position in which the physiotherapist finds him when she enters the ward. The patient is tipped head up in a position for drainage of the upper zone.

The physiotherapist working if possible with two other staff members, either two nurses, two physiotherapists or a combination should carry out the technique of manual hyperventilation with the physiotherapist applying coarse shakings to the chest and the third person aspirating the patient when necessary.

If the area is clear the bed will be tipped in the opposite direction to drain the lower zone and shaking continued. Suction is given when secretions are detected and before and after a change of position.

Following clearance of the lower zone it may be necessary to position the patient for drainage of the middle lobe or lingula.

When that side of the chest is clear, the bed will be returned to the horizontal and some of the pillows and sandbags removed to allow full range passive movements of the uppermost limbs to be given with the patient still in side lying. The patient is then turned and aspirated as soon as possible following a period of ventilation. Passive movements to the other side are given, the pillows replaced and the patient made comfortable.

The chest clearance pattern is then repeated for the second time.

This treatment should be carried out at least three times daily.

WEANING FROM A VENTILATOR

As the respiratory function of the patient starts to recover the weaning process from the ventilator begins. Often the longer the patient has been artificially ventilated the longer the weaning off process will take but this is not always the case.

. Before the process is started it is important that the patient is not under the effect of any respiratory depressive drugs and that the process is carefully explained to him.

It is important that the patient's chest is clear before he starts to breathe spontaneously and it is therefore ideal to give physiotherapy treatment a short time before the patient is tried off the ventilator. It is not wise to try him off the ventilator immediately after physiotherapy treatment especially if he has copious secretions, as he might be tired with the exertion of coughing.

Most patients find the position of half lying comfortable for the first attempts at breathing spontaneously. With the patient in this position the ventilator will be disconnected from him and a humidifier connected in its place probably with a fairly high concentration of oxygen for example 70%. It is important that a member of the staff is by the patient at the time, talking and reassuring him as well as encouraging him to breathe deeply.

The physiotherapist can play an important part during this stage reassuring and encouraging the patient who will undoubtedly be fairly anxious and uncomfortable however well prepared he has been.

Vigorous chest clearance should not be undertaken during the initial periods of spontaneous breathing as this will distress the patient and shorten his time off the ventilator. However if the patient coughs or if excessive secretions are in evidence he should be aspirated.

If the patient is comfortable and the observations stable, after half an hour an arterial blood sample will probably be taken for blood gas analysis. If the results are satisfactory the patient may be extubated if he has only been ventilated for a short period, for example, a person recovering from open heart surgery.

It is the decision of the anaesthetist as to whether a patient should be extubated or not. A patient who has received prolonged ventilation may take several days to be weaned off. Starting with short periods these will progressively lengthen as the patient gains confidence and tires less. The time he spends off the ventilator will always depend on his overall condition.

I.P.P.B. (see p. 101) can play an important part in weaning a patient from a non-triggering ventilator.

Once a patient with a tracheostomy tube has been successfully weaned off the ventilator his cuffed plastic tube will be exchanged for an uncuffed silver tube (see Fig. 5/1) with an inner speaking tube to enable him to talk. As soon as the anaesthetist is sure that the patient will no longer need suction to remove the secretions, the silver tube will be removed and a dry dressing placed over the stoma which will heal in a few days.

Physiotherapy plays an important part in this last stage in ensuring that the patient can remove his own secretions. Breathing exercises and postural drainage if necessary, should be carried out to facilitate the removal of secretions. The patient must be taught how to seal the stoma with his hand over the dressing during coughing to ensure that the secretions are coughed into the mouth and not through the stoma. No dressing can adequately seal the stoma against the high pressure of air released during a cough. As the stoma heals the need for re-inforcement by a hand over the dressing will become less until unnecessary, when the wound has healed.

BIBLIOGRAPHY

See end of Chapter 7.

Chapter 7

Intensive Care – III

by S. E. BROWN, m.c.s.p.

CHILDREN AND INTENSIVE CARE

Children in intensive care units tend to fall into three groups. One group will be the children with a congenital abnormality that needs surgical attention, for example a baby with a tracheal-oesophageal fistula or one with a congenital heart abnormality. Another group will be children who have contracted a severe medical illness, frequently respiratory distress syndrome or pneumonia. The third group will be those who have had an accident either in the home or on the roads.

The children in this last category are often found in the respiratory intensive care unit and often have head injuries sometimes combined with other injuries. They usually need assisted ventilation for varying lengths of time from overnight to several weeks.

The children described in the first two categories are often premature or newly born term babies and so are found in the neonatal unit. Patients requiring cardiac surgery are usually nursed in a separate cardiac surgery unit.

Children over the age of three years may be treated in a similar manner to adults though will need more encouragement to perform localised breathing and active mobilising exercises.

Few children under three years of age can be treated in this manner and so require a different approach to their treatment.

Neo-natal Unit

The babies in this unit are usually in either an incubator or a radiantly warmed crib for warmth. The babies in cribs are more accessible for the physiotherapist and nursing staff than the baby in the incubator who is only accessible through two portholes on either side of the lid. This lid is raised to put the child into the incubator and is then kept down so that the infant can be nursed at a fairly constant temperature.

The degree of humidity and percentage of oxygen can also be adjusted in the incubator. There are various inlets into the incubator for necessary tubes e.g. those from a ventilator and intravenous drips.

The neo-natal unit is frequently divided into medical and surgical areas for easier interchange of staff and supplies.

Cardiac Surgery Unit

Babies undergoing palliative surgery or total correction of their congenital abnormality will usually be nursed in incubators or radiantly warmed cribs. Also in this unit will be children of an older age probably up to eight or nine years old during their immediate postoperative stage before being moved onto a convalescent ward.

TREATMENT OF INFANTS

I.P.P.V.

Babies are usually intubated with a nasal uncuffed tube and receive I.P.P.V. either from a purpose-built paediatric ventilator e.g. the Bournes or Cavitron paediatric ventilators, or from a ventilator also capable of adequately ventilating an adult e.g. the Servo 900 or Phillips AV1 ventilators. Not all ventilators suitable for the ventilation of adults are suitable for small children who require a faster respiratory rate and lower pressure and volume settings.

CONTINUOUS POSITIVE AIRWAY PRESSURE (C.P.A.P.)

C.P.A.P. is increasingly used instead of mechanical ventilation in small children and also as a 'weaning off' process from a mechanical ventilator. It is used in the treatment of adults particularly in the treatment of the respiratory distress syndrome but as the adult patient has to be intubated and not many adults tolerate prolonged intubation when conscious it is not widely used.

C.P.A.P. has exactly the same effect on the patients as P.E.E.P. but refers to patients breathing spontaneously whereas P.E.E.P. refers to ventilated patients. In both cases there is a continual positive pressure in the airways throughout the respiratory cycle.

Small children tolerate intubation well, but a plastic head-box (Gregory, 1972) is now available inside which a child does not need to be intubated to receive C.P.A.P.

Most children, however, are intubated, (see Plate 7/1), and one system used is described by Pfitzner et al (1974) (see Plate 7/2). Some

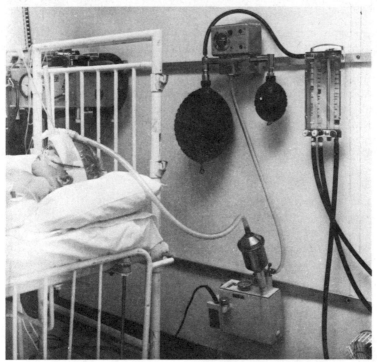

Plate 7/1   The C.P.A.P. system in use on a patient

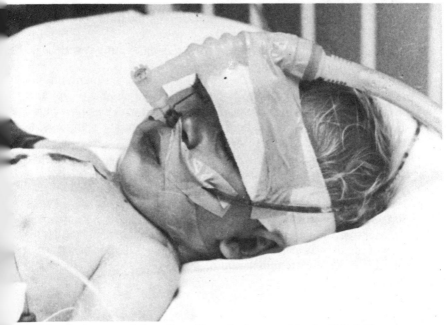

Plate 7/2   A close up of the adjustable end piece used in the C.P.A.P. system

ventilators have C.P.A.P. circuits built into them, for example the Bournes and Cavitron paediatric ventilators, so that at a flick of a switch the child is receiving C.P.A.P. rather than mechanical ventilation.

A C.P.A.P. circuit for children should contain a humidifier, preferably a heated model; a flow meter to obtain a constant flow of gas; a pressure gauge; an adjustable expiratory valve; a blow-off valve to prevent too high a pressure building up in the system and lastly a 500ml anaesthetic bag for manual ventilation should the child need immediate respiratory aid.

When C.P.A.P. is used for babies with respiratory distress syndrome or following cardiac surgery a pressure circuit is set usually between 5–10cm H_2O (0·49–0·98 kPa). A high percentage of oxygen at a fairly high flow rate is given, it may be as high as 100% oxygen initially to obtain a Pa,O_2 of 50–70mm Hg (6·65–9·31 kPa). The oxygen concentration is reduced gradually until the child is maintaining his acceptable Pa,O_2 at 40% oxygen. Then the pressure will start to be reduced.

When starting to wean the child off C.P.A.P. the pressure is reduced by 1cm H_2O (0·098 kPa) every two hours, provided that the Pa,O_2 remains satisfactory, until zero pressure is reached. If after a further period of time the condition of the child is stable and satisfactory at zero pressure the child will be extubated.

The child with respiratory distress syndrome may need physiotherapy treatment hourly while some patients following cardiac surgery will not require treatment so frequently.

Manual hyperventilation may be used during treatment with shaking or vibrating and frequent suction.

Following extubation the baby will still need frequent physiotherapy probably two-hourly at first. The child should be suitably positioned and vibrating and shaking carried out with nasopharyngeal suction if necessary to stimulate a cough and aspirate secretions.

POSITIONING

In most incubators and cribs the base on which the child is lying is easily moved for postural drainage in either the head raised or head downward position. Babies are usually nursed unclothed and have no pillows; they frequently wear mittens to prevent removal of any tubes. In order to maintain the side-lying position a small towel placed at the back of the baby is usually enough. If the baby is unable to be turned into side lying, an attempt should be made to tilt the base laterally to aid drainage.

MANUAL TECHNIQUES

Clapping, shaking and vibrating are all techniques which may be used for small children with some modifications from the technique used on adults.

Small children are far more resilient than they look and the physiotherapist treating such patients for the first time need have little fear of injuring them. Clapping is best carried out by the first two fingers of one hand only on babies, while the other hand be used to hold the child's arm out of the way and generally maintain the desired position.

Vibrating and shaking are usually carried out by the first two fingers and thumb of one hand or of both hands. If two hands are used the fingers of each hand should be positioned, one on each side of the chest wall either laterally or anteriorly and posteriorly. The fingers should perform the actual technique of shaking or vibrating while the thumbs, often touching, stabilise the action. In very small babies vibration and shaking can be done with one hand.

In none of the techniques should the palm of the hand be used in the treatment of babies. In children of over one year or 18 months, according to their size, more of the fingers may be used until children of three or over may receive a similar technique to that of adults.

Manual Hyperventilation

For small children this procedure should always be carried out by an experienced member of staff due to the danger of causing a pneumothorax from excessive pressure in the lungs. A 500ml anaesthetic bag is usually used for babies and for children over three years a one litre anaesthetic bag.

During manual hyperventilation if shaking or vibrating is synchronised with the bag-squeezing operator, chest clearance can be most effective. A third person should be available to aspirate the child when necessary.

If humidification is needed to loosen secretions during treatment saline may be introduced into the respiratory tract. A maximum of 0·5ml should be used for a small baby and to be most effective can be inserted via the suction catheter in order to prevent absorption of the liquid high in the respiratory tract (Gaskell and Webber, 1977).

The airways of an infant are so small that they can block very easily with a plug of mucus so suction must be applied quickly at frequent intervals.

If a small child without an endotracheal tube in situ needs manual hyperventilation in order to facilitate chest clearance an anaesthetic mask and bag should be used (Gregory, 1972). The child's head must be tipped backwards; an airway may be used to hold the tongue forwards; the mask should be held tightly over the nose and mouth and the bag compressed as inspiration occurs. If the actual bag compression does not coincide with the inspiratory phase of the child, air will enter the stomach which will become overinflated and possibly embarrass respiration.

MOVEMENT

Passive movements should be carried out regularly on children who are unconscious or paralysed. Small babies capable of movement usually perform adequate exercises without any prompting from the physiotherapist. Older children will need instruction in exercises and constant postural correction.

REFERENCES

Gaskell, D. V. and Webber, B. A. (1977). *The Brompton Hospital Guide to Physiotherapy*, 3rd ed. Blackwell Scientific Publications.

Gregory, G. A. et al (1972). Respiratory care of newborn infants. *Paediatric Clinics of North America* **19**, 311.

Pfitzner, J. et al (1974). Continuous positive airways pressure, a new system. *Anaesthesia* **29**, 326.

BIBLIOGRAPHY

Gregory, G. A. et al (1971). 'Treatment of the idiopathic respiratory distress syndrome with continuous positive airways pressure.' *New England Journal of Medicine*, **284**, 1333.

Gregory, G. A. et al (1975). 'Continuous positive airways pressure and pulmonary and circulatory function after cardiac surgery in infants of less than three months of age.' *Anaesthesiology*, **43**, 426.

MacDonnell, K. F. and Segal, M. S. (1977). *Current Respiratory Care*. Little, Brown and Co., Boston, U.S.A.

Norris, W. and Campbell, D. (1974). *Anaesthetics, Resuscitation and Intensive Care* – A textbook for students and residents, 4th ed. Churchill-Livingstone.

Sykes, M. K., McNichol, M. W., and Campbell, E. J. M. (1976). *Respiratory Failure*, 2nd ed. Blackwell Scientific Publications.

ACKNOWLEDGEMENTS

The author thanks all those who have helped in the preparation of her chapters, especially Dr. B. Doran, Consultant Anaesthetist, and Mrs. S. Allison, M.C.S.P., both of Manchester Royal Infirmary, and Miss D. V.

Gaskell, M.C.S.P., of the Brompton Hospital, London. Plates 7/1 and 7/2 first appeared in an article in Anaesthesia and were subsequently reproduced in the Brompton Hospital Guide to Chest Physiotherapy (3rd Ed.). The author's thanks go to Dr. J. Pfitzner, Dr. M. A. Branthwaite, Dr. I. C. W. English and Dr. E. A. Shinebourne, the Editor of Anaesthesia, and the publishers, Blackwell Scientific Publications.

Chapter 8

Thoracic Surgery – I

by D. M. INNOCENTI, M.C.S.P.

INTRODUCTION

The importance of physiotherapy in the surgical treatment of chest conditions has been gradually accepted and is now firmly established. In the early years, radical surgical treatment for tuberculosis often resulted in severe deformity. More recently much surgical progress has been made, including perfection of lung resections and open heart surgery. Concurrently, physiotherapeutic techniques have advanced and expanded, helping to make it possible for patients to return to fully active lives.

INCISIONS USED IN THORACIC SURGERY

The direction of the thoracic incision may be:

1. Oblique – lateral
2. Transverse }
3. Vertical } – anterior

Lateral Incisions

Thoracotomy. The standard unilateral method of entry into the thorax is through an intercostal space. The level of entry depends entirely on the area on which the operation is to be performed. The incision runs antero-laterally or postero-laterally (see Fig. 8/1). The former divides the lower fibres of pectoralis major, serratus anterior, and the external and internal intercostals, terminating at the anterior border of the latissimus dorsi. The latter divides the lower fibres of trapezius, latissimus dorsi, serratus anterior and the external and internal inter-costals. A high posterior continuation of the incision also divides the rhomboid major and the erector spinae.

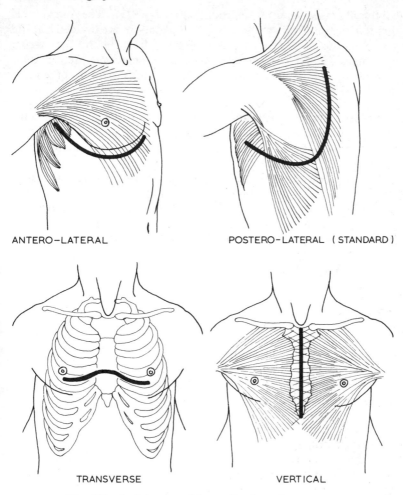

ANTERO–LATERAL   POSTERO–LATERAL (STANDARD)

TRANSVERSE   VERTICAL

Fig. 8/1   Incisions used in cardio-thoracic surgery

Anterior Incisions

For operations on the heart or mediastinum the approach is usually from the front.

a) The transverse approach is submammary and bilateral (see Fig. 8/1), through the fourth intercostal spaces and a transversely divided sternum. The pectoralis major is divided together with the external and internal intercostals. This approach is rarely used as both pleural cavities are opened. It is sometimes preferred for cosmetic reasons.

b) The vertical approach. Median sternotomy is probably the most commonly used anterior incision (see Fig. 8/1). The sternum is divided longitudinally and retracted. No muscles are divided but the action of the pectoralis major is affected because the pre-sternal aponeurosis is cut. A cosmetic incision is sometimes preferred for children or women. It is Y-shaped with the limbs of the Y at the third intercostal space.

The level of the incision and the muscles divided will determine the postoperative postural programme. Pain and abnormal muscle pull will create postoperative faults with possible deformity and limitation of movement.

The thoracotomy incision sometimes creates a scoliosis towards the operation side, i.e. a low shoulder and a high hip. The thoracoplasty operation (see p. 158) produces the opposite deformity. Due to loss of structural support the patient leans away from the affected side and compensates with a cervical shift towards the incision. Latissimus dorsi, the rhomboids, serratus anterior, trapezius and pectoralis major all exert forces on the scapula and the humerus, thus compromising shoulder movements.

DRAINAGE

Drainage of unwanted fluid and air from the thorax is necessary following both surgery and/or other trauma. Drainage may be a) closed or b) open.

a) Closed drainage. To allow drainage from the thorax but simultaneously prevent air entry, a simple air-tight system is used. A plastic tube with end and side holes is introduced into the thorax through an intercostal space and fixed with a purse-string suture. It is connected to a closed drainage bottle via a glass tube which terminates under water (see Fig. 8/2). Another short glass tube passes through the rubber bung of the bottle to allow free drainage, or to allow connection to a suction pump which aids drainage. Air and fluid will pass down the tube. The patency of the tube must be maintained by frequent attention and 'milking' to prevent or remove clots. A calibrated bottle may be used, and is the bottle of choice for cardiac surgery (see Fig. 8/3).

On free drainage the level of the fluid in the glass tube will be seen to rise on inspiration and fall on expiration, due to the alteration in intrathoracic pressure. If the fluid level ceases to swing it means either that the tubing is blocked or that the lung is fully expanded. The fluid level should *not* swing when on suction because the air pressure in the bottle is lower than the intrathoracic pressure. Bubbles denote escape of air and these increase on coughing.

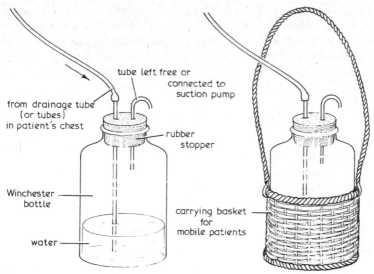

from drainage tube
(or tubes)
in patient's chest

tube left free or
connected to
suction pump

rubber
stopper

Winchester
bottle

water

carrying basket
for
mobile patients

Fig. 8/2 Diagram to show: a) closed drainage of the thoracic cavity by means of an underwater drain; b) a carrying basket

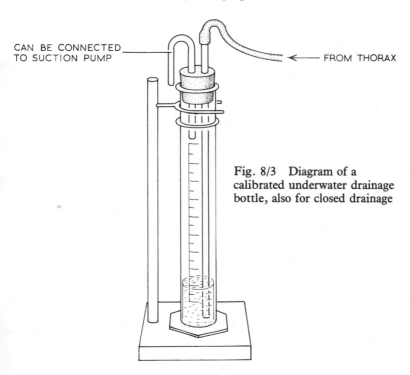

CAN BE CONNECTED TO SUCTION PUMP

FROM THORAX

Fig. 8/3 Diagram of a calibrated underwater drainage bottle, also for closed drainage

The drainage bottle must at all times remain at a lower level than the patient to prevent siphoning of fluid back into the chest. Clamping of the tubes may be necessary during difficult changes of position, but it is not necessary for the patient to remain in bed during the drainage period. Indeed patients should be encouraged to walk around carrying their drainage bottle. Many units provide suitable long-handled baskets to ease the procedure (see Fig. 8/2).

Intercostal or subcostal drainage tubes are used to drain:

1. Pleural cavity.
   a) apical – mainly air.
   b) basal – mainly fluid.
2. Mediastinum.
3. Pericardial space.

b) Open drainage is occasionally used to drain thickened and infected matter from an empyema cavity. An area of infection, which is localised by fibrosis from the remaining pleura, renders it impossible to create a pneumothorax. Pus and debris track down the tube or corrugated drain into a dressing.

PRE-OPERATIVE PERIOD

Investigations

Before surgery patients will undergo extensive investigations. All patients have chest X-rays, respiratory function tests (see p. 50), exercise tolerance tests, dental examinations, sputum culture, haematological investigations and electrocardiographic studies.

Patients with respiratory disease will possibly also undergo further tests as follows:

BRONCHOSCOPY

This procedure entails introducing a bronchoscope via the mouth to allow direct examination of the larynx, trachea, carina and the main bronchi and bronchial orifices. Suction and biopsy may be carried out during the examination. The conventional rigid bronchoscope is particularly useful for the removal of foreign bodies. A flexible fibre-optic bronchoscope may also be used either under a general or a local anaesthetic. This enables visualisation of the segmental and sub-segmental orifices of the upper lobes which are not easily seen with the rigid bronchoscope.

MEDIASTINOSCOPY

A small transverse incision is made 1·25cm (½in) above the supra-sternal notch. The strap muscles are separated and the pre-tracheal fascia entered. A finger can then be passed along the front of the trachea to the bifurcation. Abnormal paratracheal and carinal lymph nodes can thus be felt. A mediastinoscope which is a short, rigid instrument is then inserted and a biopsy taken of any abnormal lymph nodes.

The method is used either in the diagnosis of lymph node enlarge-ments in the superior mediastinum or in the assessment of operability in patients with bronchogenic carcinoma. Not all the lymph node groups which drain the lungs can be reached by mediastinoscopy.

BRONCHOGRAPHY

This is a radiographic examination in which a radio-opaque substance is introduced into the bronchial tree by means of a nasotracheal catheter or by direct injection into the trachea. The airways are outlined and any distortion, obstruction, stricture or dilatation demonstrated. The resulting radiograph is of particular interest to the physiotherapist in cases of bronchiectasis, as the affected areas are minutely delineated. Physiotherapy and postural drainage is essential prior to the investigation to clear excess secretions from the bronchial tree.

The patient should not eat or drink for approximately two hours after the examination, since the larynx has been anaesthetised and fluid may enter the lungs.

Patients with cardiac lesions may undergo the following inves-tigations:

CARDIAC CATHETERISATION

This examination is performed under local anaesthesia. A catheter is introduced into the right side of the heart through the venous system commencing at the median cubital vein. The tricuspid and pulmonary valves are traversed and the catheter finally lodged into a pulmonary artery. The left side of the heart and the aortic and mitral valves are examined. The catheter is introduced into the femoral artery or brachial artery and passed retrogradely in the aorta.

Pressures within the chambers and vessels, and pressure gradients across the valves, are measured and oxygen saturation studies are made. The cardiac output may be calculated from oxygen saturation measurements. The diagnosis of congenital abnormalities is also confirmed by catheterisation.

ANGIOCARDIOGRAPHY AND ANGIOGRAPHY

These are radiographic studies following the injection of contrast media into the heart and/or vessels to demonstrate irregularities, blockages, constrictions and aneurysms.

ECHOCARDIOGRAPHY

A non-invasive investigation whereby a beam of sound is projected into the heart from a probe held on the skin of the anterior chest wall. Sound reflections are obtained from intracardiac structures and are recorded on paper.

The technique is of most use in the diagnosis of mitral stenosis, pericardial effusion and left atrial myxoma. Recently it has been used in the evaluation of complex congenital heart disease.

Patient Assessment

The physiotherapist must become conversant with the patient's history, and examination should take account of the following:

1. Shape of chest. Deformities may be a) congenital or b) acquired.

a) Some congenital deformities affecting the thorax are: scoliosis; kyphosis; pectus carinatum (pigeon chest) – the middle portion of the sternum and the adjoining ribs protrude; pectus excavatum (funnel chest) – the lower one-third of the sternum is depressed and the ribs cave inwards to form a hollow.

b) Some acquired deformities are: barrel chest – chest held high in inspiratory position with an increased anteroposterior diameter; scoliosis or kyphosis – may be idiopathic or be secondary to disease, trauma or operation; asymmetry – due to rib flattening and impaired movement.

2. Movements of respiration

a) Thoracic upper costal ⎫ unilateral
   Thoracic lower costal ⎬ or
                 ⎭ bilateral

b) Diaphragmatic.

3. Physical signs of cardiopulmonary insufficiency. a) dyspnoea; b) orthopnoea; c) cyanosis; d) clubbing of fingers and toes; e) oedema of ankles, or sacral oedema in the bed-ridden; f) raised jugular venous pressure (if present, note whether it is sustained or whether it falls on inspiration).

4. Sputum. Note a) the type – watery; mucoid; mucopurulent; frank pus; blood stained; frank blood. b) the quantity; c) the viscosity.

5. *Joint movements.* Range of movement of thoracic spine, neck, shoulder girdle and shoulders must be ascertained.

6. *Exercise tolerance.* The distance and speed at which the patient is able to walk must be established: a) on the level; b) on slopes and c) on stairs.

7. *Special investigations.* All relevant data must be examined. The X-ray should be studied in order to compare it with the postoperative condition. Respiratory function results must be considered. The vital capacity and forced expiratory volume in one second is of special importance when lung resection is contemplated. Bronchoscopic, bronchographic, cardiac catheterisation and angiographic results should be examined.

8. *Cerebral function.* It must be appreciated that there are some definite relationships between cardiac disease and cerebrovascular accidents.

a) Atherosclerosis is a generalised disease and is an underlying cause of angina pectoris, cerebrovascular accident and intermittent claudication.

b) Emboli are frequently thrown off diseased heart valves, and from a fibrillating atrium, resulting in cerebrovascular accidents.

c) There is a definite incidence of intracranial berry aneurysm rupture occurring when there is coarctation of the aorta.

Principles of Physiotherapy

1. To explain and teach postoperative procedures: a) breathing exercises; b) arm, leg and general exercises; and c) postural awareness.

2. To teach awareness of breathing and relationships of thoracic, diaphragmatic and air movements.

3. To mobilise thoracic cage by: a) general rib movements; b) bilateral and unilateral localised rib movements; c) trunk and shoulder girdle exercises.

4. To improve diaphragmatic excursion and breathing control and ensure that there is synchronous thoracic and abdominal movement, by relaxation and localised diaphragmatic breathing exercises.

5. To clear secretions by: a) deep breathing; b) cough; c) postural drainage, percussion and shakings; d) inhalation therapy; e) intermittent positive pressure breathing.

Techniques of Physiotherapy

POSITIONS OF THE PATIENT AND THE PHYSIOTHERAPIST FOR
BREATHING INSTRUCTION

The patient's position is important in order to achieve relaxation, concentration and freedom of thoracic and abdominal movement.

The positions for the initial instructions are: a) half-lying; b) side-lying with upper arm (and possibly upper leg) supported on a pillow; c) high side-lying with the arm supported on a pillow; d) sitting in a comfortable upright chair.

Although unorthodox, it is more efficient for the physiotherapist to sit on the side of the bed when the patient is in the half-lying position. This facilitates communication with the patient and observation and control of the thorax and abdomen.

When the patient is sitting in a chair the physiotherapist should sit facing and to the side of him. With the patient in either of the side-lying positions the physiotherapist should stand behind him. This affords an unobstructed view of the patient's face and lessens the risk of cross-infection from sputum. The therapist is unencumbered by the patient's arms when controlling the thorax and abdomen and in helping him to alter position.

BREATHING EXERCISES

Very often patients are quite unaware of the relationships between thoracic and abdominal movements and air flow. A short explanation of these mechanics should be given and these factors kept in mind by the patient and the physiotherapist, as increased movement does *not* always mean increased function.

When the patient is aware of these respiratory and air movements during quiet breathing, and relaxed (it may be necessary to use the contrast method of relaxation), attention is directed towards the specific exercises. Although costal and diaphragmatic movements occur simultaneously they must be considered separately for treatment purposes.

Thoracic cage movements. Costal movements can be localised to the following areas and can be practised bilaterally and unilaterally, where necessary: i) apices; ii) lower lateral costal; iii) posterior basal.

In the past much emphasis has been placed on localised movements, but practice is now moving towards a more general pattern of movement. There is very little information on whether or not localised rib movement produces an underlying localised lung expansion. However, these exercises do have value where there is localised diminution of movement due to underlying disease or to pain.

COSTAL EXERCISES PARTICULAR TO THORACIC SURGERY

The exercises are best taught by instruction in one phase at a time, progressing to the full cycle. Air flow and movement must both be referred to, and manual resistance given on inspiration. In some cases assistance may be given at the end of expiration.

Inspiratory and expansion exercises are practised by concentrating on a gentle but full inspiration and expansion of the ribs against the physiotherapist's hands, which are placed firmly on the chest wall to guide and facilitate movement. An initial gentle intercostal stretch may be given, followed by moderate pressure as the patient tries to expand the desired area and hold the breath for a few seconds on full inspiration. Encouragement is given verbally and manually. Resistance is gradually released during expiration, which ceases at the resting point of the thorax and abdomen. The expiratory phase is not emphasised at this stage. The exercise is continued until good, easy movement and air flow are achieved.

Expiratory costal exercises. The object is maximum costal movement and expiration, to stimulate and encourage coughing. The patient tries to breathe out fully but gently, using active contraction of expiratory muscles. The physiotherapist may assist by increasing the manual pressure at the point of maximum expiration before minimally resisting the ensuing inspiration. Full expiratory exercises are a useful precursor to coughing. Full range costal breathing exercises may soon tire the patient and produce an unpleasant giddiness if protracted.

DIAPHRAGMATIC BREATHING

There is some diversity of opinion on the teaching of diaphragmatic breathing. Basically there are two schools of thought. One concentrates on epigastric and lower rib movement, swelling of the epigastrium and widening the costal angle (Gaskell and Webber, 1977). The other concentrates on allowing the whole abdomen to swell as the diaphragm descends (Innocenti, 1966).

When costal and diaphragmatic breathing exercises are mastered they should be practised in the side-lying or high side-lying position. The unilateral thoracic movement (the upper hemithorax) will be controlled by the physiotherapist's hands on the anterior and posterior aspects of the thorax. The diaphragmatic movement will be controlled and resisted by placing a hand, or hands, on the abdomen. The breathing exercises must be practised to gain control and confidence. If there is sufficient time pre-operatively, the instruction of alteration in depth and pace of breathing, and synchronisation of walking and breathing, will help very distressed patients. The synchronisation of walking and breathing can be practised in two ways, by (i) the counting method, for instance taking two steps during inspiration and three steps for expiration, (ii) consciously maintaining a regular breathing rhythm.

'*Huffing*' is a breathing exercise designed as a precursor to coughing. There are two methods:

a) A deep inspiration is taken and the expiratory phase is broken into a series of short sharp 'pants', the procedure being controlled mainly by the abdominal muscles. This is the exercise of choice for patients with increased secretions and central airway sputum problems.

b) Shallow breaths, in and out, through the mouth, gradually gaining depth and strength, are controlled by general costal movements. These are most beneficial for patients with poor thoracic excursion and peripheral patchy consolidation and/or collapse.

The irregular air flow, resulting from either method, loosens sputum and eases it towards the larger bronchi, whence it can be cleared by a cough. If there is little secretion but poor air entry, the huffing exercise and cough aids ventilation of peripheral lung tissue.

REMOVAL OF BRONCHIAL SECRETIONS

Coughing is essential to maintain patency of the airways and their dependent alveoli. In the healthy lung, secretions are continuously moved upwards by the action of the ciliated epithelium lining the main airways. In damaged lung this action is diminished or absent. Conscious coughing must therefore be taught and practised.

Cough holds. The patient must understand the importance of coughing and be assured that it will do no damage postoperatively. To ease the obviously painful manoeuvre he should be taught how to stabilise his chest when coughing alone.

The thoracotomy incision is best supported by placing the hand of the unaffected side as far round the affected ribs as possible and applying firm pressure with the hand and forearm. The other hand reinforces the hugging hold by clasping the opposite elbow and pulling it against the chest wall during the cough. The anterior thoracic incisions will best be supported by holding both hands across the sternum. Instruction should be given in the judicious use of a pillow to support the chest wall (see Figs. 8/4 and 5). This is particularly effective after cardiac surgery and increases coughing effectiveness by increasing confidence and decreasing pain.

Vibrations. Should it not be possible to clear the lungs adequately by breathing exercises and coughing, percussion, vibrations and shakings may be necessary. Percussion must be avoided in the following

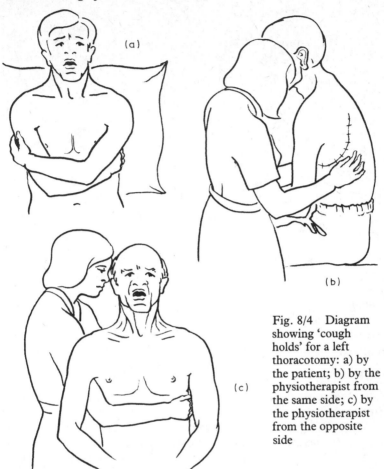

Fig. 8/4 Diagram showing 'cough holds' for a left thoracotomy: a) by the patient; b) by the physiotherapist from the same side; c) by the physiotherapist from the opposite side

instances: a) acute pneumonia; b) acute lung abscess; c) neoplasms; d) haemoptysis; e) over incision areas.

Attention should be directed to one hemithorax at a time. Vibrations and shaking are most effective if they are administered with the hands on the posterior and anterior aspects of the hemithorax and the shakings directed towards an internal focal point.

Postural drainage. The positions are shown in Chapter 11.

Inhalation therapy. This may be used in conjunction with physiotherapy in the following situations:

1. For sputum liquefaction.
2. For the relief of bronchospasm.
3. For topical treatment of infection or fungus. The finest particles

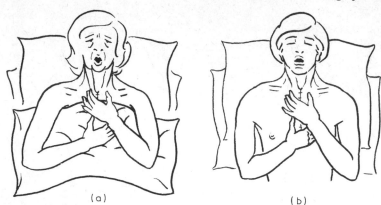

(a)   (b)

Fig. 8/5   Diagram showing 'cough holds' for a median sternotomy; a) with pillow; b) without pillow

of moisture for inhalation are produced by nebulisers and sometimes inhalation is assisted by intermittent positive pressure breathing (I.P.P.B.) (see p. 101).

Drug therapy. Systemic therapy may be instituted to lessen the viscosity of mucoid sputum. Bisolvon is such a mucolytic agent and may be administered orally in tablet or elixir form. Systemic broncho-dilator drugs may be given orally or per rectum.

GENERAL EXERCISES

Individual instruction in leg exercises should be given pre-operatively, in the lying and half-lying positions. The head and neck, shoulder girdle, arm and trunk exercises will best be taught in a class, along with postural awareness and correction. A close watch must be kept to avoid undue fatigue, especially of the cardiac patients who are fit enough to take part. Many cardiac patients should not join these exercise sessions.

Guide to a typical ward class for pre-operative and postoperative respiratory and cardiac patients.

On the first postoperative day patients in bed may attempt the neck and shoulder girdle movements, breathing and foot exercises. Trunk exercises are added about the third postoperative day. Pre-operative and fourth day postoperative patients should attempt all the exercises.

The scheme of exercises will include:

Deep bilateral costal breathing in time with instructor.

Head and neck rotation, flexion and extension.

Shoulder shrugging and bracing.

Arms bend and stretch forwards, sideways and upwards.

Diaphragmatic breathing in own time.

Foot and ankle exercises.

Alternate hip and knee flexion and extension.

Arms stretch sideways and place alternately behind neck and waist.

Trunk flexion to alternate sides.

Trunk forward flexion and extension.

Arms bend and circle elbows.

Lateral costal breathing in own time.

Trunk rotation to alternate sides with arms swinging.

Arms stretch out to sides and flex and rotate trunk to touch alternate hand to opposite foot.

Postural correction.

Diaphragmatic breathing in time with instructor.

POSTOPERATIVE PERIOD

Principles of Physiotherapy

1. To expand lung tissue by maximum inspiratory efforts with ribs and diaphragm.

2. To prevent lung collapse and/or consolidation by: a) general and localised costal and diaphragmatic breathing exercises; b) vibrations, shakings and postural drainage; c) coughing.

3. To remove excess secretions by: a) increasing rib and diaphragmatic movement; b) altering volume and speed of air flow; c) shaking, vibrations, percussion and postural drainage; d) coughing; e) suction.

4. To prevent circulatory complications by: a) foot and leg movements; b) general movements; c) deep breathing.

5. To maintain or increase mobility of thorax, head, neck, shoulder girdle and arms by: a) passive movements (for unconscious patients); b) active assisted movements; c) active movements; d) posture correction.

6. To return the patient to as full and as independent a life as possible.

A rope tied to the foot of the bed and extending to the fold of the bed-clothes aids independent movements. Most thoracic units encourage patients to dress fully as soon as all intercostal tubes are removed and to walk freely around the ward and grounds.

Patient Assessment

The physiotherapist must note:

a) The operation performed.

b) The incision.
c) Drainage tubes:
    i) number and position
    ii) amount and type of drainage.
d) Other tubes in situ:
    i) Ryle's tube
    ii) urethral catheter
    iii) intravenous lines
    iv) arterial lines
    v) endotracheal tube
    vi) tracheostomy tube.
e) Temperature.
f) Pulse.
g) Respiration:
    i) spontaneous – rate and depth
    ii) artificial – rate, pressure and volume.
h) Blood pressure.
i) Drugs prescribed, especially the type and time of administration
   of analgesics. Treatment ideally is timed to coincide with
   analgesic times as pain inhibits breathing and coughing.
j) E.C.G. pattern.
k) X-ray.
l) Blood gases.

Postoperative Cough Holds

The physiotherapist can assist the coughing manoeuvre greatly by her
encouragement and manual support, (see Fig. 8/4).

The thoracotomy incision can best be supported in the lying, half-
lying, or side-lying positions by firm pressure of the physiotherapist's
hands on the anterior and posterior aspects of the affected side of the
thorax. Probably the forward-sitting position is the most effective for
coughing, and the physiotherapist should stand on the unaffected side
of the patient. The anterior and posterior aspects of the affected side of
the thorax can be supported with the hands, whilst at the same time
the forearms will stabilise the whole chest and create a 'bear hug' hold.

The median sternotomy should be stabilised by placing both hands on
the anterior aspect of the chest. Equal pressure must be exerted to
minimise sternal movement.

Postoperative Complications

Postoperative shock, or excessively low blood pressure, is uncommon nowadays, due to adequate fluid transfusion and administration of vasopressor agents. It might occur, should there be a secondary haemorrhage.

Collapse and/or consolidation of segments or lobes of the lung are due to: a) excessive production of secretions; b) function of cilia being decreased by anaesthesia and surgical intervention; c) excessive fluid or air in the pleural cavity; d) inhibition of cough due to pain and fear; e) diminished respiratory movements; f) infection.

Cardiac arrythmia is due to surgical interference, diminished blood supply, electrolytic imbalance or hypoxia.

Carbon dioxide retention is due to inadequate ventilation.

Hypoxia may be due to ventilation/perfusion imbalance, inadequate ventilation, or both.

Deep vein thrombosis. Factors leading to deep vein thrombosis include venous stagnation, rise in platelets secondary to operation, trauma and dehydration. Movement would seem to prevent their formation. However, patients who are ambulant from the first postoperative day are still at risk. Recent work shows that prevention is only possible if blood flow is aided locally whilst the patient is on the operating table. Daily examination of the calf is necessary for early diagnosis.

Pulmonary emboli may be thrown off from a deep vein thrombosis.

Cerebrovascular accident. Emboli may be thrown off from calcified or fungoid heart valves and micro-emboli may elude the careful filter systems in the cardiopulmonary bypass system. After cardiopulmonary bypass in patients with a history of cerebrovascular accident, the recurrence of a similar incident is not uncommon.

Mononeuritis multiplex. Complete or partial motor and/or sensory peripheral nerve lesions have been noted after cardiac surgery. These are most probably due to micro-emboli (Keates, Innocenti and Ross, 1975).

Surgical emphysema is the collection of air in the interstitial spaces of subcutaneous tissues. On examination the chest, and possibly also the neck and face, appear swollen. On palpation the tissues crackle and the air can be moved under the fingers. On X-ray the tissues have a mottled appearance due to the air bubbles.

Infections may occur at any of the following sites: i) superficial incision; ii) sternum (post-sternotomy); iii) mediastinum; iv) pericardium; v) pleura; vi) bronchial stump.

Pleural effusions are due to secondary haemorrhage, infection or exudation (see p. 254). If excessive, aspiration or drainage with an intercostal tube will be necessary.

Pericardial effusions after surgery are usually due to haemorrhage. If the pericardium is left open the fluid will not restrict the heart's action.

Cardiac tamponade: should the pericardium be intact the collection of fluid within the non-elastic sac could be fatal. Fluid collecting in the pericardial cavity prevents the heart from filling during diastole. Hence cardiac output and blood pressure fall. Cardiac arrest will supervene unless emergency measures are taken and the thorax entered to incise the pericardium.

Ventilatory arrest is usually the result of total occlusion of the airway by mucus, or a foreign body.

Cardiac arrest may be total asystole or due to ventricular fibrillation (see Chapter 3).

Restricted arm and trunk movements may lead to an acquired deformity.

Renal complications occasionally precede acute failure and may necessitate peritoneal or haemodialysis.

Post bypass syndrome may complicate the recovery period. The patient feels unwell, lethargic and has a swinging pyrexia. It may be due to a pericardial and pleural reaction and is usually successfully treated with a three-day course of aspirin or steroid therapy.

Bronchopleural fistula may occur by breakdown of the bronchial stump or lung tissue. Air will pass directly from the bronchus into the pleural cavity and create or increase a pneumothorax. Bronchopleural fistula in pneumonectomy – see p. 155.

REFERENCES

Gaskell, D. V. and Webber, B. A. (1977). *The Brompton Hospital Guide to Chest Physiotherapy.* (3rd Ed.) Blackwell Scientific Publications.

Innocenti, D. M. (1966). 'Breathing exercises in the treatment of Emphysema.' *Physiotherapy*, **52**, 12, 437.

Keates, J. R. W., Innocenti, D. M. and Ross, D. N. (1975). 'Mononeuritis Multiplex.' *Journal of Thoracic and Cardiovascular Surgery*, **69**, 5, 816.

BIBLIOGRAPHY

See end of Chapter 10.

Chapter 9

Thoracic Surgery – II

by D. M. INNOCENTI, M.C.S.P.

OPERATIONS ON LUNG TISSUE

Local Resections

Local lesions of bronchiectasis, tuberculosis, neoplasms, benign tumours, fungus infections, hydatid, congenital or emphysematous cysts may be resected from the lung tissue. The standard thoracotomy incision is used for: a) *wedge resection* – a local resection; b) *segmental resection* – removal of a bronchopulmonary segment; c) *lobectomy* – removal of an entire lobe; d) *sleeve resection* – removal of upper lobe and section of the main bronchus.

It must be established that the patient has sufficient ventilatory reserve to undergo radical excision and survive the first few difficult days. Chronic lung disease may contra-indicate or defer surgery.

The unresected lung tissue expands into the vacant space, thus repositioning the airways. Should postural drainage be necessary the authentic positions may no longer suffice and individual variants must be found.

It must be recognised that the following is only a guide to treatment. Regimes will vary from hospital to hospital, and continent to continent. It is always imperative to know and abide by the surgeon's wishes and special routines.

PRE-OPERATIVE PHYSIOTHERAPY

This will follow the usual regime. Postural drainage is an important factor when much sputum is present. All patients may join the ward class. Auto-assisted shoulder elevation and the cough hold must be taught.

POSTOPERATIVE PHYSIOTHERAPY

Lateral costal and diaphragmatic breathing exercises and coughing are commenced on the day of the operation. Full active assisted shoulder elevation and abduction must be gained. Oxygen therapy is administered for the first few hours.

First postoperative day. Foot, leg, arm and shoulder girdle movements should be practised regularly through the day. The patient should be encouraged to expand the remaining lung tissue, by taking deep inspirations and holding each breath for a few seconds at full inspiration.

Resisted inspiratory costal and diaphragmatic breathing exercises, expiratory breathing exercises, shakings (if necessary) and coughing should begin with the patient in side lying, possibly with the bed tipped. Similar exercises and bilateral costal exercises should next be practised with the patient lying back on to a pillow (quarter turn up from supine). The pillow should be placed along the patient's back and the intercostal tubes arranged to rest over it. This position 'opens up' the anterior chest wall and facilitates bilateral costal movement whilst still draining the affected lung. The quarter turn forward position (quarter turn up from prone) may also be used as this allows unrestricted posterior chest movements. The patient is supported on an anteriorly placed pillow. The breathing exercises should next be repeated in the lying position. The foot of the bed is lowered and all exercises and coughing repeated in half lying.

Second postoperative day. All exercises are increased and trunk movements added to the scheme in the sitting position. The patient may sit out of bed for as long as he wishes. Drainage tubes will probably be removed.

Third postoperative day. The full ward class regime should be attempted.

Ambulation is commenced as early as possible. The presence of drainage tubes should not retard the process and as soon as suction is discontinued patients should be encouraged to walk around carrying their drainage bottle.

All exercises and postural drainage must be continued until the lungs are clear and fully expanded. Postural exercises and general activities should be progressed until discharge about the eleventh day. Young people recovering from resections for bronchiectasis need encouragement to play games in the gymnasium or grounds.

Pneumonectomy

The removal of a whole lung is commonly undertaken for excision of a carcinoma and rarely for benign disease. The other lung must be healthy and capable of supporting life. It may be impossible to maintain adequate respiration with one lung if the vital capacity is very low.

The operation may be localised or radical. Radical pneumonectomy includes excision of mediastinal glands and dissection from the chest wall or pericardium. The phrenic and recurrent laryngeal nerves may be involved, resulting in a paralysis of a hemi-diaphragm and inability to approximate the vocal cords. The latter seriously impairs the ability to cough.

Intercostal drainage is rarely used. The hemithorax is filled with fluid and air. The fluid level may need to be controlled by aspirations to prevent submersion of the bronchial stump, or a mediastinal shift. The fluid will finally organise and the hemi-diaphragm rise.

PRE-OPERATIVE PHYSIOTHERAPY

This will follow the usual routine, particular attention being paid to expansion of the base of the remaining lung and to diaphragmatic control.

POSTOPERATIVE PHYSIOTHERAPY

Oxygen therapy is administered for the first few hours. Most surgeons prefer their patients not to turn onto the unaffected side, as the fluid will submerge the bronchial stump. If the bronchial stump breaks down, thus creating a bronchopleural fistula, the fluid would drain across into the remaining lung.

Costal and diaphragmatic exercises for the remaining lung are necessary from the day of operation. *Straining* to cough should be avoided for twenty-four hours. Treatment may often be given in the half-lying or sitting position. It is only necessary to position the patient in side lying if the remaining lung requires drainage. Postural drainage will be included if there is sputum retention. As drainage necessitates lying on the incision the positioning must be carefully executed. The patient should sit forward and then turn into side sitting towards the affected side. The physiotherapist will stand behind the patient and rearrange the pillows, leaving only one on the bed. The patient's body weight must be supported at the shoulder as he lowers himself on to his elbow and then into side lying.

Although there is only one lung, bilateral costal exercises are important to retain symmetry. Breathing control and exercise tolerance can be improved by the encouragement of diaphragmatic breathing. General exercises are progressed as for a lobectomy. Recovery is often slow, due to age and the gravity of the disease.

Should a bronchopleural fistula occur from breakdown of the bronchial stump, it will be recognised by dyspnoea, irritating cough and possible expectoration of a dark fluid. The patient must sit up or be turned on to the operation side to prevent any spill-over of pleural fluid to the remaining lung.

OPERATIONS ON THE PLEURAL CAVITY

Rarely is pleural disease primary; more often it is secondary to underlying disease. Pleural reaction may be dry, or associated with fluid collection due to altered osmotic pressures (transudates) (see p. 254), or to inflammation (exudates). Causes of pleural exudates are:

   i) tuberculosis
   ii) neoplasm
   iii) pulmonary infarction
   iv) pneumonia
   v) subphrenic abscess
   vi) collagen disease.

Slow absorption of a large effusion may lead to fibrosis and subsequent lung restriction.

HAEMOTHORAX

This usually follows trauma to the chest wall which may in addition cause a pneumothorax, thus producing a haemopneumothorax. If the blood is not evacuated, organisation, pleural fibrosis and lung restriction may occur.

EMPYEMA

This is a localised collection of pus in the pleural cavity, and may result from infection of pleural fluid or spread from a lung or subphrenic abscess. It may be the result of a wound infection and must be drained.

PNEUMOTHORAX

This is a collection of air in the pleural cavity, and may be: a) traumatic; b) spontaneous; c) therapeutic.

Traumatic pneumothorax. This may be caused by: i) trauma or surgical interference of the chest wall; ii) perforation of the trachea or oesophagus; iii) rupture of peripheral emphysematous cysts during coughing or artificial ventilation.

Spontaneous pneumothorax. This is caused by the rupture of a small vesicle on the surface of the lung (see p. 258).

Therapeutic pneumothorax. Air may be introduced into the thorax to equalise intrathoracic pressures in a pneumonectomy space. The introduction of an artificial pneumothorax used to be a treatment for tuberculosis.

Operations performed on the pleural cavity are: pleurodesis; pleurectomy; decortication.

Pleurodesis

An artificial or chemical pleurisy is created by the introduction of an irritant to the pleural cavity. The ensuing pleural reaction results in the visceral and parietal pleurae becoming adherent, so preventing recurrent lung collapse.

Pleurectomy

This is performed through a standard thoracotomy incision and the parietal pleura is peeled from the chest wall. Any adhesions at the periphery of the diaphragm are freed. The visceral pleura will adhere to the chest wall, thus obliterating the pleural cavity.

Decortication

The thickened fibrotic restricting layer of visceral pleura is dissected off the lung surface. Thus the lung will expand fully and adhere to the parietal pleura.

Foreign matter and fluid are removed in pleurectomy and decortication. The chest is closed and drained with apical and basal intercostal tubes, until the lung is fully re-expanded. These tubes should never be clamped.

PRE-OPERATIVE PHYSIOTHERAPY

This follows the routine procedure. Specific instruction is given in diaphragmatic movement and unilateral costal movement.

POSTOPERATIVE PHYSIOTHERAPY

The immediate postoperative period is particularly painful and adequate analgesia must be given. The intercostal tubes must *never* be clamped. The routine postoperative regime (see p. 149) is instigated on the day of operation. Care of the drainage tubes, costal and diaphragmatic breathing exercises and coughing will be carried out with the patient in the side-lying position with the affected lung uppermost and the foot of the bed elevated. Efforts to regain maximum rib and diaphragm movement must never wane. The patient will sit out of bed on the first day and commence walking as soon as possible. All exercises are increased and postural drainage continued until inter-costal tubes and/or all excess secretions are removed. Exercises in the ward class and gymnasium, and walking, must continue until discharge about the eleventh day. All movements should be unrestricted and the posture free and upright. Vital capacity and exercise tolerance should show improvement on the pre-operative assessment. If all parameters are not satisfactory the patient should attend for out-patient physiotherapy.

OPERATIONS ON THE CHEST WALL

Resection of whole or part of one or more ribs may have to be undertaken to excise a tumour. It may be necessary to repair extensive damage with a prosthesis. Sections of one or two ribs are resected to drain an empyema space. These wounds remain open for long periods, but may eventually be allowed to close.

Thoracoplasty

An extensive resection of ribs is undertaken and the chest wall, having no scaffolding, falls inwards and obliterates the pleural cavity and/or lung tissue. The operation used to be performed in cases of tuberculosis before suitable chemotherapy was instituted and lung resection became a common practice. Results of thoracoplasty may still be seen as the operation was performed up until the early 1950s. Infected pneumonectomy spaces or persistent bronchial stump fistulae are still closed in this manner. The first rib may or may not be removed.

Pre-operatively patients are often ill and weak following previous major surgery, illness or accident.

POSTOPERATIVE TREATMENT

This commences on the day of operation. Lateral costal and diaphragmatic breathing exercises and coughing, full range active assisted shoulder movements and correction of position must be practised as soon as possible after the patient returns to the ward. The upper chest must be well supported during coughing, as there will be a paradoxical movement of the chest wall. The best position for the patient is forward sitting. The physiotherapist must hold the chest very firmly, with one hand on the back and the other over the upper part of the front of the chest.

First postoperative day. Bilateral and unilateral costal breathing exercises, diaphragmatic breathing exercises and coughing will be practised in side-lying, lying and half-lying positions. Leg, arm, shoulder girdle and head movements must be commenced. The patient will sit out of bed and walk around as soon as possible. Trunk exercises will begin on the second or third day. Posture exercises in front of a mirror are very beneficial. Intensive postural training is essential, especially in cases when the first rib has been resected.

Fractured Ribs

There will be surgical intervention only if the pleura and lungs are damaged. Pinning of multiple fractures is practised at some centres. The rib ends are approximated and fixed with medullary pins, thus reforming the rigid cage.

Major Injuries

Injuries of the chest wall occur frequently in road traffic accidents. Ribs may be dislocated or there may be numerous fractures. There is danger of the rib ends tearing the pleura and lung tissue. This results in bleeding and escape of air into tissues. A haemopneumothorax may ensue. The heart, mediastinum and great vessels are also at risk.

Multiple rib fractures result in a flail chest. Should a whole segment of ribs become detached *paradoxical breathing* will be present, which seriously compromises ventilation. On inspiration and expansion of the sound chest wall the intrathoracic pressure becomes negative and sucks *in* the disconnected portion of the chest wall. During expiration, as the sound ribs recoil, the increasing intrathoracic pressure pushes *out* the flail segment.

Not only does the flail segment move paradoxically, but so also does the air flow. As the flail chest is sucked in, air from the underlying lung is pushed into the unaffected side (should the injury be unilateral) resulting in adverse gas mixing.

TREATMENT

It is primarily necessary to maintain adequate ventilation. In massive injury an artificial airway is introduced and positive pressure ventilation established. Equal pressures are maintained intrapulmonarily, thus adequately splinting the ribs and producing a symmetrical movement. Intermittent positive pressure ventilation via a tracheostomy may be necessary for up to three weeks or until the chest wall is stable. The treatment of the chest is described in the section on ventilators.

SPECIFIC TECHNIQUES FOR TREATING RIB FRACTURES

Excess secretions within the lung and pleural cavities must be evacuated. Pain and risk of further damage prevents any shaking
manoeuvre at the site of injury. However, indirect vibration is particularly effective in these circumstances.

Methods. a) Institute shaking and percussion to the unaffected side
during drainage of the affected side.

b) The shoulder girdle may be shaken down rhythmically onto the
chest wall by clasping both hands over the shoulder of the damaged
side. This is particularly effective when the whole of the lower chest is
involved.

c) Shakings over the actual area can be performed, if necessary,
when the section is firmly splinted by a sustained high intrathoracic
pressure. This situation occurs if the patient coughs whilst tracheal
suction is in progress.

Congenital Deformities

PECTUS CARINATUM (PIGEON CHEST)

The sternum projects forward and is held in a prominent position by
the ribs and costal cartilages.

Operation is undertaken to improve ventilatory capacity or (more
commonly) for cosmetic reasons. The offending costal cartilages are
removed and the sternum split horizontally and depressed. Fixation is
established by suturing together both pectoralis major muscles in the
mid-line.

PECTUS EXCAVATUM (FUNNEL CHEST)

The sternum is depressed in its lower end and with the in-turning
costal cartilages forms a depression of varying degree. Ventilatory and
cardiac function may be impaired and operation is performed to
relieve this and for cosmetic purposes.

The costal cartilages are mobilised and the sternum split horizontally and may be held in its corrected position by a metal bar, or by
a rib which has been resected for the purpose. More recently, for
cosmetic reasons, a pre-formed plastic prosthesis is placed subcutaneously which greatly improves the contour of the chest.

Postoperative physiotherapy follows the routine procedure for maintaining clear airways, lung expansion and preventing lung collapse. It
is advisable to nurse the patient in the lying position and to avoid the

half-lying or kyphotic position. Side lying should also be avoided if possible. Shoulder girdle, arm exercises and postural correction are of particular importance. All exercises should be practised bilaterally to maintain symmetry.

Scoliosis and Kyphosis

Causes of scoliosis are: i) congenital; ii) idiopathic; iii) paralytic; iv) traumatic.

The reason for operation may be to correct deformity, to alter the growth potential, or for cosmetic purposes.

Operations which may be undertaken on the spine are posterior spinal fusion, multiple wedge resections, distraction or compression rods, or other compression forces on the convexity.

Cosmetic operations undertaken may be sub-total scapulectomy or costectomy.

Physiotherapy is of great importance to maintain adequate ventilation, increase muscle power and re-educate a good postural pattern. The vital capacity and the maximum voluntary ventilation (see p. 50) may be severely affected, as is the gas transfer and work of breathing. The patient will probably be nursed in a plaster bed or split plaster jacket for up to three months.

BIBLIOGRAPHY

See end of Chapter 10.

Thoracic Surgery – III

by D. M. INNOCENTI, M.C.S.P.

CARDIAC SURGERY

Modern techniques include closed and open procedures.

Closed heart surgery does not interfere with the circulation through the heart and the internal defect is corrected without direct vision. A small incision is made in the myocardium through which an instrument or finger is passed.

Open heart surgery necessitates interfering with the circulation through the heart to obtain an unobstructed view of the lesion. The circulation and gaseous exchange is carried out by a heart-lung machine to maintain viability of all body tissues.

EXTRACORPOREAL CIRCULATION

Heart operations sometimes take a few hours. During this time the surgeon requires an empty and quiet heart. The process of blood circulation and oxygenation must be undertaken artificially. Venous blood is siphoned and gravity-drained from cannulae in the inferior and superior venae cavae or from the right atrium. The blood is oxygenated, cooled or heated, filtered and pumped back into a) the aorta (just above the aortic valve), or b) the femoral artery.

As the blood flow is taken on to bypass, the ventricular pressures fall and the heart stops pumping. At some centres the heart is made to fibrillate by an electric shock to prevent unwanted contractions. After the operation the heart may contract spontaneously as the intracardiac pressure increases with blood-flow. It may be necessary to promote the return to normal rhythm with a D.C. shock and local drug therapy.

The coronary arteries may remain unperfused without damage to the myocardium for up to 40 minutes at normal temperature, or longer with a hypothermic heart. It may be necessary to perfuse them with separate cannulae if the operation is prolonged.

OXYGENATORS

Bubble oxygenators. Oxygen is bubbled into the bottom of an oxygenating tube, which contains the venous blood. The blood is arterialised as the oxygen bubbles rise. Excess gas is eliminated in the debubbling chamber and the blood filtered before entering the arterial line.

Membrane oxygenators. The natural process of oxygenation of blood occurs across a semipermeable membrane. In membrane oxygenators the blood film and the oxygen are separated by a stationary or rotating semipermeable membrane. Problems of size have not yet been overcome, and this machine is not yet in general use.

THE PUMPING MECHANISM

This must be capable of moving blood volumes of up to five litres/minute against pressures of up to 180mm Hg. The natural flow is pulsatile. The artificial flow is constant.

Filters are placed in the circuit to remove fibrin strands and debris.

Bubble traps are made of silicone-coated meshwork and are a necessary safety device to prevent air emboli from entering the circulation.

Heat exchangers maintain the normal physiological temperature against excessive heat loss in the circuit. They rapidly cool and re-warm the blood when necessary. As oxygen requirements are greatly reduced in cool tissues, difficult or long operations may be performed under hypothermia.

PRE-OPERATIVE PHYSIOTHERAPY

This follows the regime outlined on p. 143. It is particularly important to watch for signs of distress when positioning the patient. Many are unable to lie down due to heart failure. A knowledge of the drips, drains, leads and the possible need for ventilation is given to the patient. Those undergoing open heart surgery must know that the first few days will be spent in the intensive care unit.

POSTOPERATIVE PERIOD

Following a closed procedure, the patient will return directly to the ward. The regime is similar to the pulmonary scheme. The lung secretions will probably be less but general progress may be a little slower.

Following open heart surgery, the patient will return to the intensive care unit and may or may not be artificially ventilated. Continuous oxygen therapy will be in progress and in some cases Entonox will be administered. (Entonox is a mixture of nitrous oxide and oxygen which is used in the immediate postoperative hours for its analgesic and sedative effect.) The patient will be attached to:

a) an oscilloscope which shows the electrocardiograph;
b) venous lines for intravenous infusions, drug therapy and central venous pressure recordings;
c) an arterial line to which is attached a transducer or manometer which records the arterial pressure;
d) rectal and peripheral temperature probes;
e) urethral catheter;
f) Ryle's tube;
g) drainage tubes;
h) pacemaker leads.

Guide to Physiotherapy Progression Following Cardiopulmonary Bypass

Certain operative procedures and postoperative treatments are discussed in this section, but it must be emphasised that it is only possible to generalise. Each patient must always be assessed individually and at each treatment. Techniques must vary with the patient's condition and the surgeon's wishes.

Postoperative treatment and positioning is entirely dependent on the surgeon's wishes. Some do not wish their patients to commence physical treatment on the day of operation, nor to alter position for twenty-four hours. Others like to institute the first treatment as soon as the patient is co-operative, and allow alterations of position for physiotherapy and nursing procedures after the first few hours.

Treatment of Patients with Intra-Aortic Counterpulsation Therapy

The treatment may be given as described, but special care must be taken on two counts:
a) The E.C.G. electrodes referring to the balloon machine must not be disturbed, as the interference will adversely affect the pumping mechanism.

b) The balloon catheter must not be compressed at the point of entry in the femoral artery.

Treatment of Patients on Artificial Ventilation

Specific treatment of the chest during artificial ventilation and suction techniques are discussed in the section on intensive care (see Chapters 5 and 6).

Treatment of Patients Breathing Spontaneously

Special attention must be given to the cardiovascular state throughout the treatments.

DAY OF OPERATION

i) Breathing exercises and coughing. The patient is nursed flat or in half lying and general deep breathing must be encouraged by firm but gentle pressure of the physiotherapist's hands on the lower costal area. Huffing and coughing will be practised but it is rare for the patient to expectorate at this stage.

ii) Active plantar and dorsiflexion of feet.

iii) Passive or active-assisted knee flexion and extension, hip abduction and adduction approximately 6 to 10 times.

iv) Passive or active-assisted shoulder elevation and abduction approximately 6 to 10 times.

FIRST POSTOPERATIVE DAY

First treatment will be given as above and unilateral expansion exercises added. The physiotherapist supports the sternum with one hand, and gives gentle resistance with the other over the requisite area. Unilateral shakings over the lower lateral and posterior aspects of the chest are also instituted to loosen secretions.

It will be necessary to support the incision and drainage sites during coughing.

Second treatment will be as for the first, but the patient should tolerate more breathing exercises, shakings and coughing.

Third treatment. All limb exercises should now be active-assisted or active. The patient may be turned for treatment, if his condition permits. The nurse in attendance will help to move and position the patient comfortably in side lying. Care of pressure areas and the change of bed linen will probably take place at these turning sessions.

The physiotherapist resists inspiratory efforts and assists expiratory efforts by manual pressure on the anterior and posterior aspects of the

hemithorax under treatment. Shakings are given and huffing practised in this position. Adequate support must be given during coughing. If the patient's condition allows, the treatment is carried out on
both sides.

The time spent in the side-lying position depends on the patient's
cardiovascular and pulmonary condition. The latter is assessed by the
daily morning X-ray and regular blood-gas measurements.

SECOND POSTOPERATIVE DAY

Transfer to the general ward may occur any time after 24 hours and
depends on the condition of the patient's respiratory and cardiovascular systems. The physiotherapy is continued along previous
lines. All limb exercises should now be active. Breathing, shaking and
coughing exercises will continue in the lying and side-lying positions.
It may be necessary to posturally drain a specific lung area and to add
percussion over the back if sputum becomes particularly tenacious or
if early consolidation is present. Coughing may be more successful if
the patient is supported in forward sitting or the incision is supported
by a pillow (see Fig. 8/5a).

THIRD, FOURTH AND FIFTH POSTOPERATIVE DAYS

Chest physiotherapy will continue two or three times a day, depending entirely on the X-ray appearances, blood-gas measurements, lung
expansion and sputum production. It may be necessary to tip the bed
for treatment if there are excess secretions, if the patient's condition
allows.

Most surgeons like their patients to sit out of bed on the third or
fourth day and start walking about on the fourth or fifth day. General
arm and trunk exercises will now be done in the class.

Stair climbing may be commenced as soon as the patient is ready.
This may be as early as the fifth day. About six stairs should be
attempted the first time and the number increased over the next few
days.

OPERATIONS

Heart operations will be considered in two sections:

Acquired disorders.
Congenital disorders.

ACQUIRED DISORDERS

The Pericardium

Pericardectomy is performed to relieve the symptoms of chronic constrictive pericarditis. The pericardium is fibrotic and sometimes calcified due to previous tubercular infection. The constricted heart is unable to expand in diastole with resultant diminished cardiac output.

Incision: median sternotomy.

Closed procedure. The calcific and fibrotic pericardium is completely dissected and removed.

Postoperative physiotherapy. The routine postoperative treatment will commence on the day of the operation. Progress may be slow as exercise tolerance will be impaired due to the prolonged period of myocardial restriction. The patient will get out of bed about the third day and be discharged during the third week.

The Myocardium

Aneurysms may result from previous myocardial infarction. If high intracardial pressures are maintained during the early post-infarction days there is risk of stretching the young fibrotic tissue. This ballooning of the wall of a cardiac chamber compromises the cardiac output and there is risk of rupture.

Infarcted tissue creates an akinetic area within the myocardium. If this is large the cardiac output is diminished. Cardiac failure may supervene.

Cardiomyopathy. In some myopathies the muscle may be greatly hypertrophied or the chambers enlarged. A forceful contraction becomes impossible, resulting in a diminished cardiac output.

Incision: median sternotomy.

Open procedure. Operations on the myocardium may involve: i) resection of aneurysm; ii) resection of infarcted tissue; iii) selective myocardial resection.

Pre- and postoperative physiotherapy. The treatment will follow the routine scheme, but progression will be slow as exercise tolerance is diminished due to protracted illness.

The Valves

The four valves lie in the same plane and one or more may become diseased causing them to become stenotic or incompetent (see p. 336).

Operations on the valves are carried out under direct vision with a cardiopulmonary bypass, except for mitral valvotomy which is very successfully performed by a closed technique in certain circumstances. Valve surgery aims to repair or replace the deficient valve.

Valve Repair

CLOSED MITRAL VALVOTOMY

Incision: left thoracotomy through the fifth intercostal space.

Closed procedure. The heart is entered through the auricular appendage of the left atrium. The commissures of the valve are split with the finger or by special dilators. Rarely is this a permanent cure, but it affords good relief from symptoms. A further valvotomy or valve replacement may have to be undertaken in later life.

Pre- and postoperative physiotherapy follow the same routine as for thoracotomy. The progression of exercises may be a little slower than for lung resection. Discharge from hospital is on about the fourteenth day.

OPEN VALVOTOMY

This may be performed on the mitral, pulmonary or aortic valves. The commissures of the valves are split under direct vision with the patient on cardiopulmonary bypass.

ANNULOPLASTY

This is a method of correcting a regurgitant valve by decreasing the size of the valve ring with sutures and securing Teflon.

VALVULOPLASTY

The cusps of a moderately involved valve may be sutured or refashioned to produce an effective closure. In some selective instances repair or reconstitution of chordae tendinae is undertaken.

Incision: median sternotomy.

Pre- and postoperative physiotherapy will follow the routine cardiac scheme. After operation the patient is returned to the intensive care unit for the first 24 to 48 hours before transfer to the general ward. Discharge will be about the fourteenth day.

Valve Replacement

This is commonly undertaken as the treatment for incompetent or stenotic valvular lesions. Some mechanical prostheses in use are:

a) *Starr-Edwards.* A mechanical ball and cage device made of

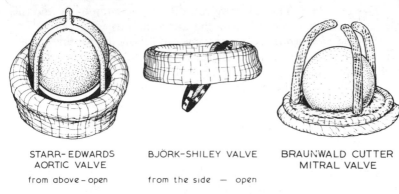

STARR- EDWARDS   BJÖRK-SHILEY VALVE   BRAUNWALD CUTTER
AORTIC VALVE   MITRAL VALVE

from above - open   from the side — open

Fig. 10/1   Artificial heart valves

stainless steel. The early steel ball type is being replaced by a silicone ball type (see Fig. 10/1).

b) Björk-Shiley. A free-floating plastic disc suspended in a Stellite cage (see Fig. 10/1).

c) Braunwald-Cutter. A mechanical ball and cage device in which the prongs of the cage are not closed (see Fig. 10/1).

Some biological prostheses in use are:

a) Carpentier-Edwards. A bioprosthesis, comprised of a porcine aortic valve, which has been preserved in a buffered gluteraldehyde solution and fitted on a flexible frame (see Fig. 10/2a).

b) Allograft. A human valve, treated with antibiotics and stored in a nutrient solution, may be fitted to a flexible frame, or sutured directly into place (see Fig. 10/2b).

Incision: median sternotomy.

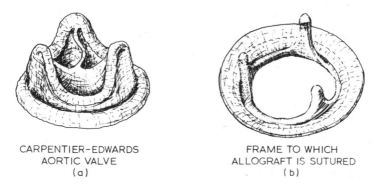

CARPENTIER-EDWARDS   FRAME TO WHICH
AORTIC VALVE   ALLOGRAFT IS SUTURED
(a)   (b)

Fig. 10/2   Diagram showing a bioprosthetic heart valve and frame to which the allograft is sutured

Open procedure. The defective valve is excised completely and the prosthesis sutured securely into the valve annulus.

Pre- and postoperative physiotherapy will follow the routine bypass scheme. Patients will be discharged, either to their home or to a convalescent home, in the second or third week.

Note: The words allograft and homograft are interchangeable.

The Vessels

Grafts

Patients suffering from intractable angina or who have survived myocardial infarction may be found, by coronary angiography, to have operable occlusions of the coronary arterial system.

AORTOCORONARY ARTERY BYPASS GRAFT

This is perhaps the most recent advance in cardiac surgery, superseding the Vineberg operation of implantation of the internal mammary artery into the myocardium.

Incisions: median sternotomy and interrupted incisions along the course of the long saphenous vein.

The procedure is carried out under cardiopulmonary bypass. Part of the saphenous vein is removed and reversed to obviate the valves. One end is anastomosed to the aorta, just above the aortic valve, the other anastomosed distal to the farthest block. Three or four grafts may be undertaken at one session.

Pre- and postoperative physiotherapy will follow the routine bypass scheme. Discharge will be in the second or third week.

Resection and Anastomosis

Thoracic Aortic Aneurysms

Aneurysms of the aorta are results of trauma, hypertension, inflammation, coarctation or atherosclerosis. Aneurysms of the ascending aorta are often associated with Marfan's Syndrome. They may be saccular or fusiform.

Dissecting aneurysm. Should the tunica intima rupture, the blood will flow between the intimal and medial arterial coats. The flow into connecting arteries will be compromised as the blood will bypass any arterial junction (see p. 267).

Symptoms. An initial episode of acute pain is not always present. Symptoms are mainly attributable to pressure on surrounding structures.

a) Venous engorgement from pressure on the superior vena cava, brachiocephalic vein or the right atrium.

b) Dyspnoea, cough or stridor from pressure on the trachea, bronchi or lung tissue.

c) Dysphagia caused by pressure on the oesophagus.

d) Alteration of speech and difficulty in coughing from pressure on the recurrent laryngeal nerve.

e) Renal failure due to altered perfusion of renal arteries.

f) Back pain.

The roots of the innominate, subclavian and common carotid arteries may be occluded by clot or dissection. It is common for the aneurysm to rupture, fatally, into the pericardium, trachea or oesophagus.

Incision: is dependent on the site of the lesion, but usually it is a median sternotomy for ascending aortic aneurysm and a thoracotomy for descending aortic aneurysm.

Procedure. The aneurysm is resected and the aortic ends anastomosed or reconstituted with a Dacron graft. If the vessels arising from the arch of the aorta are involved, they will be implanted into the graft. Repairs of aneurysms of the ascending aorta and aortic arch are carried out on cardiopulmonary bypass. Hypothermia is necessary if the cerebral circulation is affected. Venous blood is taken from the right atrium and returned to the femoral artery. Repairs of the descending aorta do not necessitate cardiopulmonary bypass.

Pre- and postoperative physiotherapy. Minimal pre-operative treatment is given to teach breathing exercises and the postoperative routine. There is great risk of rupture, so the patient is kept as quiet as possible. Postoperative treatment will follow the routine bypass scheme with discharge about the third week.

Pulmonary Embolectomy

Massive or repeated embolus may obstruct so much of the pulmonary vasculature that an adequate circulation cannot be maintained. Urgent operation may then be necessary.

Incision: median sternotomy.

Procedure. The operation is carried out on cardiopulmonary bypass. The pulmonary artery is incised vertically and the embolus is lifted out. A sucker is passed into the right and left pulmonary arteries to ensure clearance of as many embolic fragments as possible.

It may be necessary to ligate the inferior vena cava to prevent further embolic incidents. This will be performed through a lateral abdominal incision.

Pre- and postoperative physiotherapy. The operation being an emergency procedure, there will be no pre-operative physiotherapy. Postoperative treatment will follow the routine bypass scheme.

Cardiac Myxoma

This is a rare condition of specific tumour formation within the cardiac chambers which most commonly arises in the left atrium. It is mobile and obstructs the mitral valve. The signs and symptoms are those of intermittent mitral valve disease. It may throw off emboli.

Incision: median sternotomy or left antero-lateral thoracotomy.

Open procedure. The heart is entered through the left atrium and the myxoma resected away from its root on the atrial wall. Alternatively, the right atrium is entered and the septum divided and removed with the pedicle and myxoma. The septum will be repaired or patched with Dacron.

Pre- and postoperative physiotherapy follow the routine bypass scheme. Discharge will be between ten days and three weeks.

Heart Block

This is a condition where there is interference in the normal conducting system of the heart. There are various degrees of the condition which may be due to:

    i) Coronary artery disease
    ii) Myocarditis
   iii) Valve disease
   iv) Rheumatic fever
    v) Diphtheria
   vi) Congenital disorder
  vii) Surgical interference

In complete heart block the atria and ventricles work independently. The pulse rate is slow, usually between thirty and forty beats per minute. There is risk of attacks of unconsciousness during which the patient's pulse stops. Convulsions may occur if unconsciousness is prolonged. When the pulse returns the patient regains consciousness and may have a characteristic flush. Such periods of unconsciousness are termed Stokes-Adams attacks.

PACEMAKERS

An electrical device which artificially paces the heart is being increasingly used to correct the condition of heart block. There are two methods of inserting a permanent internal artificial pacemaker system:

1. Transvenous system. A cardiac catheter with a wire core and electrode tip is passed transvenously and embedded into the myocardium at the apex of the right ventricle. The pacemaker box is implanted subcutaneously in the axilla or epigastrium and connected to the electrode wire.

2. Epicardial system. Should the previous method be unsuccessful, it is necessary to perform a left thoracotomy and pericardotomy. Small electrodes are sutured to, or screwed into the epicardium and connected by screened wires to the pacemaker box, implanted subcutaneously as above.

A temporary pacing system may be necessary and will be fixed transvenously through the basilic vein or subclavian vein. The wires will be attached to an external pacemaker box.

Internal and external pacemaker systems may work on a fixed rate, on demand, or be atrial triggered.

Fixed rate pacemakers discharge at regular fixed intervals. The atrial and ventricular contractions will not be synchronised.

Demand pacemakers may operate in two ways. One type is linked to the interval between ventricular contractions. A ventricular contraction is sensed by the pacemaker, but should the next contraction be delayed the pacemaker will produce an impulse. The second type produces stimuli regularly. A spontaneous ventricular contraction will be sensed and the stimulus superimposed upon it (this will be ineffective as the myocardium will have depolarised). Should a ventricular contraction not take place the impulse will produce a contraction.

Atrial triggered pacemakers produce a near normal situation. An electrode situated in the right atrium relays the atrial impulse via a lead to the pacemaker box. The pacemaker then produces a stimulus which is relayed via a second wire and electrode to the right ventricle. As the atrial rate varies, so will the ventricular rate.

Postoperative physiotherapy. For transvenous implants – routine chest care with complete mobilisation after twenty-four hours. For epicardial implants – routine post-thoracotomy scheme.

SURGICAL TREATMENT OF TACHYCARDIAS

Certain ventricular tachycardias and some cases of Wolf-Parkinson-White syndrome can be effectively treated by an operation when drug treatment has failed. Some patients who have recurrent attacks of ventricular tachycardia and who have a left ventricular aneurysm may be cured of their tachycardia by excision of their aneurysm.

In recent years with the development of electrical mapping of the epicardium in the operating theatre it has been possible precisely to identify the course of a re-entry circuit in W-P-W syndrome. The surgeon can then interrupt a part of this circuit by cutting myocardial fibres and thus prevent development of a tachycardia.

CONGENITAL DISORDERS

In order to help to understand these, a brief outline of the development of the heart is given here.

Development of the Heart

The heart is formed between the 21st and 40th days of embryonic life. Two symmetrically developing endothelial tubes fuse, commencing at the bulbar or arterial end, to form a tubular heart. As the tube grows in length, two grooves appear in the surface, which subdivide it into three primitive sections or chambers. The arterial end is called the bulbus cordis, the central chamber the ventricle, and the venous end the sinuatrial chamber. The groove between the ventricle and the sinuatrial chamber indicates the position of the atrioventricular canal.

The tube continues to increase in length. The middle portion grows more rapidly than the ends, resulting in the formation of a U-shaped loop, termed the bulboventricular loop (the right limb of the loop is formed by the bulb and the left limb by the ventricle).

The venous end of the tube (the common atrium) is pushed into an S-shaped curve and so lies above and behind the ventricular portion. A fold appears at the venous end of the atrium, dividing the chamber, to form the sinus venosus. Meanwhile, paired endothelial tubes arise to form the dorsal aortae, which grow down to the pericardium and join with the bulbus to form the truncus arteriosus.

The venous drainage is established by the union of an anterior cardinal vein from the head end of the embryo with a posterior cardinal vein from the tail end. This vessel then opens into the sinuatrial chamber by draining into the sinus venosus. The umbilical arteries and veins develop. These veins terminate in the sinuatrial chamber and will eventually drain into the right atrium.

The atria are formed from the common chamber.

The communication between the atrium and the ventricle (the atrioventricular canal) becomes divided by the formation of the atrioventricular endocardial cushions. These swellings grow from the centres of the ventral and dorsal walls of the canal, join together (thus forming the septum intermedium of His), and leave the right and left atrioventricular orifices, within which the mitral and tricuspid valves form.

The division between the right and left atria is formed by the growth of two septa (see Fig. 10/3).

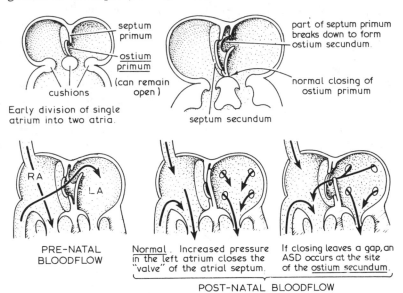

Fig. 10/3   Diagram illustrating the development of the atrial septa and showing how an atrial septal defect can occur

The first septum, or septum primum, grows from the upper and dorsal part of the atrial wall down towards the endocardial cushions. It is necessary in the fetal heart for the two atria to communicate. The free passage of blood is maintained below the advancing edge of the septum. This communication is termed the ostium primum, and is low down, near to the atrioventricular canal. This hole decreases in size and finally closes as the septum encroaches on the endocardial cushions. To maintain an inter-atrial communication the dorsal part of the septum breaks down. This communication is termed the ostium secundum (foramen ovale) and is high up in the septum.

The second septum, or septum secundum, is formed by inflection of the muscular atrial wall, and it overlaps the septum primum at its periphery, leaving the centre free.

Whilst the septum is developing, a pulmonary vein opens into the left atrium and subsequently expands into the four pulmonary veins.

The ventral walls of the atria bulge forwards, one on each side of the bulbus cordis, to form the atrial chambers.

The separation of the ventricles and of the truncus arteriosus into the aortic and pulmonary trunks are interrelated. Four endocardial cushions grow at the distal end of the bulbus (ventral, dorsal, right and left). The right and left cushions join to form the distal bulbar septum, which divides the orifice into ventral or pulmonary and dorsal or aortic sections. The four cushions eventually form the aortic and pulmonary valves.

Right and left spiral ridges appear within the truncus arteriosus and fuse together forming the spiral aortopulmonary septum (thus dividing the truncus arteriosus into the pulmonary trunk and the aorta). The proximal end of the septum fuses with the distal bulbar septum. The distal end of the aortopulmonary septum fuses with the aortic arches; thus one pair of arches fuse with the pulmonary trunk and the others with the aorta.

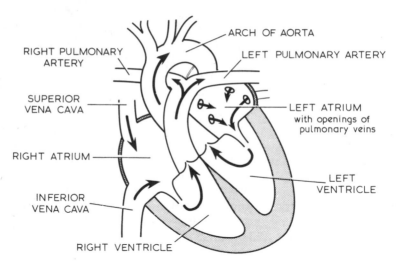

Fig. 10/4   The normal anatomy of the heart

The separation of the ventricles occurs in three stages:

a) A muscular ridge projects into the ventricle to form the muscular septum, and fuses with the dorsal atrioventricular endocardial cushion, at its right extremity.

b) Right and left bulbar ridges fuse to form the proximal bulbar septum, and divide the bulbus cordis into pulmonary and aortic channels, which will continue up into the truncus arteriosus. The proximal bulbar septum fuses with the ventricular septum and the right extremity of the fused atrioventricular cushions.

c) The atrial septum fuses with the centre of the atrioventricular cushions and the ventricular septum with the right extremity. Hence, there is a portion of cushion dividing the right atrium from the left ventricle. It is this tissue which forms the membranous portion of the ventricular septum.

The mitral and tricuspid valves develop at the atrioventricular orifices by proliferation of endothelial tissue. The aortic and pulmonary valves develop from the four endocardial cushions at the distal end of the bulbus cordis.

The heart rotates to the left before birth and this rotation affects the final positions of the aorta, pulmonary trunk and valves, relative to each other. The normal anatomy of the heart is shown in Fig. 10/4.

At the bedside it is often useful to divide congenital cardiac disorders into three main physiological groups:

	HAEMODYNAMIC PROBLEM	EXAMPLES
Group 1	Hypoxaemia (Decreased pulmonary blood flow)	Tetralogy of Fallot Transposition of great vessels (complicated forms) Pulmonary atresia
Group 2	Volume overload (Increased pulmonary blood flow)	Ventricular septal defect Atrial septal defect Persistent ductus arteriosus Transposition of great vessels Total anomalous pulmonary venous drainage
Group 3	Pressure overload (Increased pressure in heart chambers behind obstruction)	Pulmonary stenosis Aortic stenosis Coarctation of aorta

Corrective operations for most of the above conditions are open procedures on cardiopulmonary bypass. The two exceptions are persistent ductus arteriosus and coarctation of the aorta.

All conditions may be isolated lesions or they may be combined with other defects. Each lesion will be considered separately in this text.

Coarctation of the Aorta

This is a constriction located at any site but most commonly just distal to the origin of the left subclavian artery (see Fig. 10/5); many tortuous collateral vessels develop chiefly over the scapular region. It

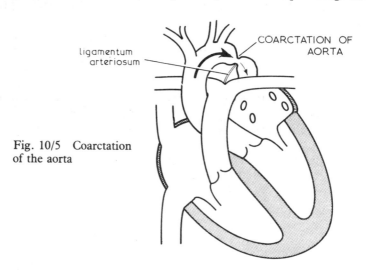

ligamentum
arteriosum

COARCTATION OF
AORTA

Fig. 10/5   Coarctation
of the aorta

may be due to contraction at the time of obliteration of the ductus arteriosus, or more possibly to embryonic malformation at the junction of the third, fourth and sixth aortic arches.

Haemodynamics. Proximal hypertension: the blood pressure in the head and arms is elevated and increases on exercise. There is distal hypotension and delayed femoral pulses. Blood flow to the lower half of the body is maintained through collateral vessels.

Symptoms. Patients may be asymptomatic or there may be headache, dizziness, tinnitus, epistaxis and palpitations due to increased blood pressure in the head and neck. Cold feet and possible claudication in the lower limbs are the result of decreased blood flow to the lower part of the body.

Incision: left postero-lateral thoracotomy through the fourth intercostal space.

Closed procedure. The coarctation is dissected and the ligamentum arteriosum or persistent ductus is ligated and divided. Due to the presence of large collaterals, care is required to prevent haemorrhage. The aorta is opened longitudinally over the constriction and a Dacron onlay patch anastomosed to its margin.

Pre- and postoperative physiotherapy. Routine post-thoracotomy regime. The incision may extend very high posteriorly and special attention must be paid to posture and arm movements. Physiotherapy must not be vigorous and tipping avoided. The blood pressure must not rise excessively, as it will put undue strain on the anastomosis site. Discharge is during the second or third week. Vigorous exercise should be avoided for a few months.

Pulmonary Stenosis

This is a congenital defect of fusion of the valve commissures, possibly in association with infundibular stenosis. It is probably due to failure of complete rotation of the left dorsal ridge during separation of the aorta and pulmonary artery.

Haemodynamics. The pulmonary circulation is decreased and the work of the right ventricle increased. This may result in right ventricular hypertrophy and diminished cardiac output, which is the main problem in severe cases.

Symptoms. Exertional dyspnoea, fatigue and possibly systemic venous congestion; hypoxaemia and cardiac failure in infants.

Incision: median sternotomy.

Open procedure. The valve is exposed via the anterior aspect of the pulmonary artery and the commissures are cut. If the annulus is constricted it is cut through vertically and a Dacron or pericardial gusset inserted. It may be necessary to replace the valve.

Infundibular resection. The right ventricle is entered and the obstructing infundibular muscle and fibrosis is resected or the infundibulum is incised and a Dacron or pericardial gusset inserted.

Pre- and postoperative physiotherapy. Routine bypass scheme with discharge in the second or third week.

Aortic Stenosis

Left ventricular outflow obstruction may be caused at three levels, a) valvular, b) subvalvular, or c) supravalvular. The majority of patients with valvular stenosis do not develop symptoms until the valve becomes calcified around the age of 40 to 50.

Haemodynamics. The narrowed valve orifice subjects the left ventricle to a pressure overload. As a result left ventricular hypertrophy develops.

Symptoms. Mild – asymptomatic; severe – fatigue, syncope, effort dyspnoea and angina.

Incision: median sternotomy.

OPEN PROCEDURES

Valvular stenosis. Valvotomy is performed by entering the ascending aorta and incising the commissures.

Subvalvular stenosis. If the obstruction is due to a fibrous diaphragm arising from the ventricular septum, it may be approached through a low aortic incision and a through-valvular excision will be undertaken. When muscular sub-aortic stenosis is present, it may be corrected by selective myomectomy through a right or left ventricular incision.

Supravalvular stenosis. This is relieved by suturing an elliptical Dacron gusset into a vertical incision through the constricted portion of the aorta.

Pre- and postoperative physiotherapy. Routine bypass scheme with discharge in the second or third week.

Persistent Ductus Arteriosus

The ductus arteriosus, which connects the left pulmonary artery to the descending thoracic aorta just beyond the origin of the left subclavian artery, should have contracted, closed and fibrosed into the ligamentum arteriosum in a few days from birth. Occasionally it persists and blood will flow from the aorta into the pulmonary system (see Fig. 10/6).

Haemodynamics. As a result of recycling of the shunted blood, the left side of the heart eventually becomes overloaded.

Symptoms. Asymptomatic or exertional dyspnoea. There is risk of subacute bacterial endocarditis and pulmonary hypertension.

Incision: left postero-lateral thoracotomy through the fourth-intercostal space.

Closed procedure: ligation of ductus arteriosus.

Pre- and postoperative physiotherapy. Routine thoracotomy scheme with discharge at about the eleventh day.

Atrial Septal Defect

Ostium secundum. This is a defect in the middle area of the septum. It is due to failure of fusion of the septum secundum to the septum primum to obliterate the foramen ovale. This is the most common and simplest to correct (see Fig. 10/3).

Ostium primum. The defect occurs low down in the septum and is sometimes associated with malformed mitral and tricuspid valves. It is due to defective formation of the interatrial septum as it fuses to the

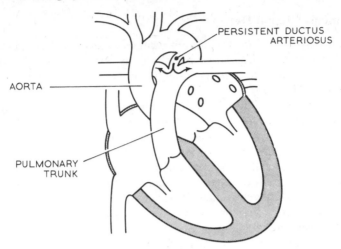

Fig. 10/6   Persistent ductus arteriosus

endocardial cushions. The operation is more complicated, because of the proximity of valves, coronary sinus, and the atrioventricular node.

Sinus venosus. This is a defect occurring high in the septum near to the orifice of the superior vena cava.

Haemodynamics. There is a left to right shunt and if the defect is large it may function as a common atrium.

Symptoms. Secundum lesions may be asymptomatic or show mild exertional dyspnoea as the blood flows from the left to the right atrium, thus overloading the pulmonary system. Primum defects may produce extreme dyspnoea due to left ventricular failure if the mitral valve is involved.

Incision: a median sternotomy or an anterior right thoracotomy, through the fourth intercostal space.

Open procedure. The heart is entered through the right atrium.

The secundum type is closed by direct suture. The primum type is repaired by insertion of a Dacron patch. If the mitral valve is involved it will be repaired first. Great care is taken to avoid damage to the atrioventricular bundle, which runs near to the operation site.

The sinus venosus type is associated with anomalous drainage of the pulmonary veins from the right upper lobe into the right atrium. The defect is repaired with a Dacron patch which redirects the venous drainage into the left atrium.

Pre- and postoperative physiotherapy. Routine bypass scheme with discharge between ten days and three weeks.

Ventricular Septal Defect

This is perhaps the most common form of congenital heart disorder and involves the muscular or membranous portions of the septum. The defect may occur independently or be associated with other lesions (see Fig. 10/7).

Haemodynamics. The size of the shunt depends upon the size of the defect and the ratio between the resistance to flow into the aorta and pulmonary artery. In small defects the pulmonary blood flow may be only 1·5 × systemic flow. In larger defects the ratio increases until eventually pulmonary hypertension develops and the flow across the defect begins to fall. In extreme pulmonary hypertension the flow will reverse as the right ventricular (R.V.) pressure is now greater than the left ventricular (L.V.) pressure. Both ventricles are subjected to a volume overload.

Symptoms. Patients with small defects may be asymptomatic. Large defects may cause exertional dyspnoea and right ventricular failure with systemic venous congestion.

Relief may be temporary in infants or complete after the age of three or four years.

TEMPORARY OPERATION

Relief is obtained by pulmonary artery banding (Muller & Dammann, 1952).

Incision: median sternotomy or left thoracotomy through the fourth intercostal space.

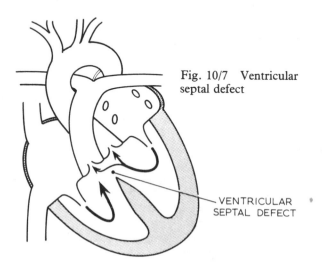

Fig. 10/7   Ventricular septal defect

VENTRICULAR
SEPTAL DEFECT

Closed procedure. The pulmonary artery is identified and its lumen restricted by a Teflon band. If the ductus arteriosus is persistent it is ligated and dissected.

REPAIR OF THE DEFECT

Incision: median sternotomy.

Open procedure. The heart is entered through the right ventricle, or the right atrium. If the defect is small it can be repaired by primary suture. Larger defects are repaired with a Dacron patch.

Pre- and postoperative physiotherapy. Routine bypass scheme with discharge between eleven days and three weeks.

Tetralogy of Fallot

This is perhaps the most common form of congenital heart disease with cyanosis. There is (1) a high ventricular septal defect, (2) a pulmonary stenosis, which may be valvular, infundibular or a combination of the two, (3) an anomalous position of the aorta, and (4) hypertrophy of the right ventricle (see Fig. 10/8).

The anomaly results in a right to left interventricular shunt due to the right outflow tract obstruction and high right ventricular pressure. There is systemic cyanosis and risk of syncope. The child is usually undersized, has clubbing of fingers and toes, exertional dyspnoea and a spontaneous desire to squat. There is an acyanotic group of patients with the same anatomical abnormalities, but without severe pulmonary stenosis and therefore minor shunting.

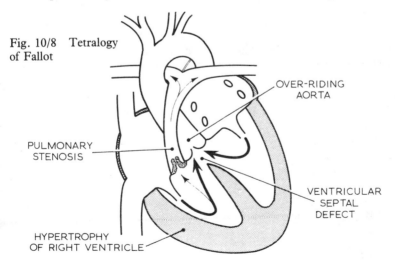

Fig. 10/8 Tetralogy of Fallot

OVER-RIDING AORTA

PULMONARY STENOSIS

VENTRICULAR SEPTAL DEFECT

HYPERTROPHY OF RIGHT VENTRICLE

The condition is probably due to the misalignment of the spiral ridges in the embryonic heart. This would account for the dextra-posed aorta, small pulmonary trunk and abnormal valves and ventricular septal defect. The secondary hypertrophied right ventricle is due to outflow obstruction.

Correction may be palliative in the early years. Total correction is preferred before school age.

ANASTOMOTIC PALLIATIVE TREATMENT

Blalock's anastomosis. Anastomosis of the pulmonary artery to the left subclavian artery (Blalock, 1945).

Incision: left postero-lateral thoracotomy through the fourth inter-costal space.

Waterston's anastomosis. Anastomosis of the ascending aorta and the right pulmonary artery (Waterston, 1962).

Incision: right antero-lateral thoracotomy through the fourth inter-costal space.

PALLIATIVE OR FIRST STAGE CORRECTION BY CLOSED PULMONARY VALVOTOMY

An expanding dilator (Brock, 1948) or valvulotome is introduced into the outflow tract of the right ventricle and the pulmonary valve is dilated.

TOTAL CORRECTION

Incision: this depends on previous palliative surgery. A median ster-notomy or submammary incision will be used following a Waterston or Blalock procedure, and if there has been no previous intervention.

Open procedure. Existing anastomoses are closed prior to the intracardial total correction to avoid 'flooding' of the lungs when cardiopulmonary bypass is established. The right ventricle is opened and a pulmonary valvotomy and/or infundibular resection carried out. The ventricular septal defect is repaired either by primary suture or by the insertion of a Dacron patch. The position of the Dacron patch will correct the position of the over-riding aorta.

Pre- and postoperative physiotherapy. Routine bypass scheme. After correction there may be considerable alveolar oedema. It may be necessary to prolong artificial ventilation with the use of P.E.E.P. (see p. 111), and to wean the patient off the ventilator with the use of C.P.A.P. (see p. 130). Breathing exercises with emphasis on inspi-ration are particularly important. Fine shakings and percussion seem to be helpful in the resolution of the peripheral lung involvement. Discharge is at about three weeks.

Complete Transposition of the Great Vessels

The aorta arises from the right ventricle, the pulmonary artery arises from the left ventricle. The two circulations, pulmonary and systemic, instead of being in series are in parallel. Thus venous blood circulates round the body while oxygenated blood circulates round the lungs. For the child to survive there must be a communication between the two circulations. Possible communications are persistent ductus arteriosus, atrial septal defect or ventricular septal defect (see Fig. 10/9).

Symptoms. There may be cyanosis, syncope and dyspnoea.

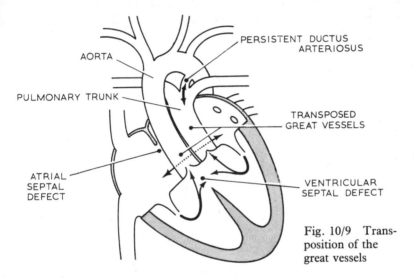

Fig. 10/9 Transposition of the great vessels

PALLIATIVE OPERATIONS

Incision: right lateral thoracotomy through the fifth intercostal space.

a) The atrial septum is excised (Blalock & Hanlon, 1950), or ruptured (Rashkind & Miller, 1966), to create an atrial shunt.

b) The pulmonary artery may be banded to protect the pulmonary system from overloading, if there is a large ventricular septal defect (Sterne et al, 1965).

CORRECTIVE OPERATIONS

A. Physiological. 1. Inflow tracts may be altered by transposing the pulmonary veins into the right atrium and the inferior vena cava into the left atrium. It may be necessary to use Dacron grafts (Baffes, 1956).

2. All inflow and outflow tracts may be retained but the venous return is redirected by excising the existing atrial septum and creating an artificial atrial septum fashioned from the pericardium. The pulmonary venous return in the left atrium is directed towards the tricuspid valve and right ventricle. The systemic venous return in the right atrium is entrained to the mitral valve and the left ventricle. Ventricular septal defects and anastomosis will be corrected (Mustard, 1964).

B. Anatomical. The pulmonary artery and aorta are switched round so that oxygenated blood now enters the systemic circulation. The coronary arteries are reimplanted (Ross, Rickards and Somerville, 1976).

Pre- and postoperative physiotherapy. Routine post bypass scheme. Discharge is at about three weeks.

The following conditions are improved by reconstructive or palliative surgery:

Pulmonary Atresia

The pulmonary valve or trunk is malformed or deficient. The pulmonary blood flow is maintained by other communications, e.g. atrial and ventricular septal defects and a persistent ductus arteriosus.

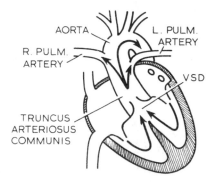

Fig. 10/10   Truncus arteriosus communis

Truncus Arteriosus Communis

A common pulmonary systemic trunk arises from the ventricles. There will be a ventricular septal defect and the trunk may or may not have two valves (see Fig. 10/10).

Tricuspid Atresia

The tricuspid valve is deficient and the right ventricle may be malformed. The pulmonary flow is maintained through atrial and ventricular septal defects and a persistent ductus arteriosus.

Single Ventricle

This is a chamber which receives blood either from a common A.V. valve or from both A.V. valves. Both arterial trunks arise from this single chamber. Frequently there is an appendage to the chamber which is rudimentary and is called an outlet chamber. It is now possible in some patients to insert an artificial septum made of Dacron or pericardium and thus separate the pulmonary and systemic circulations.

Total correction of some cases of pulmonary atresia, tricuspid atresia, truncus arteriosus, and single ventricle can be achieved by the use of a valved conduit. This is a Dacron tube with a homograft or heterograft valve sewn into it. Depending on the site of obstruction the conduit is anastomosed between the right atrium or right ventricle and the pulmonary artery.

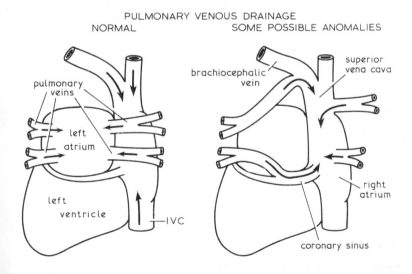

Fig. 10/11   Pulmonary venous drainage to show the normal and some of the possible anomalies

Anomalous Pulmonary Venous Drainage

All or some of the pulmonary veins may drain into the superior vena cava, the coronary sinus or directly into the right atrium. Sometimes the veins join behind the left atrium and are channelled into the brachiocephalic vein. Rarely drainage is into the inferior vena cava (see Fig. 10/11).

REFERENCES

Baffes, T. G. (1956). 'A new method for surgical correction of transposition of the aorta and pulmonary artery.' *Surgery, Gynaecology and Obstetrics*, 102, 227.

Blalock, A. and Hanlon, C. R. (1950). 'The surgical treatment of complete transposition of the aorta and the pulmonary artery.' *Surgery, Gynaecology and Obstetrics*, 90, 1.

Blalock, A. and Taussig, H. B. (1945). 'The surgical treatment of malformations of the heart in which there is pulmonary stenosis or pulmonary atresia.' *Journal of the American Medical Association*, 128, 189.

Brock, R. C. (1948). 'Pulmonary valvulotomy for the relief of congenital stenosis. Report of three cases.' *British Medical Journal*, 1, 1121.

Muller, W. H. and Damman, J. F. (1952). 'The treatment of certain congenital malformations of the heart by the creation of pulmonic stenosis to reduce pulmonary hypertension and excessive pulmonary flow. A preliminary report.' *Surgery, Gynaecology and Obstetrics*, 95, 213.

Mustard, W. T. (1964). 'Successful two-stage correction of transposition of the great vessels.' *Surgery*, 55, 469.

Rashkind, W. and Miller, W. W. (1966). 'Creation of atrial septal defect without thoracotomy. A palliative approach to complete transposition of the great arteries.' *Journal of the American Medical Association*, 196, 991.

Ross, D. N., Rickards, A. and Somerville, J. (1976). 'Transposition of the great arteries; logical anatomical arterial correction'. *British Medical Journal*, 1, 1109.

Sterns, L. P., Ferlie, R. M. and Lilleheic, W. (1965). 'Cardiovascular surgery in infancy. Ten year results from the University of Minnesota Hospitals.' *American Thoracic Surgery*, 1, 519.

Vineberg, A. M. (1952). 'Treatment of coronary artery insufficiency by implantation of the internal mammary artery into the left ventricular myocardium.' *Journal of Thoracic Surgery*, 23, 42.

Waterston, D. J. (1962). 'Treatment of Fallot's tetralogy in children under one year of age.' *Rozhledy v Chirurgii*, 41, 181.

BIBLIOGRAPHY

Barnard, C. N. and Schrires, V. (1968). *The Surgery of the Common Congenital Cardiac Malformations*. Staples Press.

Belcher, J. R. and Sturridge, M. F. (1972). *Thoracic Surgical Management*, 4th ed. Baillière Tindall.

Brooks, D. K. (1967). *Resuscitation*. Edward Arnold Ltd.

Emery, E. R. J., Yates, A. K. and Moorhead, P. J. (1973). *Principles of Intensive Care*. Unibooks, English Universities Press Ltd.

Gibbon, J. H. Jr., Sabiston, D. C. Jr. and Spencer, F. C. (Eds.) (1976). *Surgery of the Chest*, 3rd ed. W. B. Saunders Co., Philadelphia, London and Toronto.

Harris, E. M., Nautze, J. M., Seelye, E. R., Simpson, M. M. and Taylor, M. F. (1972). *Intensive Care of the Heart and Lungs*. Blackwell Scientific Publications.

Keen, G. (1975). *Chest Injuries*. John Wright and Sons Ltd.

Killen, D. A. and Gobbel, W. G. Jr. (1968). *Spontaneous Pneumothorax*. Little, Brown and Co., Boston.

Spurrell, R. A. J. et al (1975). 'Surgical treatment of ventricular tachycardia after epicardial mapping studies.' *British Heart Journal*, **37**, 115.

ACKNOWLEDGEMENT

The author wishes to thank the members of the Surgical Thoracic Unit at Guy's Hospital, London, for their continuing interest.

Chapter 11

Introduction to the Treatment of Medical Chest Conditions

by D. V. GASKELL, M.C.S.P.

COMMON CLINICAL MANIFESTATIONS IN RESPIRATORY DISEASE

Cough

Coughing is a forced expiration against a closed glottis. A high pressure of air is built up in the trachea and major airways and the sudden opening of the glottis is followed by an explosive discharge producing the characteristic noise. It is one of the commonest signs of respiratory disease and will be stimulated by the presence of excessive secretions in the respiratory tract or by other irritations of the nerve endings in the larynx, trachea, bronchi or even the pleura. Many smokers regard a morning cough as normal.

Sputum

The normal adult forms about 100ml of mucus from his respiratory tract daily. This blanket of mucus is removed by the action of the cilia which beat upwards in the direction of the larynx, and carries with it any small particles deposited on the mucosal lining of the lung. Excess mucus, or failure of the normal process of removal, will stimulate the cough reflex and mucus will be expectorated as sputum.

Sputum may be mucoid, black or grey, blood-stained or contain plugs or casts. Mucoid sputum is clear or white. Black or grey sputum may be mucoid but flecked with black or grey deposit due to various causes such as cigarette smoke, atmospheric pollution, coal dust etc. Purulent sputum may contain a variable amount of pus, it is usually yellow, but may become green and foul-smelling. If there is only a small amount of pus present, sputum is described as mucopurulent.

Blood-stained sputum varies from slight streaking to gross haemoptysis when the patient coughs pure blood. Blood-stained sputum must always be reported to the physician in charge of the patient and should always be investigated. It occurs in bronchiectasis, cystic fibrosis and in some cases of simple bronchitis; but it may be an early sign of carcinoma or pulmonary tuberculosis. Rusty blood-stained sputum is a feature of lobar pneumonia.

Plugs and casts may be found in the sputum of patients with pulmonary eosinophilia as in asthma and aspergillosis.

It is very important for the physiotherapist to observe the type of sputum expectorated by the patient and to note any change in its appearance or quantity.

Some patients have particularly thick and viscid sputum, which is often noticeable in the early stages of an infection when the patient has a fever and may be slightly dehydrated. Care should be taken not to nurse the patient in a dry atmosphere, the intake of fluid should be encouraged and if oxygen is being given it should be humidified. Thick secretions can also be moistened by extra humidification, which can range from simple steam inhalations to the use of ultrasonic nebulisers. If intermittent humidification is being given, it is helpful if the physiotherapist can treat the patient immediately afterwards.

Dyspnoea

This is an awareness of difficulty in breathing which may be due to a variety of causes. It may vary considerably in degree. After exercise normal healthy people may have rapid breathing (tachypnoea) and experience mild transient dyspnoea which may not be distressing. Dyspnoea can be observed in patients suffering from severe emphysema. Breathlessness precipitated by lying flat and relieved by sitting up is known as orthopnoea.

Wheeze

This is a musical sound mainly heard on expiration and caused by airways obstruction. Airways obstruction may be caused by narrowing of the bronchial lumen due to bronchospasm, oedema of the bronchial mucosa or excessive secretions; it is the combination of these factors together with the normal shortening and narrowing of the bronchus on expiration which causes the wheeze. A typical wheeze can be heard in asthmatic patients. More rarely a wheeze may be caused by bronchial stenosis or a foreign body.

A wheeze can be greatly exaggerated if the patient forces his expiration.

Stridor

This is a musical sound mainly heard on inspiration and is caused by obstruction in the trachea or larynx.

Chest Pain

This is frequently due to pleuritic pain which is sharp and stabbing in character and worse on coughing or deep breathing when the patient may 'catch' his breath. It is usually localised but may be referred to the abdominal wall, or with diaphragmatic pleurisy to the tip of the shoulder. There are other causes of chest pain including fractured ribs, intercostal nerve root pain, costochondritis, intrathoracic neoplasms, pulmonary embolus, and coronary insufficiency. If in doubt as to the cause of chest pain, the physiotherapist should always discuss the matter with the physician before carrying on with the treatment.

Cyanosis

This means 'blueness'. It is caused by hypoxaemia (lack of oxygen) and is not always easy to judge unless it is severe. Cyanosis may also be associated with hypercapnia (increased carbon dioxide concentration in arterial blood).

Finger Clubbing

This is the filling in of the angle between the skin and the base of the nail. Later there is increased curvature of the nails and the pulps of the fingers become enlarged.

In pulmonary disease this is usually associated with chronic septic conditions such as lung abscess, severe bronchiectasis, cystic fibrosis or with neoplasm. It may also be associated with other diseases or may be familial with no underlying cause.

DIAGNOSTIC PROCEDURES

Radiography

Examination of postero-anterior and lateral chest films will be carried out and compared with any previous X-rays. If necessary the physician may order tomography when films taken of the lungs are focussed at different depths, or fluoroscopy or screening which allows examination of the heart, lungs and diaphragm in the dynamic state. A bronchogram may be performed. This is the introduction of a radio-opaque substance into the bronchi which outlines the bronchial tree and may reveal bronchiectasis (see p. 222). Various other investigations such as a barium meal may also be ordered.

Examination of Bronchial Secretions

Sputum examination is of great value in the diagnosis and treatment of chest disease. Pathological investigation of the sputum may include microscopic examination for malignant cells or bacteria, culture for identification of bacteria and determination of their sensitivity to antibiotics.

Diagnostic Skin Tests

These will include tuberculin testing and allergy reactions.

Bronchoscopy (see p. 140).

Pulmonary Function Studies

These will give much valuable information (see Chapter 23).

Pleural and Lung Biopsy

These are carried out via thoracoscopy or small thoracotomy incisions.

OBSTRUCTIVE AIRWAYS DISEASE

The flow of air through the lungs may be reduced by obstruction in the airways. Common causes of this are excessive secretions, bronchospasm, or oedema of the bronchial mucosa. Frequently a combination of all three is found, as in acute asthmatic attacks.

Airways obstruction may also be the result of scar tissue narrowing or kinking the bronchi, as can happen in chronic bronchitis, or it may follow the destruction of the elastic honeycomb structure of the lung as in some cases of emphysema. The bronchi lose the support of the surrounding lung and tend to collapse in expiration.

Air flow through the bronchi can be assessed either by measurement of the peak expiratory flow (P.E.F.) using a Wright's Peak Flow

Meter, or the forced expiratory volume in one second ($F.E.V._1$) which is normally 70 to 80% of the forced vital capacity (F.V.C.).

Reversible Airways Obstruction

In some cases $F.E.V._1$ and peak flow measurements improve after the patient is given a bronchodilator. Reversibility of airways obstruction is a hopeful sign; a bronchodilator or steroid regime may overcome bronchospasm and give relief.

Such cases often have mucus hypersecretion and respond well to appropriate physiotherapy. Asthma and early chronic bronchitis are diseases in which airways obstruction is usually reversible.

Irreversible or Fixed Airways Obstruction

Irreversibility is demonstrated when administration of a bronchodilator fails to secure any improvement in the peak flow or $F.E.V._1$. This shows that the airways have suffered structural damage; little improvement can be expected from drugs, and physiotherapy is directed towards improving the efficiency of respiration in the face of the defect.

Severe chronic bronchitis, generalised bronchiectasis, and severe emphysema provide examples of this condition. A degree of reversibility may be found superimposed on a fixed obstructive defect. Alleviation of the reversible element may bring about improvement and is always worth trying.

RESTRICTIVE PULMONARY DISEASE

Air flow in the lungs may be hindered in the absence of any bronchial disease. Ankylosing spondylitis or kyphoscoliosis may cause abnormalities of the rib-cage which restrict expansion of the lung. Restrictive defects may also be caused by diffuse interstitial pulmonary fibrosis (fibrosing aiveolitis), pleural fibrosis, widespread post-tuberculous fibrosis and pulmonary oedema. In this latter group of conditions, it is a change in pulmonary compliance (stiffness) that restricts the expansion of the lung.

Patients with restrictive lung disease may need to breathe more rapidly (tachypnoea) to satisfy their respiratory needs, because the lung volumes are reduced and they cannot take deep breaths. Diseases of the lung itself often interfere with the alveolar wall, adding difficulties of gas transfer to those of pulmonary restriction.

RESPIRATORY FAILURE

When the lungs cannot maintain an adequate gas exchange, respiratory failure is said to exist. Campbell has suggested that a PO_2 below 60mm Hg (7·98kPa) at rest or a PCO_2 above 49mm Hg (6·52kPa) should be used to define respiratory failure.

It may be caused by depression of the respiratory centre by poisons, drugs, anoxia, head injuries, or cerebral disease; by failure of the respiratory muscles as in poliomyelitis, acute polyneuritis and myasthenia gravis; by loss of functioning lung tissue as in extensive pneumonia, pulmonary collapse, pneumothorax, following resection of lung tissue, or crush injury of the chest wall; by obstructive airways disease as in status asthmaticus or in acute exacerbations of chronic bronchitis. Patients with chronic lung disease are particularly prone to respiratory failure.

The aims of the treatment are to maintain clear airways and to ensure adequate alveolar ventilation whilst treating the underlying cause. If the failure is associated with a normal or low PCO_2 oxygen therapy will not present any problems, but if the patient is in *hypercapnic respiratory failure* with a low PO_2 and a high PCO_2 oxygen therapy must be very carefully controlled as the free use of oxygen may remove the patient's only remaining ventilatory drive. A safe method of giving controlled oxygen is by means of a Ventimask. There are five types which supply 24%, 28%, 35%, 40% and 60% concentrations of oxygen respectively.

Physiotherapy has a vital role to play in the removal of secretions and the maintenance of adequate ventilation, by means of postural drainage, effective coughing and deep breathing.

It may be necessary to consider some form of assisted ventilation, either by means of intermittent positive pressure breathing (I.P.P.B.) or by intubation and artificial ventilation. Some patients may require a tracheostomy but many physicians are reluctant to consider this when the patient has a long history of chronic lung disease.

COR PULMONALE

In 1961 the World Health Organization offered the following definition of cor pulmonale:
'Hypertrophy of the right ventricle resulting from diseases affecting the function and/or the structure of the lung, except when these pulmonary alterations are the result of diseases that primarily affect the left side of the heart or of congenital heart disease.'

Cor pulmonale most commonly occurs in association with

long-standing pulmonary disease such as chronic bronchitis, bronchiectasis or with diffuse fibrosis of the lungs following pneumoconiosis etc. It may be seen in long-standing kyphoscoliosis and also following obstruction of the pulmonary vascular bed by pulmonary emboli. It is rarely seen in primary emphysema.

It is frequently precipitated by a respiratory infection causing hypoxia and carbon dioxide retention superimposed upon chronic pulmonary disease. Initially CO_2 retention produces an increase in cardiac output and systemic arteriolar dilatation resulting in a bounding pulse.

Dilatation of cerebral vessels may produce headache, raised intracranial pressure and papilloedema. The pulmonary arterioles constrict in response to hypoxia; this effect combines with the increased cardiac output to produce pulmonary hypertension which may be further aggravated if many of the pulmonary blood vessels are obliterated by disease. In the later stages of the disease pulmonary hypertension becomes severe (reaching systemic levels) and right ventricular failure develops as a result of the enormous work load and continuing hypoxia.

Clinical Features

In addition to signs of the original disease, the patient is cyanosed, the extremities warm and the pulse full. The jugular venous pressure is raised, the liver enlarged and dependent oedema will be present. An electrocardiogram may show the large, sharply pointed P-waves of right atrial hypertrophy and there may be signs of right ventricular hypertrophy. As the cardiac output falls, the extremities become cold and the pulse small; venous congestion and oedema increase. The chest X-ray reveals cardiac enlargement and dilatation of the main pulmonary arteries.

Treatment

The main aim of treatment is to improve the alveolar ventilation. This will be by means of bronchodilators, oxygen therapy, physiotherapy and antibiotics. Diuretics with potassium supplements will be given for the cardiac failure. Digitalis therapy is seldom of great use. Once the underlying pulmonary condition starts to respond to treatment, the cardiac condition will improve.

PHYSIOTHERAPY

Treatment should be vigorous and aimed at clearing the airways of excess secretions and improving alveolar ventilation. I.P.P.B. is often helpful as many patients are slightly confused and unable to co-operate fully. Some patients tolerate postural drainage well but if the patient becomes cyanosed and distressed during this procedure, they may be more comfortable in a modified position. Oxygen therapy should be continued during physiotherapy and the mask only removed when the patient wishes to expectorate.

Treatments should be short and frequent; care should be taken not to tire the patient.

Ideally treatment should be carried out for about 20 minutes every two hours for the first 48 hours. If persistent hypoxaemia, hyper-capnia and acidosis are shown on arterial blood gas analysis, the patient should be roused, given I.P.P.B., and encouraged to cough at intervals during the night.

When the patient's condition improves, treatments can be cut down and continued along the lines for the original disease.

CLINICAL ASSESSMENT OF THE CHEST

The physician will examine the patient's chest by means of inspection, palpation, percussion and auscultation. The physiotherapist may like to repeat this examination at intervals during the course of treatment.

Inspection

The patient's pattern of breathing should be observed. Many patients have a characteristic pattern. In asthma, chronic bronchitis and emphysema they may have an over-inflated chest and most of the respiratory movements occur in the apical region; they may even have paradoxical movement of the lower ribs. An abdominal 'bounce', due to a sudden increase in obstruction, may be present in severe emphy-sematous patients (see p. 237); these patients may also breathe out with 'pursed lips'. It has been suggested that the resultant back pressure may prevent collapse of airways and subsequent air trapping. Many patients use the accessory muscles, varying from a slight con-traction of the sternomastoids to the use of trapezius and elevation of the shoulder girdle with every inspiratory effort.

The rate of respiration should be observed as the patient may be noted to be dyspnoeic either at rest or after the effort of undressing. Note of cyanosis or clubbing should also be made.

Palpation

Any chest deformities should be observed and a physiotherapist may often note decreased movement by placing her hands on either side of the thorax and asking the patient to take a deep breath.

It is sometimes helpful to take chest measurements. The resting measurement should be recorded, followed by full expiration and full inspiration. The measurements should be taken at three levels, at the fourth costal cartilage, at the level of the xiphoid process, and at the level of the ninth costal cartilage. This will often reveal an over-inflated upper chest with poor basal movement, particularly in asthma, chronic bronchitis, and emphysema. If a peak flow meter or vitalograph are available, it is helpful to measure the peak flow or F.E.V.$_1$ before and after physiotherapy.

PHYSIOTHERAPY IN THE TREATMENT OF MEDICAL CHEST CONDITIONS

Postural Drainage

Postural drainage consists of placing the patient in various positions designed to drain secretions from the different segments of the lungs by means of gravity. This can be further assisted by vibrations or shaking on expiration and clapping over the chest wall. Postural drainage will drain secretions from the periphery of the lung to the larger airways, from where they can be coughed up more easily.

The length of time spent in each position will vary from patient to patient and will depend on the type and quantity of sputum being expectorated. Each individual patient must be carefully considered, X-rays should be studied and if a bronchogram is available it is of considerable help when working out postural drainage positions.

It may be necessary to spend an average of 15 to 20 minutes in each position and occasionally longer. Ideally the patient should remain in each position until that particular area has been cleared, which may necessitate draining different areas at alternate treatments. The most badly affected area should always be drained first. Postural drainage should never be carried out immediately after a meal.

If a patient has reversible airways obstruction, it is often helpful to give a bronchodilator about 15 minutes before postural drainage, as coughing can aggravate bronchospasm particularly in asthmatic patients. If secretions are very thick and tenacious, a mist or steam inhalation may be given beforehand.

During postural drainage the patient should be encouraged to take deep breaths and to cough at intervals. By this means, the collateral airdrift between the alveoli can be made use of in order to remove secretions from smaller airways. The patient should remain clothed during treatment as percussion over the bare chest wall is painful. Any tight or extra warm clothing should obviously be removed.

POSTURAL DRAINAGE POSITIONS

Upper Lobe

APICAL BRONCHUS (Fig. 11/1)

The patient should sit upright, with slight variations according to the position of the lesion which may necessitate leaning slightly backwards, forwards or sideways. This position is usually only necessary for infants or patients being nursed in a recumbent position, but occasionally may be required if there is an abscess or stenosis of a bronchus in the apical region.

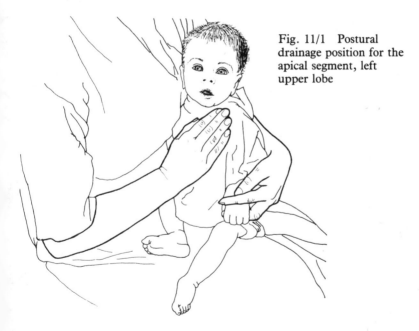

Fig. 11/1 Postural drainage position for the apical segment, left upper lobe

POSTERIOR BRONCHUS

(*a*) *Right* (Fig. 11/2). The patient should lie on his left side horizontally, and then turn 45°on to his face, resting against a pillow with another supporting his head.

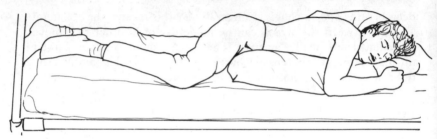

Fig. 11/2 Postural drainage position for the posterior segment, right upper lobe

(*b*) *Left* (Fig. 11/3). The patient should lie on his right side turned 45° onto his face with 3 pillows arranged to raise the shoulders 12 inches (30cm) from the bed.

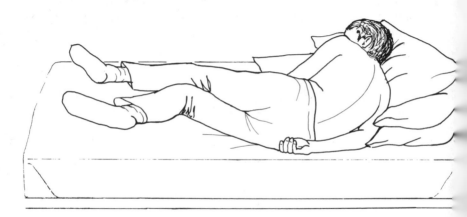

Fig. 11/3 Postural drainage position for the posterior segment, left upper lobe

ANTERIOR BRONCHUS (Fig. 11/4)
The patient should lie flat on his back with his knees slightly flexed.

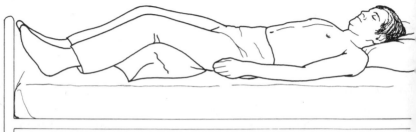

Fig. 11/4 Postural drainage position for anterior segments, upper lobe

Middle Lobe

LATERAL BRONCHUS

MEDIAL BRONCHUS

The patient should lie flat on his back with his body quarter turned to the left maintained by a pillow under the right side from shoulder to hip. The foot of the bed should be raised 14 inches (35cm) from the ground (Fig. 11/5).

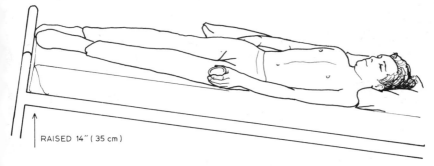

RAISED 14" (35 cm)

Fig. 11/5   Postural drainage position for the right middle lobe

Lingula

SUPERIOR BRONCHUS

INFERIOR BRONCHUS

The patient should lie flat on his back with his body quarter turned to the right maintained by a pillow under the left side from shoulder to hip.

The foot of the bed should be raised 14 inches (35cm) from the ground.

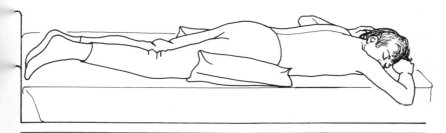

Fig. 11/6   Postural drainage position for the apical segments, lower lobes

Lower Lobe

APICAL BRONCHUS (Fig. 11/6)

The patient should lie flat on his face with a pillow under his hips.

MEDIAL BASAL (CARDIAC) BRONCHUS (Fig. 11/7)

The patient should lie on his right side with a pillow under his hips and the foot of the bed should be raised 18 inches (46cm) from the ground.

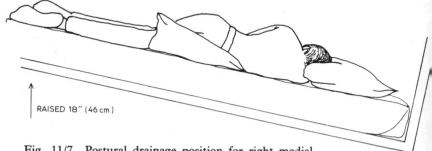

RAISED 18" (46 cm)

Fig. 11/7   Postural drainage position for right medial basal segment and left lateral basal segment

ANTERIOR BASAL BRONCHUS (Fig. 11/8)

The patient should lie flat on his back with the buttocks resting on a pillow and the knees bent; the foot of the bed should be raised 18 inches (46cm) from the ground.

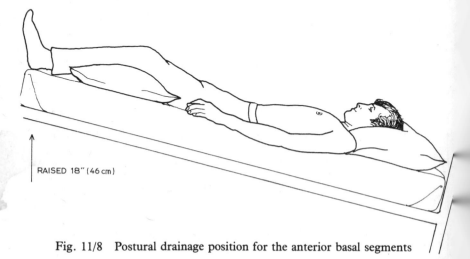

RAISED 18" (46 cm)

Fig. 11/8   Postural drainage position for the anterior basal segments

LATERAL BASAL BRONCHUS (Fig. 11/9)

The patient should lie on the opposite side and the foot of the bed should be raised 18 inches (46cm) from the ground. It is helpful to place an extra pillow under the patient's hips.

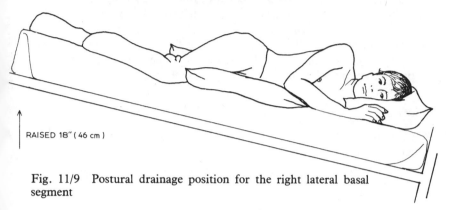

RAISED 18″ (46 cm)

Fig. 11/9   Postural drainage position for the right lateral basal segment

POSTERIOR BASAL BRONCHUS (Fig. 11/10)

The patient should lie flat on his face with a pillow under the hips, the foot of the bed should be raised 18 inches (46cm) from the ground.

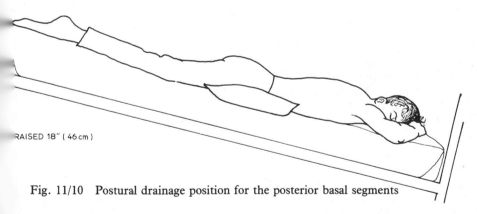

RAISED 18″ (46 cm)

Fig. 11/10   Postural drainage position for the posterior basal segments

Inhalations Given in Association with Postural Drainage

Bronchodilators, steam inhalations, mist therapy and mucolytic agents should always be given *before* postural drainage. Inhalations of antibiotics or antifungal agents should be given *after* postural drainage.

Bronchography

Before a bronchogram the patient should be given postural drainage if there appear to be excessive secretions which would prevent adequate filling of the bronchi.

After a bronchogram patients with bronchiectasis or cystic fibrosis will be given postural drainage in order to clear the radio-opaque medium from the bronchi; in other conditions some will be removed by the action of the cilia, the rest will be absorbed by the blood stream. The physiotherapist should discuss with the radiologist whether physiotherapy is required following bronchography.

Modified Postural Drainage

Certain patients may be too dyspnoeic to tolerate postural drainage, particularly those with severe bronchospasm or emphysema. It is better to turn this type of patient onto alternate sides for short periods of time without tipping the bed. Some will tolerate lying flat, others prefer to be propped up with several pillows. Shaking, vibrations and clapping may be given in this position.

Postural Drainage at Home

Many patients with chronic chest disease will need to carry out postural drainage at home. This can often present problems as it may be necessary to tip the bed and this is not always possible. This problem can be overcome by placing a 6 inch (15cm) thick pile of newspapers or magazines tied tightly together on the bed and placing pillows on top of this. The patient can lie over this in varying positions and thus drain most areas of his lungs.

Young patients can drain the posterior basal areas by lying over the side of the bed with their forearms resting on the floor, but this position cannot be maintained for any length of time.

Babies and small children can be given postural drainage over their mother's knee.

Before a patient is discharged from hospital the physiotherapist should instruct him in how to carry out postural drainage at home adapting to the various situations. The timing factor should be taken into consideration as it is not always possible to spend as long on drainage in the home. The patient should be encouraged to spend as long as is practical until the worst of the secretions have been cleared, e.g. 15 to 20 minutes, possibly less.

Contra-indications to Postural Drainage

1. Recent haemoptysis. Once the bleeding has stopped, postural drainage may usually be resumed but permission should always be sought from the physician first. It is better not to percuss for a day or so.
2. Severe hypertension.
3. Certain cardiac arrythmias.
4. Following recent head injuries.
5. If there is regurgitation of gastric juices as in hiatus hernia.
6. Tension pneumothorax.
7. Severe surgical emphysema.
8. Aneurysm or obstruction of main blood vessels.
9. Pulmonary oedema.

BREATHING CONTROL

The term 'Breathing Exercises' is misleading as it implies that the patient is physically exerting himself. In fact, many patients suffering from respiratory disease are already expending far too much effort on respiration and need to be taught how to control their breathing, hence the title of this controversial section.

There are several different techniques of teaching breathing control and there is still some controversy about the precise action of certain respiratory muscles and about the mechanics of breathing (Campbell, Agostoni & Newsom Davis, 1970). Physiotherapists must be prepared to change the rationale of their techniques as more experiments are performed in this field. They must also be prepared for disappointing results of certain lung function tests before and after treatment. Although the patient with emphysema may have obviously improved and his exercise tolerance increased, the $F.E.V._1$ may remain disappointingly low but the F.V.C. may improve. This type of patient may show improvement in his respiratory pressure volume relationship (Innocenti, 1966). Patients with asthma will often show improvement in their $F.E.V._1$ after effective treatment. As more sophisticated lung function tests are developed, it is to be hoped that the effects of breathing control will be more fully understood.

Diaphragmatic Breathing

The diaphragm is the main respiratory muscle and the physiotherapist must have a thorough knowledge of its action before attempting to teach this technique to patients.

One method of teaching diaphragmatic breathing concentrates on forward movement of the whole abdominal wall. A second technique combines forward movement of the upper abdominal wall with some lateral movement of the lower ribs.

POSITION OF THE PATIENT

Diaphragmatic breathing is usually taught in a relaxed half-lying or sitting position, particularly if the patient is short of breath due to chest disease. In the supine position the domes of the diaphragm will be elevated due to the weight of abdominal viscera and this may be distressing to patients suffering from dyspnoea.

When treating the majority of cases, the patient should be well-supported with pillows or cushions and should be sitting straight, the iliac crests should be level as faulty posture could cause distortion of chest movement.

TECHNIQUE

The physiotherapist should explain to the patient the aims of the treatment and should point out the faults in his pattern of breathing; the use of a mirror may help. It may be helpful to demonstrate diaphragmatic breathing to the patient before actually getting him to try it himself.

The patient should try to relax as much as possible first, then the physiotherapist should place her hands lightly on the upper abdomen overlapping the anterior costal margins. The patient should start by breathing out and at the same time relax the upper chest; if he is doing this correctly, the physiotherapist will feel the upper abdomen and anterior costal margins sink down and in. When the patient is ready to breathe in, he should be told to 'try to get air in round his waist' and if he does this correctly, the upper abdomen will bulge forward slightly and the anterior costal margins will move up and out. Many patients make the mistake of trying to take too deep a breath in and will expand the apical areas; this will inhibit diaphragmatic movement.

Some patients find it very difficult to learn diaphragmatic breathing and many reverse the abdominal movement at first. It is vital to remember that the expiratory phase is completely passive; any forcing and prolonging of expiration will tend to increase airways obstruction.

Once the patient has mastered the technique, he should put his own hands in the correct place and feel his respiratory movements. He should be instructed to practise several times a day on his own (see Fig. 11/11).

Some physiotherapists prefer to place a hand lower on the abdomen when teaching diaphragmatic breathing commencing with a breath

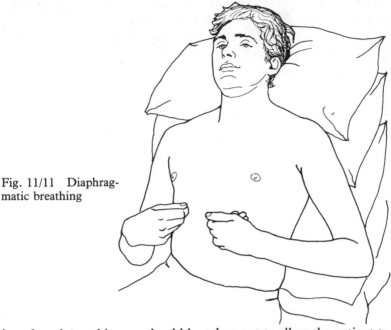

Fig. 11/11 Diaphrag-
matic breathing

in; when doing this care should be taken not to allow the patient to
contract the abdominal wall on expiration as movements of the
abdomen can occur that are not associated with breathing.

Use of Diaphragmatic Breathing During Attacks of Dyspnoea

If patients can be taught how to control their breathing during an
attack of dyspnoea, this can be of great benefit to them.

The patient should be put into a relaxed position and encouraged to
practise diaphragmatic breathing. The *rate* of respiration does not
matter at this stage, it is the pattern of breathing that is important.
Every effort should be made to relax the upper chest and to get the
patient to do gentle diaphragmatic breathing at his own rate. As the
patient gains control of his breathing he should be encouraged to slow
down his respiratory rate.

There are five different positions that the patient can adopt when in
distress.

1. HIGH SIDE LYING (Fig. 11/12A)

Five pillows are used to prop the patient up in bed, one of which is
placed under the patient's side between the waist and axilla in order to
wedge him up in bed and to keep his spine straight.

2. FORWARD LEAN SITTING (Figs. 11/12B and 12C)

The patient sits at a table resting the upper part of his chest against several pillows or the child sits or kneels with the upper chest supported on pillows.

3. RELAXED SITTING (Fig. 11/12D)

This is an unobtrusive, useful position that can be taken up easily.

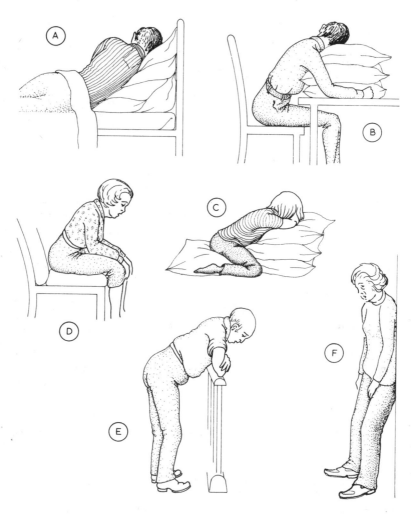

Fig. 11/12　Various positions that the dyspnoeic patient can adopt

4. FORWARD LEAN STANDING (Fig. 11/12E)

The patient can lean forward against an object of suitable height.

5. RELAXED STANDING (Fig. 11/12F)

The patient can lean back against a wall. The shoulders should be relaxed.

Localised Basal Expansion

This type of breathing is a useful method of trying to mobilise the lower chest and may make better use of the basal areas of the lungs. It should not be performed during attacks of dyspnoea as it requires extra effort. It can be taught bilaterally or unilaterally and is a 'trick' movement. Some authorities state that it utilises the 'bucket-handle' movement of the ribs, but there is a certain amount of controversy about this, although it seems to be agreed that the movement is caused by the contraction of the outer fibres of the diaphragm when the central tendon is fixed.

When treating chest disease it is better to start off by teaching unilateral basal expansion, otherwise the patient is inclined to exaggerate the movement of the upper chest.

POSITION OF PATIENT

It is best to start with the patient in half lying or sitting well supported so that he is unable to move his spine and thus simulate movements of the chest wall. Once the patient has mastered the correct technique he can sit upright and practise in front of a mirror.

TECHNIQUE

The physiotherapist should place the palm of her hand in the mid-axillary line at about the level of the eighth rib; her fingers should be well round the posterior aspect of the thorax. The patient should relax and breathe out allowing his lower ribs to sink down and in; at the end of expiration the physiotherapist should give firm pressure with her hand and instruct the patient to push with his ribs against her hand as he breathes in. Pressure should be released at the end of maximum inspiration.

If the aim of treatment is to re-expand lung tissue, the emphasis should be on holding the maximum inspiration for a short time before breathing out again, but if the patient has air trapping, the emphasis should be on relaxation during expiration.

The patient should be taught how to give pressure himself (see Fig.

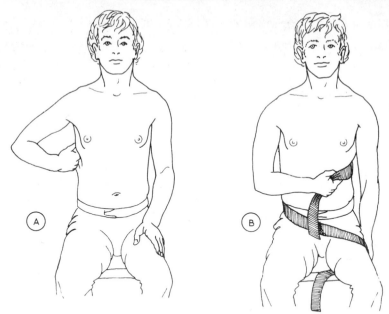

Fig. 11/13   A patient applying pressure to perform localised breathing exercises: a) with the back of the hand; b) with a webbing strap

11/13A) and some find it helpful to use a webbing band (see Fig. 11/13B). Some patients may have a stiff wrist or shoulder, in which case the back of the fingers or pressure by the opposite hand may be used.

The patient should be instructed to practise about 8 deep breaths at a time, then to rest before repeating 8 more, and so on. About 24 breaths at a time should be practised.

If the patient complains of dizziness, he is probably hyperventilating and should be told to pause longer between each breath.

Apical Expansion

This type of expansion is only necessary following certain types of thoracic surgery or when there is deformity of the chest wall or an apical air pocket following spontaneous pneumothorax. It is not always necessary to teach apical expansion if there is disease in the upper lobe; a typical example of this is in cystic fibrosis when there is often involvement of the upper lobe but the patient is already over-expanding the upper chest.

POSITION OF THE PATIENT

The patient should be in a well-supported half-lying or sitting position. The physiotherapist should place her fingertips beneath the clavicle and encourage the patient to expand his chest upwards against her hand on inspiration. The patient can then be taught to give pressure himself with the opposite hand. This exercise should be taught unilaterally as it is only used for localised conditions.

If there is a persistent apical air pocket it is sometimes helpful to lie the patient flat on the unaffected side and tip the foot of the bed during breathing exercises.

Breathing Control on Stairs and Hills

Many patients with chest disease become very distressed when walking upstairs and up hills. If they can be taught to breathe in rhythm with their steps, this will often help them a great deal.

Each individual will vary, for example, some patients find it helpful to breathe out for two steps and in for one step, others prefer an even count. This does not matter so long as the patient breathes rhythmically with his steps. Many patients either hold their breath or breathe in an unco-ordinated manner on stairs and hills.

Once a suitable rhythm has been established, the patient should be encouraged to breathe with the diaphragm whilst walking. It should be impressed upon him that if he is half-way up a flight of stairs and is becoming distressed, it is better to stop and rest rather than trying to go on and having to sit down for 10 minutes afterwards to recover.

Other Types of Breathing Control

The physiotherapist can help breathless patients in other ways. Many complain of distress when they bend down – whenever possible they should kneel to do the task; if it is something like fastening shoe laces, they should breathe out as they bend forward.

GENERAL EXERCISE

It is a well-known fact that many patients suffering from chronic pulmonary disease benefit from physical conditioning. It is also well known that asthma may be induced by means of exercise, although the exact mechanism still remains obscure. Bearing these factors in mind, physiotherapists should be prepared to change their approach to exercise in the treatment of patients with pulmonary diseases as more research is done in this field.

Children enjoy classes and for young patients with cystic fibrosis or bronchiectasis, an energetic class with plenty of running and jumping helps to loosen secretions before postural drainage. As these patients grow older, they prefer to take an active part in sport at school and they should be encouraged to do this as it is a boost to their morale to be able to compete with their contemporaries.

At one time most patients with asthma were encouraged to attend classes. These consisted of fairly vigorous general and posture exercises interspersed with breathing control. In view of the recent work on exercise-induced asthma, swimming is obviously the best type of exercise for asthmatics, but if circumstances are such that the only way of treating these patients is in a class, the following precautions should be taken.

1. The peak flow or $F.E.V._1$ should be measured before the class. Those patients with a particularly low reading should not take part in the class that day and should be treated individually.

2. The more vigorous exercises should not last for more than three minutes at a time and should be interspersed with breathing control.

Older patients with chronic bronchitis or emphysema do not do well in classes and should be treated individually. Although relaxed shoulder girdle and trunk movements may help to a certain extent, most benefit will be gained by a graduated exercise programme. Levison and Cherniack (1968) found that the respiratory muscles of these patients consumed 35% to 40% of the total oxygen uptake compared to 10% to 14% in normal individuals, therefore there was only 60% to 65% of the oxygen available for exercising non-respiratory muscles. After training in breathing control, many of these patients will be able to tolerate graduated exercise reasonably well, but patients who develop either premature ventricular contractions or marked cyanosis during exercise may need supplementary oxygen. The type of exercise given will vary according to the facilities available; some hospitals will exercise the patients by means of bicycles and treadmills, others by means of graduated walks and increasing the number of stairs climbed each day (McGavin, Gupta, Lloyd and McHardy, 1977).

Each individual patient must be carefully assessed and exercised within his limitations. It is hoped that further research will reveal more about the effects of exercise in certain types of pulmonary disease and that physiotherapists will be able to apply these findings to their work.

REFERENCES

Campbell, E. J. M., Agostoni, E. and Newsom Davis, J. (1970). *The Respiratory Muscles — Mechanics and Neural Control*. Lloyd-Luke (Medical Books) Ltd.
Innocenti, D. M. (1966). 'Breathing Exercises in the Treatment of Emphysema.' *Physiotherapy*, **52**, 437.
McGavin, C. R., Gupta, S. P., Lloyd, E. L. and McHardy, G. J. R. (1977). 'Physical rehabilitation for the chronic bronchitic.' *Thorax*, **32**, 307.
World Health Organization (1961). 'Chronic Cor Pulmonale.' *W. H. O. Tech. Rep. Ser.*, No. 213, 14.

BIBLIOGRAPHY

See end of Chapter 14.

Chapter 12

Pulmonary Infections

by D. V. GASKELL, M.C.S.P.

PNEUMONIA

The term pneumonia indicates an inflammation of the substance of the lungs.

The classification of pneumonia can be based on the anatomical distribution of the disease and on the nature of the infecting organism.

1. LOBAR PNEUMONIA

This is a pneumonic consolidation confined to one or more lobes of the lung. It is due to infections by specific organisms which are blood-borne, the main one being the virulent pneumococcus of which there are several different types. More rarely, it may be caused by *Staphylococcus aureus* or Friedlander's (*Klebsiella pneumoniae*) bacillus.

2. BRONCHOPNEUMONIA

This is a consolidation occurring in patches around infected peripheral bronchi. It may be confined to a small area or it may be widespread throughout the lung. It is often caused by inhaled air-borne organisms such as streptococci, haemophilus influenzae and non-epidemic strains of pneumococci. In its early stages tuberculosis starts as a localised patch of bronchopneumonia, but widespread tuberculous bronchopneumonia may occur.

3. VIRAL PNEUMONIA

This may be complicated by secondary bacterial infection.

4. INHALATION PNEUMONIA

This may vary from a small area of consolidation to severe suppurative infection following inhalation of infected material.

5. PNEUMONIA SECONDARY TO DISEASE OF THE BRONCHI

This is often associated with bronchial carcinoma or bronchiectasis.

LOBAR PNEUMONIA

This is the classical type of pneumonia and may occur at any age. It is most frequently associated with infection by the pneumococcus.

The pathology of lobar pneumonia is briefly summarised as follows. The first stage of spreading inflammatory oedema proceeds to the second stage of red hepatisation in which the affected lobe is firm, airless and red in colour, often with petechiae (minute haemorrhages) beneath the pleura. Bronchi in the affected lobe may also be plugged with fibrin. The alveolar capillaries are congested with blood and the alveoli are filled with red blood cells and fibrin. The third stage is that of grey hepatisation when the lung shows a greyish-yellow appearance; prior to this the bronchial arteries are blocked proximal to the affected lobe but they appear to open up at this stage. The alveolar capillaries become less congested during the stage of grey hepatisation and the pulmonary arteries may become thrombosed. The neutrophils phagocytose the pneumococci but apparently do not kill them. As resolution occurs the alveoli are invaded by macrophages which engulf both the leucocytes and their contained pneumococci.

The onset of the disease is often preceded by an upper respiratory tract infection. The patient rapidly becomes ill with an abrupt rise in temperature, with shivering and occasionally vomiting. At the same time pleuritic pain frequently develops over the affected lobe and the patient's respirations become rapid, shallow and sometimes grunting. There may be a dry painful cough at this stage but the patient will soon start to cough up 'rusty' sputum due to particles of altered blood from the areas of red hepatisation. Cold sores (Herpes simplex) often develop at this stage.

The face will be flushed and possibly cyanosed. The respiration rate is raised and there will be diminished movement on the affected side with pain on deep inspiration. Within the first 24 to 48 hours signs of consolidation will appear, there will be dullness to percussion over the affected lobe and bronchial breathing will be present; there may be signs of pleural rub or even pleural effusion.

The diagnosis will be confirmed by an X-ray. In the days before antibiotics were available, the patient remained very ill for 5 to 10 days, then, if he survived, the temperature would subside rapidly by 'crisis' or more slowly by 'lysis'. Nowadays, this process is nearly always cut short by effective use of antibiotics, the patient's condition beginning to improve within 48 hours of starting treatment. As the signs of consolidation disappear, the sputum will become more purulent and the pleuritic pain less. It is possible for the condition to resolve without sputum production.

Treatment

The question of whether the patient should be treated in hospital will depend on the severity of disease and the care available at home. The general practitioner can abort many attacks of lobar pneumonia by the prompt use of antibiotics in the early stages of the disease. If the patient requires admission to hospital, treatment consists of general management, control of pleuritic pain, antibiotics, the use of oxygen and appropriate physiotherapy.

Occasionally a patient may be first seen at a very advanced stage of the disease. This may be due to late referral or to an overwhelming infection. In this case the correct antibiotic is vital and the sputum should be examined immediately. Occasionally in pneumonia complicating severe influenza, the larynx and trachea may be blocked by sloughed mucous membrane and bronchoscopy followed by tracheostomy may be required.

As soon as the patient's temperature has subsided he should sit out of bed and his activities should be gradually increased. Younger patients will recover more quickly than those over the age of 60.

Full recovery may be delayed by complications:

1. *Delayed resolution*. If resolution is delayed for more than 2 or 3 weeks, the possibility of an underlying condition such as carcinoma or bronchiectasis must be suspected and investigated. The sputum should also be examined for tuberculosis. Slow recovery should be anticipated in patients suffering from diabetes, cirrhosis of the liver, chronic alcoholism or nephritis.

2. *Pleural effusions* may occur but usually subside within a week or two of treatment.

3. *Empyema* can occur if the effusion becomes purulent.

4. *Cardiac failure*, possibly complicated by cardiac arrythmia, may occur in elderly patients.

5. *Pericarditis, endocarditis and meningitis*, can occur.

Physiotherapy

The aims of treatment are to assist in the removal of secretions and to regain expansion in the affected area.

Early in the disease, during the stage of red hepatisation, the physiotherapist may not be able to help much and vigorous treatment will only aggravate pleural pain.

Some physicians will not order treatment until the patient starts to expectorate; others prefer the physiotherapist to see the patient from the beginning.

If treatment is ordered in the early stage of the disease, gentle diaphragmatic breathing and localised basal expansion, holding the breath on full inspiration, should be started. The patient should be encouraged to cough but if the lung is still consolidated, this may not be productive in which case the physiotherapist should not force the patient to cough unnecessarily; I.P.P.B. may be helpful in aiding removal of secretions in severe cases.

Once the stage of grey hepatisation starts, the patient will be able to expectorate. Postural drainage should be given for the affected area. If there is severe pleuritic pain, only gentle vibration should accompany it but percussion may be started as soon as the pain improves. Diaphragmatic breathing and localised basal expansion should be continued and treatment carried out two or three times a day.

As the X-ray improves and the sputum decreases, the treatment can be cut down. Breathing exercises should be continued until discharge from hospital and older patients may need help with ambulation.

BRONCHOPNEUMONIA

Bronchopneumonia is very common, particularly in the aged. It is very often associated with chronic bronchitis and may also occur postoperatively, particularly in heavy smokers.

The initial symptoms are those of acute bronchitis, but the patient gradually becomes more ill and more breathless and cyanosis increases. It can be differentiated from bronchitis by the presence of patchy bronchial breathing and by the presence of patchy shadows on the X-ray.

The temperature, pulse and respiratory rate will be raised and there may be signs of carbon dioxide retention. The patient may sound 'bubbly' and have difficulty in getting rid of his secretions which will be purulent. There will usually be basal crepitations but the signs of consolidation will be minimal.

In patients with advanced chronic bronchitis, an attack of bronchopneumonia may precipitate cor pulmonale. Treatment will be similar to that of lobar pneumonia but particular care must be taken over the use of sedatives and oxygen. The principles of oxygen therapy will be the same as those in acute exacerbations of chronic bronchitis.

Physiotherapy

Unlike lobar pneumonia, patients with bronchopneumonia have secretions from the early stages of the disease and should have vigorous physiotherapy immediately. Many of these patients have underlying chest disease and will go into respiratory failure unless prompt action is taken.

Postural drainage with percussion and chest shaking should be given for the appropriate area. The patient may be dehydrated and if the secretions are very thick, steam inhalations or mist therapy may help to loosen tenacious sputum.

If the patient is drowsy and will not cough effectively, I.P.P.B. in conjunction with postural drainage is often helpful. If there is associated bronchospasm a bronchodilator may be ordered. If the patient will not cough despite these vigorous measures, it may be necessary to perform nasopharyngeal suction in order to clear excessive secretions. Occasionally some patients are very difficult to suck out via the nose and in this case it may be helpful to insert a Magill airway and suck out the pharynx.

Initially, two-hourly treatment may be necessary and if the patient is verging on respiratory failure, it may be necessary to continue treatment during the night. As the patient improves, postural drainage will be cut down and gradually discontinued. Diaphragmatic breathing and localised basal expansion are taught and early ambulation encouraged.

VIRUS PNEUMONIA

Typical outbreaks of virus pneumonia may be seen in the armed forces or in general practice in the absence of superimposed bacterial infection. The patients are often not ill enough to require admission to hospital. The disease starts with the usual symptoms of general malaise followed by a cough which may be paroxysmal. If pain is present it is usually retrosternal rather than pleural. Physical signs in the chest may be scanty. X-ray may reveal an area of consolidation with a ground glass appearance and varying distribution.

Treatment

A virus pneumonia usually resolves within two weeks without specific treatment, although tetracycline sometimes seems to help. If the condition fails to improve, the diagnosis of carcinoma or pulmonary infarct should always be borne in mind.

Physiotherapy

Breathing exercises may be ordered for these patients if they are admitted to hospital. Postural drainage is only necessary if they have secretions present.

INHALATION PNEUMONIA

These bronchopneumonias are mainly caused by inhalation of food or juices from the upper gastro-intestinal tract. They are particularly liable to occur in infants and old people, those with bulbar neurological lesions, those under sedation and during or after anaesthesia or alcohol intoxication. They may also occur due to achalasia of the cardia, pharyngeal diverticulum, hiatus hernia and oesophageal strictures.

Clinically, inhaled vomit may give rise to haemorrhagic pneumonia with gross pulmonary oedema. These patients may be gravely ill and may even require intubation and artificial ventilation.

Smaller amounts of inhalation may occur in bulbar palsies and diseases of the oesophagus and the patient may present with recurrent cough and sputum. Once the cause of the pneumonia has been recognised its treatment may prevent further pneumonia.

Physiotherapy

Prompt treatment by means of postural drainage and possibly I.P.P.B. is vital. If pulmonary oedema has occurred, physiotherapy may not be indicated until this has resolved.

LUNG ABSCESS

A lung abscess is a necrotic, suppurative, cavitated lesion mainly due to infection by pyogenic organisms. It is also associated with tuberculosis, fungal infections, necrosis in malignant tumours and infected cysts.

Causes

Inhalation of infected material is a common cause. This material usually comes from the upper respiratory tract and may come from infected teeth, dental extraction or tonsillectomy. Foreign bodies or vomit may also be inhaled. The infected material is inhaled into a bronchopulmonary segment leading to a pneumonia which breaks down to form an abscess. The contents are coughed up leaving an abscess cavity usually infected with a mixed group of organisms. Lung abscess may also be secondary to bronchial carcinoma and other forms of obstruction, or following pulmonary emboli.

An abscess may develop in the course of staphylococcal pneumonia, Friedlander's pneumonia or tuberculosis. Rare causes include actinomycosis, infected hydatid cyst and extension of amoebic abscess of the liver through the diaphragm.

The site of the abscess is influenced by gravity. If infected material is inhaled by an unconscious patient the abscess will occur in the most dependent part of his lung, i.e. if he is on his back the apical segments of the lower lobes or the posterior segment of his right upper lobe are frequent sites for abscess formation.

Signs and Symptoms

Symptoms frequently appear within three days of inhalation of infected material. Malaise and fever are accompanied by cough and pleuritic pain. At this stage the disease is often mistaken for pneumonia and antibiotics are started. In the absence of treatment the disease progresses with fever, pleurisy and possibly dyspnoea and cyanosis. This worsens over a period of about 10 days after which the patient characteristically coughs up a large amount of pus which may be foul-smelling and frequently contains blood. Other cases may be less obvious in their onset.

There will be dullness to percussion and sometimes bronchial breathing; a pleural rub may also be heard.

Chest X-rays will reveal the segment of lung involved. To begin with, the affected segment will be opaque but when discharge of the abscess has occurred, a cavity will be seen containing a fluid level. The X-ray of a breaking-down peripheral carcinoma is characteristic: the walls of the cavity are thick and irregular.

Treatment

This will consist of antibiotics and accurate postural drainage. If the response to treatment is not satisfactory or drainage is not occurring freely, a bronchoscopy should be performed to exclude any obstruction such as a carcinoma. Very rarely resection of the area may be necessary.

Physiotherapy

This will consist of accurate postural drainage. The X-rays, particularly lateral views, must be studied carefully in order to establish the exact position of the abscess. If a fluid level is visible the patient is likely to have copious, foul-smelling sputum when drainage is instituted; in this case his condition will improve rapidly and the abscess will quickly reduce in size. Treatment should be carried out two or three times daily, until sputum is negligible and the X-ray shows healing of the abscess. Breathing exercises are not necessary as the aim of the treatment is removal of secretions from the abscess cavity.

Postural drainage may not be immediately effective; the orthodox postural drainage positions may require adaptation in case the abscess has caused distortion of the bronchi. Gentle vibration may assist drainage, but percussion should not be attempted as there is always the possibility of haemoptysis occurring. If postural drainage is not effective after two or three days, the physician will probably consider a diagnostic bronchoscopy.

BRONCHIECTASIS

Bronchiectasis is a dilatation of the bronchi usually associated with obstruction and infection.

Causes

Bronchiectasis can be congenital but in most patients it is an acquired condition. It may follow inadequately treated pneumonia, particularly that associated with whooping cough (pertussis) or measles in which the mucus is thick and viscid causing obstruction and small areas of collapse. At this stage in the illness permanent bronchiectasis can be prevented if the obstructing plugs can be removed by vigorous physiotherapy.

Bronchiectasis may also develop when infection occurs distal to a bronchial obstruction caused by bronchial carcinoma, adenoma or external pressure from primary tuberculous glands. It may be associated with pulmonary infection which heals by fibrosis as in tuberculosis. It seems possible that bronchiectasis may follow bronchiolitis in infants and it commonly develops from the suppurating bronchiolitis in cystic fibrosis.

Mechanism and Changes

If a bronchus is obstructed air cannot reach the smaller airways and alveoli distal to the block. The air within them is gradually absorbed and all the smaller branches and alveoli collapse. The larger bronchi, which are held open by C-shaped cuffs of cartilage, remain patent. Should obstruction persist and infection supervene, certain changes follow because the products of inflammation are unable to escape along the airways. The alveoli undergo pneumonic consolidation which may lead to destruction of their walls and replacement by scar tissue. The smaller bronchi and bronchioles are obliterated, the inflamed large bronchi lose their rigidity and elasticity and tend to dilate. It is thought that the dilatation is partly due to the damming back of secretions and partly to shrinkage of the surrounding lung tissue caused by fibrosis.

The effects of these changes can be clearly seen in a bronchogram which will reveal varying degrees of dilatation of larger bronchi and failure to fill of smaller bronchi and bronchioles (see Fig. 12/1).

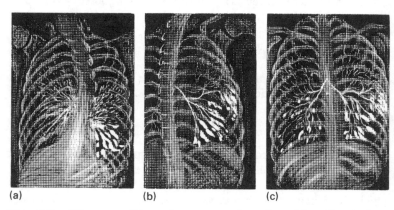

(a)   (b)   (c)

Fig. 12/1   Diagrams of bronchograms to show bronchiectasis: a) shows involvement of left lung; b) shows involvement of middle and lower lobes; c) shows involvement of both lungs

Signs and Symptoms

Cough and sputum are classical symptoms of bronchiectasis. The cough is often associated with change of position since this causes accumulated secretions to leave the cavities and come in contact with healthy bronchial mucous membrane and thus stimulate the cough reflex.

The sputum is usually purulent and in advanced cases several hundred millilitre (ml) may be coughed up in 24 hours.

Haemoptysis of varying severity may occur. Oddly enough the most severe haemoptysis is found in patients with relatively little previous history of cough and sputum. The middle lobe is the most common site of severe bleeding which may follow erosion of an artery by a 'broncholith' – a nodule of calcium derived from a lymph gland affected in a primary tuberculous complex. When haemoptysis is the only symptom the condition is sometimes known as a 'dry bronchiectasis'.

On examination of the respiratory movements some flattening of the thoracic wall over the diseased lobe may be noticed and movement may be diminished in this area, which is a sign of fibrosis. Usually vital capacity is also decreased.

The general condition of the patient will vary considerably depending on the extent of the disease. Some patients look ill, have clubbing of the fingers, dyspnoea and copious quantities of sputum, while others are well apart from repeated chest infections following upper respiratory tract infection.

Complications

Repeated attacks of pneumonia are liable to occur either in the affected area or due to 'spill-over' of infected sputum into other areas of the lung. Cerebral abscess was a classical complication but is rarely seen these days. Pleural effusion and empyema are relatively rare in previously diagnosed bronchiectasis, but underlying bronchiectasis is not uncommon in chronic empyema, presumably the original infected collapse giving rise to both conditions. Many patients have associated sinusitis and some physicians feel that this is the cause of the condition, infected material being inhaled into the lungs during sleep. Other physicians feel that the infection affects the respiratory tract as a whole.

Prognosis

If the material causing an obstruction is expectorated before changes actually occur then air will enter the collapsed area of lung and full restoration to normal should take place, but if the obstruction is not relieved early permanent damage occurs.

In the period before the use of antibiotics the prognosis of severe bronchiectasis was poor but with modern medical and surgical treatment, the prognosis has improved. Long-term survival will depend on the amount of lung destruction and the amount of generalised bronchitis. If the disease is very localised the patient may be cured by surgery. In the majority of patients symptoms may be reasonably well controlled, but not abolished, by means of antibiotics and postural drainage.

Most patients are able to lead a reasonably normal life apart from chronic cough and sputum, and more frequent respiratory infections than other people.

Treatment

The main object of treatment is to relieve the obstruction before permanent damage occurs. Thus efficient treatment of measles and whooping cough, removal of possible sources of infected material, and very careful prophylactic treatment to prevent postoperative lung collapse are all important.

Once bronchiectasis is established, prevention of accumulation of secretions will prevent further deterioration of the patient's general condition, subsequent complications and spread into other areas of the lung.

Conservative treatment consists of antibiotics and physiotherapy. If the disease is very localised or if there are repeated severe haemoptyses, surgery may be contemplated in order to resect the affected area.

Physiotherapy

In the conservative treatment this consists of clearing the cavities by accurate postural drainage, percussion and deep breathing exercises; training the patient in how to keep the cavities clear by postural drainage at home; encouraging better use of all areas of the lung by breathing exercises (see Chapter 11); and encouraging exercise and sport in the younger patient. For patients with 'dry bronchiectasis' whose main symptom is haemoptysis, postural drainage will be of limited value.

If resection is to be undertaken, pre- and postoperative physiotherapy on the lines indicated in Chapter 9 is essential.

CYSTIC FIBROSIS

Cystic fibrosis is an hereditary disease affecting the exocrine glands. The main abnormalities are increased secretion of mucus and a high sodium chloride content of sweat. Most of the clinical abnormalities are related to obstruction by viscid mucus; the lungs, paranasal sinuses, pancreas and intestine are particularly affected. Bronchial obstruction by viscid mucus leading to secondary infection and lung damage is the commonest cause of death.

The disease is transmitted by a recessive gene and it has been calculated that 1 in 20 of the population of the United Kingdom may carry this.

Clinical Features

One of the earliest manifestations of the disease is acute intestinal obstruction at birth resulting from meconium ileus, which occurs in about 10% of cases. Others may present with symptoms suggesting pancreatic insufficiency, these include failure to thrive despite a good appetite, frequent large, foul-smelling stools and a protuberant abdomen. Many present with respiratory symptoms varying from recurrent cough to severe pneumonia. The cough is characteristically paroxysmal and violent. Following repeated infections, bronchiectasis will develop and there may be finger clubbing. Thick purulent sputum will be expectorated. There may be associated airways obstruction and cor pulmonale may develop during the course of a severe infection or in the terminal stages.

Diagnosis

Early diagnosis is of vital importance and any child or young adult with chronic or recurrent respiratory infection should be suspected of having cystic fibrosis, especially if relevant gastro-intestinal symptoms are present. The sodium chloride content of the sweat must be estimated; in children suffering from cystic fibrosis the concentrations of both sodium and chloride are over 70mEq/litre in the sweat. This test is less reliable in adults.

Prognosis

The natural history of the disease is very variable. At one time it was unusual for children with cystic fibrosis to survive over the age of 14. However in recent years early diagnosis and prophylactic treatment have considerably improved the prognosis with many patients surviving into their twenties and thirties.

Treatment

Many of these patients are treated at special centres where the staff have experience in the treatment of the disease and are able to instruct the parents in the care of the child.

Intestinal obstruction caused by meconium ileus will require surgical treatment but otherwise treatment will consist of maintaining nutrition, encouraging drainage of the respiratory tract and the control of pulmonary infection.

A high calorie and high protein diet with some restriction of fat and starch should be given with supplements of pancreatin and vitamins A, D and E. Additional salt and fluid should be given in feverish states or in hot weather, to replace the loss in the sweat.

Prevention and treatment of pulmonary complications by means of antibiotics and effective bronchial drainage are of vital importance. Mist therapy may be given in order to reduce the viscosity of the sputum. If airways obstruction is present a bronchodilator may be given. Emphasis should be placed on prophylactic treatment in the early stages of the disease. For patients with established lung damage, treatment should be guided by the clinical response.

Physiotherapy

Physiotherapy has a vital role to play in the treatment of cystic fibrosis. As soon as the diagnosis has been confirmed, a regime of postural drainage must be instituted and the patient and his relatives should be instructed in how to carry out postural drainage at home. This should be done once or twice daily for up to 30 minutes at a time depending on the amount of secretions present. If the X-ray shows that specific segments of the lung are involved, the appropriate postural drainage positions should be used. Otherwise the basal areas and mid-zones should be drained each day.

Patients with cystic fibrosis should be encouraged to take as much active exercise as possible; this will not only help to loosen secretions but will also boost their morale when they find they can compete in sports and games.

Breathing exercises should also be taught as some patients develop chest deformities. They should include diaphragmatic breathing and localised basal expansion. Apical expansion is not necessary.

During acute exacerbations physiotherapy must be stepped up. The patient may be admitted to hospital for intensive treatment and postural drainage may be given up to six times a day for 45 minutes at a time. It is often better to drain different areas of the lung at different sessions, e.g. the basal areas may be drained at one session and the mid-zones at the next session. If secretions are particularly tenacious, humidification should be given before or during treatment. If reversible airways obstruction is apparent, a bronchodilator given before postural drainage may be helpful.

On rare occasions, if the patient is not in the terminal stages of the disease, I.P.P.B. may be of help in clearance of secretions. Because these patients have a tendency to pneumothorax the inspiratory pressures should be kept low. The course of treatment should be short (5–14 days) because I.P.P.B. has been shown to increase residual volumes in these patients if used for long periods of time (Matthews et al., 1964).

In the terminal stages of the disease, treatment should be according to the patient's tolerance and it may not be possible to clear the chest completely each time. Treatments will be shorter and should not cause unnecessary distress to the patient.

Most physicians like patients with cystic fibrosis to visit the physiotherapy department when they come to the out-patient clinic; in this way the physiotherapist can check that the patient is carrying out his treatment correctly at home and can discuss any relevant problems with the patient and his relatives.

PULMONARY TUBERCULOSIS

Infection with the tubercle bacillus in an individual who has not previously experienced contact with the organism is called primary tuberculosis; re-infection after the primary lesion is called post-primary tuberculosis. Miliary tuberculosis is produced by acute diffuse dissemination of tubercle bacilli via the bloodstream.

In most countries in the western hemisphere, infection is almost entirely with the human bacillus, which is spread by droplet infection. In less economically developed countries, milk still serves as a vehicle for infection with the bovine organism causing primary abdominal tuberculosis.

People vary greatly in their susceptibility to the disease. Susceptibility may be inborn, but the disease is not hereditary. Resistance may be lowered by malnutrition, overwork and lack of sleep. The risks of infection are increased by proximity, either from overcrowded housing or by individual exposure.

The Role of the Physiotherapist

Physiotherapy per se is not indicated in the treatment of tuberculosis but the physiotherapist may well be asked to treat patients with active pulmonary tuberculosis either because of associated conditions or because of complications which have arisen through reactions to certain drugs.

There is no danger to the physiotherapist provided she observes certain simple rules:

1 A mask and gown should be worn *only* if indicated by the ward sister or consultant.

2 The physiotherapist should position herself so that the patient does not cough directly into her face.

3 The physiotherapist should wash her hands immediately after treating the patient.

4 If, accidentally, sputum has soiled her uniform, the physiotherapist *must* change it at once and *before* treating the next patient.

In hospitals where patients are regularly treated for pulmonary tuberculosis, the physiotherapist will have a medical examination, to include chest radiograph and either a Mantoux or Tine test. Any physiotherapist who is unhappy about treating a patient with active pulmonary tuberculosis should discuss the matter with the consultant in charge of the case.

Any physiotherapy which may be prescribed will be entirely at the discretion of the individual consultant, but physiotherapists may be asked to treat the following tuberculous conditions:

Tuberculous Pleural Effusion or Empyema

Once medical treatment has been instituted by means of aspiration and anti-tuberculous drugs, there is no risk of physiotherapy causing spread of the disease and it has an important part to play in the prevention of chest deformity and the loss of respiratory function due to calcification and thickening of the pleura.

The patient should be given localised expansion exercises to all areas of the affected side of the chest, attention being paid to the apical area even though the effusion is usually in the posterior basal area.

Belt exercises are often helpful and the patient should be encouraged to practise several times a day.

If severe chest deformity occurs, the patient should lie on his unaffected side with two pillows under his thorax in order to open out the ribs on his affected side. He should take up this position for half an hour at a time at least four times a day and should be encouraged to practise intermittent expansion exercises whilst in this position.

Treatment should be continued until chest expansion is equal and the X-ray has improved.

Middle Lobe Syndrome

Physiotherapy is often ordered for children with a collapsed middle lobe due to pressure from primary tuberculous glands. Although results are frequently disappointing it is worth persevering with postural drainage, vibrations and breathing exercises as some children obtain benefit from it. The physiotherapist should frequently review the situation with the physician, particularly if no improvement has been obtained after about two weeks' treatment.

Tuberculous Bronchiectasis

Some patients have associated bronchiectasis and will require postural drainage for the affected area. It is wiser not to percuss the chest owing to the danger of haemoptysis and the physiotherapist should always stand behind the patient when he is coughing. Treatment should be given two or three times daily according to the amount of sputum.

Associated Asthma or Bronchitis

Physiotherapy may be ordered for asthmatic or bronchitic patients with tuberculosis, when the treatment will be on the same lines as that for ordinary asthma or bronchitis (see Chapter 13), except that I.P.P.B. should not be given if there are any signs of cavitation, as this would be detrimental to healing. Bronchodilators should be given by means of a simple nebuliser.

Surgical Procedures

Occasionally, a thoracoplasty may be performed (see p. 158) and in these cases physiotherapy is very valuable. Still more rarely, a localised resection may be performed – usually a segmental resection to excise an encapsulated cavity which will not completely heal.

Pre- and postoperative physiotherapy is as for other thoracic surgical procedures (see p. 143).

Peripheral Neuritis

Many alcoholic patients contract pulmonary tuberculosis. In addition, one of the drugs (isoniazid) which is frequently used in the treatment of tuberculosis is a known neurotoxic and can cause peripheral neuritis. There are thus two reasons why some of these patients are found to be suffering from quite severe peripheral neuritis leading to gross ataxia and inability to perform fine finger movements. Physiotherapy for these is indicated and can provide some very rewarding results. Frenkel's exercises are particularly useful.

REFERENCE

Matthews, L. W., Deershuk, C. F., Wise, M., Eddy, G., Nudelman, H., and
Specter, S. (1964). 'A therapeutic regimen for patients with cystic fibrosis.'
Journal of Pediatrics, **65**, 558.

BIBLIOGRAPHY

See end of Chapter 14.

Chapter 13

Chronic Bronchitis, Emphysema and Asthma

by D. V. GASKELL, M.C.S.P.

CHRONIC BRONCHITIS

The following definition of chronic bronchitis was approved by a committee of the World Health Organization in 1961:

'Chronic bronchitis is a chronic or recurrent increase above the normal in the volume of mucous secretion sufficient to cause expectoration, when this is not due to localised bronchopulmonary disease. The words "chronic" or "recurrent" may be further defined as "present on most days during at least three months of each of two successive years".'

Causes

Cigarette smoking and atmospheric pollution are two factors that are the main cause of hypersecretion. Infection is probably most important in causing irreversible lung damage.

Changes

The fundamental pathological change is hypertrophy of the mucus glands in the walls of the bronchi and an increase of goblet cells in the epithelial lining of the bronchial tree. This causes an excessive production of mucus (see Fig. 13/1).

At the same time, the cilia are unable to discharge the excessive mucus and have no more than a churning action upon it. These factors add to the obstruction of the airways.

The excessive mucus in the bronchi predisposes the patient to infection. Where this is limited to the large- and medium-sized bronchi, serious impairment of respiratory function is unlikely. If it

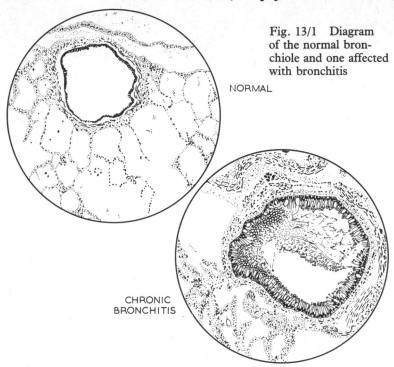

Fig. 13/1   Diagram of the normal bronchiole and one affected with bronchitis

NORMAL

CHRONIC BRONCHITIS

extends to the periphery of the lung and causes acute bronchiolitis and bronchopneumonia, the lobules may fail to resolve the exudate and may be replaced by fibrosis and contractures. Thus repeated infections over the years progressively reduce the number of patent airways and the area of effective alveolar surface.

The contraction of several lobules causes adjacent healthy lobules to expand and the individual alveoli become larger since many of them have previously been involved in acute inflammation and their weakened walls tend to rupture. In addition the scarred and distorted bronchioles often become kinked on expiration and cause air trapping. These mechanisms lead to the development of secondary emphysema.

Signs and Symptoms

Characteristic symptoms are cough, sputum, wheeze and dyspnoea. The patient may complain of increasing disability following a recent infection, but on close questioning he will usually reveal that he has had a smokers' cough for many years.

As the disease develops the cough gradually becomes more continuous and frequently a bout of coughing occurs when the patient lies down. Upper respiratory tract infections tend to 'go down to the chest', when the sputum becomes purulent and increases in volume. To begin with the exacerbations may be fairly mild but later they cause increasing wheeze and dyspnoea and last for longer periods.

At a relatively early stage the patient's cough is exacerbated by fog and symptoms become worse during foggy weather.

There is considerable variation in individuals as to whether cough, sputum, wheeze or dyspnoea are the predominant symptoms.

Some patients may have a certain amount of reversible airways obstruction whilst in others it may be mainly irreversible due to a predominant emphysematous factor.

In the early stages of the disease the patient's general condition may be fairly good but in the later stages he may develop cor pulmonale and may appear blue and bloated. If the chronic bronchitic patient develops bronchopneumonia he may go into acute hypercapnic respiratory failure.

Clubbing of the fingers is unusual but may be seen if polycythaemia is present or it may be due to additional complicating factors such as bronchial neoplasm or bronchiectasis.

In the later stages of the disease the chest is often barrel-shaped with kyphosis, increased anteroposterior diameter, horizontal ribs, prominent sternal angle and wide subcostal angle. It is seldom that this appearance can be reversed once it is established.

Movement of the chest wall is restricted and may be confined to the upper thorax. The patient may have to use the accessory muscles of respiration. In the advanced stages of the disease, if there is a marked emphysematous factor, there may be paradoxical movement of the lower part of the chest wall. (The lower costal margin is pulled inwards on inspiration due to the pull of the low, flattened diaphragm.)

On auscultation rhonchi are widespread particularly at the bases of the lungs. In milder cases they may only be present on forced expiration. If emphysema is present the breath sounds will be diminished.

Treatment

In the early stages of the disease, prophylactic treatment is extremely important. Once chronic bronchitis is established there is no possibility of a permanent cure and the most that can be done is to try to prevent further damage and alleviate the patient's symptoms.

Sources of bronchial irritation should be reduced to a minimum and the patient must be persuaded to give up smoking. It may be advisable for him to stay indoors during foggy weather.

Antibiotics will be ordered during acute exacerbations and the physician will impress upon the patient the importance of starting these at the very first sign of an upper respiratory tract infection. Some patients may be put on to long-term antibiotics, bronchodilator drugs and occasionally corticosteroids. Diuretics may be ordered for patients in cardiac failure.

In acute exacerbations controlled oxygen therapy is of vital importance, particularly in those patients with a permanently raised P_{CO_2}.

Physiotherapy

Physiotherapy is of benefit in all stages of the disease.

In the early stages of chronic bronchitis the patient should be given postural drainage for the basal areas of the lungs. As many of these patients are older, this is more comfortably done in alternate side lying with the foot of the bed raised 12–18 inches (30–45cm) from the floor. In hospital this should be done at least twice a day for up to 30 minutes at a time; vibrations and shaking on expiration will often help in removal of secretions. It is important for the physiotherapist to teach the patient how to drain his chest at home and if the bed cannot be tipped, a comfortable drainage position should be devised; he should be encouraged to carry out postural drainage morning and evening until his chest seems clear (this may take about 10 minutes on each side). It is important to fit in this regime with the patient's life and he is far more likely to carry out postural drainage regularly if it is only for a fairly short period at a time.

Breathing control should be taught in the early stages of the disease in the hopes that chest deformity will be prevented. Many of these patients will have poor basal expansion. The patient should be taught diaphragmatic breathing in all the relaxed positions, also localised basal expansion. If an exercise regime is to be started, many patients are able to improve their exercise tolerance quite considerably at this stage.

In the later stages of the disease, treatment will have to be modified to a certain extent. Most patients with chronic bronchitis will still tolerate postural drainage although there may be extensive lung damage. Many of these patients benefit from I.P.P.B. given in conjunction with postural drainage. A bronchodilator may be used in the nebuliser as there is often a degree of reversible airways obstruction and the secretions are more easily mobilised and expectorated due to the more effective aeration of the lungs by the ventilator. Vibrations and shaking should be given on expiration. Treatment should be given two or three times daily. At this stage in the disease the patient will have developed faulty breathing habits and may well have the typical barrel-shaped chest. Although it may be impossible to reverse the chest deformity, the pattern of breathing may be altered by means of breathing control and the patient can be taught what to do when in distress (see p. 207). Controlled breathing on stairs and hills is important. If an exercise regime is started it should be modified according to the patient's tolerance (see p. 211).

During acute exacerbations the chronic bronchitic may go into hypercapnic respiratory failure and prompt treatment will be required. If the secretions can be removed and effective alveolar ventilation restored, the patient's condition will improve. Many of these patients are drowsy and unresponsive and it is helpful to use I.P.P.B. with a mask instead of a mouthpiece. The patient should be turned onto his side and the foot of the bed elevated. If he has severe secondary emphysema he may not tolerate being tipped and should just be rolled onto his side. Help will be required to hold the mask over the patient's face and it may be necessary to hand-trigger the I.P.P.B. machine. It is important to observe the chest wall movement and the patient's level of consciousness (see p. 105).

Once effective ventilation has been established, shaking and vibrations should be given on the expiratory phase and often the patient will start to cough and expectorate spontaneously and his colour will improve. If there has been no response after 10 to 15 minutes, nasopharyngeal suction should be considered. Care must be taken not to overtire the patient and controlled oxygen should be given whenever the I.P.P.B. mask has been removed. Treatment should be carried out for about 20 minutes at two-hourly intervals for the first 48 hours. If a bronchodilator is being given, this should be used for alternate treatments at four-hourly intervals.

The patient should be carefully observed for any signs of increased drowsiness after treatment and if so, the matter must be reported to the physician as it may be necessary to run the I.P.P.B. machine off air with added controlled oxygen.

During the night, it may be possible to cut down the number of treatments between 10 p.m. and 6 a.m., but it is usually necessary for the nursing staff to rouse the patient to give him I.P.P.B. and encourage him to cough at least once during this period. After 48 hours many patients will show marked improvement and the number of treatments may be cut down. If the patient does not improve the physician will have to decide whether to intubate and ventilate him, but many physicians are reluctant to take this step when patients have severe chronic bronchitis. If the patient is intubated, treatment will be as described in Chapters 5 and 6.

EMPHYSEMA

'Emphysema is a condition of the lung characterised by increase beyond the normal in the size of airspaces distal to the terminal bronchiolus, i.e. the acinus' (Reid, 1967).

There are several pathological classifications of emphysema. The two main types are:

Panacinar emphysema when there is dilatation or destruction of the acinus. This has been graded according to the size of the holes.

Grade I   – holes up to 1mm in diameter
Grade II – holes up to 1–3mm in diameter
Grade III – holes up to 3–5mm in diameter
Grade IV – holes over 5mm in diameter

Patients who die from primary or idiopathic emphysema are found to have panacinar emphysema of at least Grade III severity throughout most of the lungs.

Centriacinar or centrilobular emphysema when the dilatation is more proximal and affects the alveoli arising from the respiratory bronchioli.

Causes

Emphysema commonly occurs in association with obstructive airways disease (see p. 193) and is also related to occupational lung disease (see p. 244). This is known as secondary emphysema.

More rarely it develops as a primary disease without any previous history of chest disease. It seems possible that in some patients a genetic factor might be responsible for the development of primary emphysema not related to chest disease or smoking. Eriksson has described three members of a family developing emphysema at an early age, all of whom had dysproteinaemia with a marked reduction of α_1-antitrypsin (Eriksson, 1964).

Signs and Symptoms

Lung function tests will show a low F.E.V.$_1$ which does not improve following the administration of a bronchodilator, thus demonstrating irreversible airways obstruction. The residual volume will be increased and the pressure volume loop will show an abrupt swing to a positive intrathoracic pressure on expiration. These are both indications of air trapping.

The X-ray will show a low flat diaphragm (below sixth rib anteriorly) and a large retrosternal translucent area, due to excess air in the lungs. Bullae may be visible. Cardiovascular changes such as a narrow vertical heart (less than 11·5cm), prominence of the pulmonary trunk, large hilar vessels and small lung vessels will be seen.

Owing to the loss of elasticity in the lung, the patient finds it difficult to breathe out, but paradoxically, the more effort he makes to breathe out the more distressed he becomes. This is because forced and prolonged expiration will cause earlier shut-down of diseased airways and consequent air trapping. The work of breathing will also be increased; some patients may have learnt the trick of 'pursed lip' expiration, which causes a certain amount of back-pressure and may prevent shut-down of the airways.

Many emphysematous patients are breathless at rest and have been described as 'pink puffers' because cyanosis is not usually noticeable as in the chronic bronchitic or 'blue bloater'. By major effort, the emphysematous patient is able to ventilate sufficient alveoli to keep his blood gases normal, so that he appears pink. The absence of hypoxaemia tends to preserve a normal pulmonary artery pressure and spares him from cardiac failure.

On examination, the thorax may appear over-inflated, basal expansion diminished and the chest elevated by the accessory muscles of respiration; there may even be paradoxical movement of the lower ribs due to the pull of the flattened diaphragm, the whole pattern of breathing appears unco-ordinated and every breath out is an effort. In some patients it will be noticed that on expiration the jugular veins fill and the inward movement of the abdomen on expiration is interrupted by a 'flick' or 'bounce' as the outward flow of air is suddenly checked by the increase in obstruction.

Treatment

This will be mainly palliative in the prevention and treatment of infection. The patient should be taught to breathe with the minimum amount of effort and to make the best use he can of his remaining healthy lung tissue by means of physiotherapy.

Occasionally surgical treatment may be considered if a patient has a large bulla compressing areas of healthy lung tissue. The ultimate success of plication or resection of large bullae will depend on the severity and extent of disease in the remaining lung tissue.

Physiotherapy

The aims of treatment are to teach the patient to breathe with the minimum amount of effort and to try to establish a co-ordinated pattern of breathing. Aid in removal of secretions may be necessary.

The patient must first be taught to control his breathing. A simple explanation of the mechanics of breathing should be given and the faults in his breathing pattern should be pointed out to the patient. He should be placed in a comfortable, well-supported half-lying or sitting position and encouraged to relax his upper chest and shoulders. Gentle, controlled diaphragmatic breathing should then be taught with emphasis on completely relaxed expiration (Gandevia, 1963). The rate of breathing should not be slowed down as the patient would then tend to lose control and revert to an unco-ordinated pattern. If abdominal 'bounce' is noted the patient should be encouraged to shorten his expiratory phase and breathe in a little sooner (Innocenti, 1966). When the patient has gained a certain amount of control he should be shown the various relaxed positions to adopt when in distress. Many patients suffering from orthopnoea find it more comfortable to sleep in the high side-lying position.

The next progression will be to teach the patient controlled breathing with walking and how to breathe on climbing the stairs. Certain patients with very severe emphysema may be unable to walk without oxygen and may be supplied with a portable oxygen cylinder. This type of very disabled patient may find it easier to walk with a high walking frame.

If the patient has excess secretions he must be taught how to cough effectively and modified postural drainage may be necessary. Many patients with emphysema become very distressed by conventional postural drainage positions. Some patients will tolerate lying flat without the bed tipped, whilst others will only be able to lie on their side propped up by several pillows. Shaking on expiration should be given in a suitable position and effective coughing encouraged. Many emphysematous patients cough ineffectively due to shut-down of the airways and have distressing paroxysms of coughing. They should be told to breathe in after every two or three coughs and in this way will avoid shut-down of the airways.

It may also be helpful to use I.P.P.B. in order to aid expectoration. It is worth trying this with a bronchodilator at first and then measuring the F.E.V.$_1$ and F.V.C. before and after I.P.P.B. to see if there is any degree of reversibility present. If severe over-inflation or bullae are present, it is wiser to use a simple nebuliser.

Having taught the patient breathing control and aided expectoration, the next aim of physiotherapy will be to attempt a certain amount of lateral basal expansion, thereby trying to produce a more normal synchronised movement of the thoracic cage. Some physiotherapists feel that this is unnecessary, but it is often worthwhile to persevere with localised basal expansion although it will take some time to achieve. Hooper of Melbourne (1967) has demonstrated this effect by means of cineradiography.

Some physiotherapists like to teach thoracic mobility and posture exercises to emphysematous patients, in which case the emphasis should be on relaxed movements in co-ordination with breathing. Any form of bending forward should be avoided as this will cause distress.

COMPENSATORY EMPHYSEMA

This may occur when a section of a lung contracts by fibrosis or collapse or is removed surgically. The rest of the lung expands to fill the space by over-inflation. This is known as compensatory emphysema and is not associated with any defect of function.

ASTHMA

The term 'asthma' refers to the condition of people with widespread narrowing of the airways which changes in its severity over short periods of time and which is not due to cardiac disease.

Three factors contribute to this bronchial obstruction: contracture of the bronchial muscle – true bronchospasm; oedema of the mucous membrane; plugging with viscid mucus.

Causes

It is generally accepted that the bronchi of patients suffering from asthma are 'hypersensitive'.

Cases of asthma have been divided into two main groups:

1. The extrinsic type, where there is a recognisable antigen, which is associated with a history of eczema, hay fever, urticaria etc. This type commonly occurs in children and young people with a family history of allergy. Reaction to external allergens can be demonstrated by skin tests, when a weal develops within 10 minutes of the intradermal injection of the allergen.

2. The intrinsic type where no antigen is recognised. This type usually occurs in people of 40 years or over who have no personal or family history of allergy. The disease is often associated with infections.

Although these two groups of asthma differ broadly in many

respects, the division is a provisional one as allergic factors may in due course be demonstrated in the intrinsic group.

Though the precipitating factors are mainly allergy and infection, attacks may also be caused by vigorous exercise, atmospheric pollution and other non-specific factors.

Psychological factors must also be taken into account. Although it is doubtful whether psychological stress alone causes asthma there is little doubt that such distress exacerbates asthma in certain patients. In these patients treatment is not likely to be satisfactory unless the situation is appreciated and the patient handled with sympathetic understanding, tact and firmness, and the difficulties eased as much as possible.

Symptoms

A classical attack of asthma is rapid in onset. The patient has difficulty in breathing out and this results in an audible wheeze. In very severe attacks the airways obstruction may become so severe that there is no longer an audible wheeze.

The frequency and duration of attacks vary considerably. If a very severe attack has continued for more than 24 hours, it is described as status asthmaticus and the patient will require admission to hospital.

Cough frequently occurs during asthma attacks and may be distressing and non-productive in the early stages. Once the bronchodilatation has been achieved, the patient is often able to cough up plugs of tenacious sputum and will experience considerable relief.

Many patients suffering from asthma develop a barrel-shaped chest due to over-inflation of the lungs, but even long-standing chest deformity may be reversed if the asthma is effectively dealt with. In the very young child with chronic asthma the sternum may be drawn inwards or there may be Harrison's sulcus. Older children tend to develop pigeon chest or the same type of barrel-chest as adults. They also frequently have poor posture. Fortunately even gross deformities may reverse to a surprising degree if the chronic asthma is relieved by treatment.

Investigations

Various investigations are carried out including tests for hypersensitivity and respiratory function tests. Examination of the blood and sputum for eosinophils is also helpful.

The most valuable respiratory function test is the forced expiratory volume in one second ($F.E.V._1$) and the forced vital capacity

(F.V.C.). This can be measured at the bedside by means of a portable spirometer. A vitalograph or vitalor is often used. These are valuable means of assessing the patient's response to treatment.

Treatment

Treatment is by means of bronchodilators and sometimes cortico- steroids. An antibiotic may be prescribed if infection is present.

If a particular allergen has been identified, it is sometimes possible to avoid it or at least reduce exposure to it. In the case of house dust, it is particularly important to avoid accumulation of dust by making changes in the furnishing of the patient's bedroom and cleaning it very thoroughly. The mattress should be vacuum-cleaned every day. There is controversy over the value of desensitisation, some allergists feeling that it is helpful in certain cases.

Sodium cromoglycate (Intal) is of use in inhibiting the patient's reaction to allergy and as a result of its prophylactic use, many asthmatic children are able to lead a much more normal life with very little loss of schooling.

Physiotherapy

The physiotherapist will be asked to treat asthmatic patients whose condition will vary from severe status asthmaticus to those patients who have no symptoms at all at the time of treatment. In the former situation the aims of treatment will be to achieve bronchodilatation and to assist in the removal of secretions, whereas in the latter situation the physiotherapist should teach the patient what to do when he has an asthma attack, assist in removal of any secretions present and try to teach a more efficient pattern of breathing. Obviously there will be many patients varying between these two extremes.

When a patient is admitted in status asthmaticus bronchodilators will be given in order to relieve bronchospasm and a very effective means of delivering these drugs is by I.P.P.B. If this equipment is available, the physiotherapist is often asked to treat the patient at this stage. The F.E.V.$_1$ or peak flow should be measured first and the patient should sit comfortably upright in bed and use the I.P.P.B. machine until the nebuliser is empty. Apart from encouraging the patient to breathe with his lower chest whilst using the machine the physiotherapist should not attempt other measures at this stage. If I.P.P.B. is not available a simple nebuliser should be used. The physiotherapist should then put the patient in a high side-lying position and encourage gentle diaphragmatic breathing in the patient's own time. He will not be able to breathe slowly at this stage.

As the bronchodilator takes effect, the patient will be able to breathe more easily and may start to cough spontaneously. About 15 minutes after administration of the bronchodilator (either by I.P.P.B. or other means) the physiotherapist should treat the patient in high side lying, gently vibrate the chest on expiration and encourage the patient to cough. Frequently he will expectorate tenacious sputum containing plugs and will experience rapid relief. The F.E.V.$_1$ or peak flow will demonstrate the improvement. However, some patients are unable to expectorate and if they persist in trying at this stage, the airways obstruction will become worse. Apart from making the patient comfortable and encouraging gentle diaphragmatic breathing, the physiotherapist should leave this type of patient until the drugs start to take effect. I.P.P.B. with a bronchodilator can be repeated at four-hourly intervals. As the patient's condition improves he will be able to lie flat and even be tipped in order to remove secretions.

Breathing control is of importance; it can be a great help to a patient during a mild attack of asthma. He should be told to get into a relaxed position (see p. 208) and to try to breathe gently with his diaphragm, expiration should not be forced. In between attacks patients should practise this type of breathing and should also include basal expansion exercises. Many children with asthma develop quite severe chest deformities and faulty patterns of breathing; these deformities will disappear if the asthma is treated effectively. Breathing exercises will help to improve the faulty breathing habits.

Certain patients with asthma, particularly children, have secretions present at all times; in this situation, it is helpful if the patient carries out postural drainage each day in order to prevent accumulation of secretions. The physiotherapist should explain how to do this at home.

Many patients have exercise-induced asthma and research is being done in this field at the present time. If asthma patients are treated in classes, more vigorous exercises should not be done for more than three minutes at a time and should be interspersed with gentle breathing exercises. Asthma is less likely to be induced by swimming (Fitch & Morton, 1971) and this is a very effective form of exercise for these patients.

FUNGAL INFECTIONS OF THE LUNG

The main fungal infections of the lung (pulmonary mycoses) encountered in Britain are aspergillosis, candidiasis, actinomycosis and cryptococcosis.

Aspergillosis

This is the commonest fungal disease affecting the lungs. The Aspergillus thrives on decaying vegetation in warm, humid conditions and releases spores particularly through the winter months. *Aspergillus fumigatus* is the most common species responsible for aspergillosis in man. There are four different types.

ASYMPTOMATIC ASPERGILLOSIS

Many bronchitics have a few spores in their sputum. This is due to poor sputum clearance and the ubiquity of the spores. No special treatment is necessary.

ASPERGILLOMA

A solid ball of fungus (mycetoma) may grow in a pre-existing cavity. It commonly forms in an old tuberculous cavity and less frequently in cavities caused by lung abscess, pulmonary infarction etc. Radiographically a crescent of air may be seen over the ball of fungus which can be shown to change its position with changes of posture.

Some patients may be asymptomatic, others may have recurrent haemoptyses or repeated infections with thick purulent sputum.

Aspergilloma is often left untreated as there is always the risk of spread of infection during surgery and bronchopleural fistula may result. However, lobectomy may be undertaken if recurrent severe haemoptyses occur.

DISSEMINATED ASPERGILLOSIS

There may be spread of the disease into the lung and pleura with progressive destruction of the lung tissue; it may also spread to other organs. The patient is very ill and there is a poor prognosis. Treatment may be by amphotericin B given intravenously or pneumonectomy may occasionally be considered.

BRONCHOPULMONARY ASPERGILLOSIS WITH ALLERGIC MANIFESTATIONS

Some patients become allergic to the Aspergillus and about $2\frac{1}{2}$ hours after exposure the bronchi and bronchioles become acutely inflamed, oedematous and haemorrhagic. Transient pulmonary infiltrates develop associated with fever, wheezing and eosinophilia. Bronchial casts, often brown in colour, may be coughed up from which *Aspergillus fumigatus* can be cultured. Obstruction of bronchi by mycelium can result in collapse of a segment or lobe or rarely, a lung.

Repeated attacks can cause bronchiectasis or the disease may spread into the alveoli and cause diffuse pulmonary fibrosis.

Treatment will be by means of various antifungal agents. Allergic bronchopulmonary aspergillosis may persist for years with episodes of wheeze, fever, eosinophilia and radiographic evidence of transient consolidation and collapse. Some patients will recover spontaneously, others develop severe chronic asthma and may need corticosteroids and bronchodilators in order to overcome symptoms.

PHYSIOTHERAPY

The aims of treatment will vary according to the patient's symptoms. Vigorous postural drainage will be necessary in order to remove bronchial casts, often an exhausting procedure for the patient and the physiotherapist. If wheezing is the main problem, treatment will be similar to that of asthma consisting of I.P.P.B., assisted coughing and breathing control. Treatment may be necessary three times a day.

Frequently the patient will be wheezy but will also have patchy areas of consolidation. I.P.P.B. with bronchodilators should be given first in order to relieve spasm, this should be followed by postural drainage for affected areas with fairly vigorous shaking of the chest; if the patient will not tolerate the correct postural drainage position it should be modified. Some patients will be having antifungal inhalations and if so, these should be given after physiotherapy when it is hoped the airways will be reasonably clear.

OCCUPATIONAL LUNG DISEASE

Damage to the lungs by dusts or fumes or noxious substances inhaled by workers in certain specific occupations is known as 'occupational lung disease'.

Coal Miners' Pneumoconiosis

This is a special type of pneumoconiosis due to the prolonged inhalation of coal dust, rather than rock dust which produces silicosis. It is most prevalent in the South Wales coalfields and there are two types.

1. Simple Pneumoconiosis. The X-ray shows diffuse reticulation at first. Later small scattered nodules up to 5mm in diameter develop, often with surrounding emphysema. The disease is only progressive if the worker remains exposed to dust.

2. Progressive Massive Fibrosis. The X-ray shows large dense shadows mostly in the middle and upper zones with surrounding emphysema. At one time it was thought that this was due to a tuberculous infection superimposed on a simple pneumoconiosis, but it is now thought that fibrosis caused by an enhanced immune reaction occurs followed by the deposition of immune globulin in the pneumoconiotic lungs.

CLINICAL FEATURES

The diagnosis of pneumoconiosis should be suspected in a man who complains of increasing breathlessness on exertion and who has worked in the coal mines for several years. It is common for the patient to be a cigarette smoker and to have associated chronic bronchitis. If sputum is present it is usually mucoid but it will become purulent during infective exacerbations. It may become jet black when lesions cavitate. Once progressive massive fibrosis is established the disease is progressive even if the patient is no longer exposed to coal dust. In advanced cases, the patient becomes grossly disabled and death from cor pulmonale is common. Pulmonary tuberculosis may develop as an added complication.

TREATMENT

There is no specific treatment for pneumoconiosis and the most important aspect of its management is prevention. This implies effective dust suppression, the early recognition of dust retention by means of routine radiography and when necessary, the provision of alternative employment in areas of low dust concentration to prevent progress of the disease.

PHYSIOTHERAPY

Physiotherapy will be similar to that used in the treatment of chronic bronchitis and emphysema. If the patient has an infection every effort should be made to assist in the removal of secretions. If there is extensive fibrosis, I.P.P.B. may be helpful in assisting the patient to cough. In the advanced stages of the disease, all that the physiotherapist can do is to try to teach the patient to breathe with the minimum amount of effort and to assist in effective coughing.

Silicosis

Silicosis is due to inhalation of fine particles of free silica. It occurs in coal mines, in the granite and sandstone industries, in metal foundries, in various metal grinding processes and in the pottery industry.

CHANGES

The earliest is the development of fine fibrotic nodules around the particles of silica throughout the lungs. As the disease develops, these nodules increase in size and finally there are large areas of fibrosis. Tuberculosis may be a complication.

CLINICAL FEATURES

Symptoms do not usually develop until after several years of exposure to the dust. The chronic form of the disease usually presents with progressive dyspnoea on exertion, accompanied by unproductive cough and recurrent bouts of bronchitis. Occasional haemoptysis may occur. If tuberculosis supervenes there is deterioration in the general condition accompanied by increase in cough and sputum, pyrexia and loss of weight. Eventually the patient becomes very disabled and death occurs from bronchopneumonia, tuberculosis or cor pulmonale.

TREATMENT

There is no specific treatment and since silicosis continues to progress after exposure to the dust has ceased, it is vital to diagnose the disease early and remove the patient from further contact with the dust. All workers exposed to silica dust should have regular chest X-rays.

PHYSIOTHERAPY

The treatment will be as for chronic bronchitis and emphysema. The aims will be to help in removal of secretions by means of postural drainage and possibly intermittent positive pressure breathing and to teach the patient to breathe with the minimum amount of effort.

Asbestosis

This is a form of pneumoconiosis due to the inhalation of asbestos dust, causing a progressive fibrosis of the lungs, particularly the lower lobes. The main symptoms are cough and dyspnoea. Asbestos bodies can be found on microscopy of the sputum.

Preventative measures are similar to those used in silicosis.

Carcinoma of the bronchus is a common complication and malignant mesothelioma of the pleura also occurs.

Various other occupational diseases such as *Farmer's lung* and *Bird Fancier's lung* will be encountered by physiotherapists treating chest disease. Details can be found in textbooks dealing with chest disease and physiotherapy will be directed towards assistance with expectoration and teaching the patient to breathe with the minimum amount of effort. I.P.P.B. may also be of help.

DIFFUSE FIBROSING ALVEOLITIS

This is alternatively known as diffuse interstitial lung disease, diffuse interstitial pulmonary fibrosis, Hamman-Rich syndrome.

It is a condition of unknown aetiology characterised by a diffuse inflammatory process beyond the terminal bronchiole. Essential features are cellular thickening of the alveolar walls showing a tendency to fibrosis and the presence of large mononuclear cells within the alveolar spaces.

Clinically the outstanding characteristic is progressive and unremitting dyspnoea. Clubbing of the fingers is common. The disease is often fatal, in the subacute form originally described by Hamman and Rich this may be within six months, in the commonest chronic form within a few years.

The only effective treatment is with corticosteroid drugs. Other treatment is purely palliative. Oxygen is given in high concentrations, as patients with fibrosing alveolitis do not retain carbon dioxide. In the later stages secondary infection may require treatment. Heart failure may be temporarily improved with diuretics and digitalis. Appropriate sedation should be given in the terminal stages.

PHYSIOTHERAPY

This will be purely palliative but may be of help during infections when I.P.P.B. and chest vibration may help in the removal of secretions. Positions for dyspnoea and breathing control during walking can also be taught to the patient in the early stages of the disease in the hope that they might help a little.

REFERENCES

Eriksson, S. (1964). 'Pulmonary emphysema and α_1-antitrypsin deficiency.' *Acta Medica Scandinavica*, 175, 197.
Fitch, D. and Norton, A. R. (1971). 'Specificity of exercise in exercise-induced asthma.' *British Medical Journal*, 4, 577.
Gaskell, D. V. (1966). 'Acute exacerbations in chronic bronchitis.' *Physiotherapy*, 52, 431.
Grant, R. (1970). 'The physiological basis of increased exercise ability in patients with emphysema after breathing and exercise training.' *Physiotherapy*, 56, 541.
Hooper, A. E. T. (1967). 'Physical therapy for an emphysematous patient.' *Proceedings of the Fifth W.C.P.T. International Congress*, pp. 119–33. Australian Physiotherapy Association.
Innocenti, D. M. (1966). 'Breathing exercises in the treatment of emphysema.' *Physiotherapy*, 52, 437.

Reid, Lynne (1967). *The Pathology of Emphysema*. Lloyd-Luke (Medical Books) Ltd.

Webber, B. A., Shenfield, G. M. and Paterson, J. W. (1974). 'A comparison of three different techniques for giving nebulised albuterol to asthmatic patients.' *American Review of Respiratory Disease*, **109**, 293.

World Health Organization (1961). 'Chronic Cor Pulmonale.' *W.H.O. Tech. Rep. Ser.*, No. 213, 14.

BIBLIOGRAPHY

See end of Chapter 14.

Pulmonary Embolism, Lung Tumours and Diseases of the Pleura

by D. V. GASKELL, M.C.S.P.

PULMONARY EMBOLISM

A pulmonary embolus most commonly arises from a deep vein thrombosis in the leg or pelvis. More rarely it may arise from an intracardiac thrombosis following atrial fibrillation or cardiac infarction.

CLINICAL FEATURES

It may present in different ways and it is important to distinguish between the signs of massive pulmonary embolism and pulmonary infarct.

Massive Pulmonary Embolism

This is defined as obstruction to more than 50% of the major pulmonary artery branches.

A large pulmonary embolism may cause sudden death; the classical description of an elderly, possibly obese patient around the tenth postoperative day calling for a bedpan and suddenly collapsing is well known. If the embolism is not immediately fatal, the patient becomes suddenly shocked and will complain of central chest pain, there will be distressing dyspnoea but not orthopnoea, and cyanosis and profuse sweating. The blood pressure will fall and the jugular venous pressure will rise; 60–85% of the cross-sectional area of the pulmonary arteries have to be occluded before the systemic blood pressure falls and only massive emboli can cause such acute obstructive pulmonary hypertension. There will be sinus tachycardia and a gallop rhythm. Pulmonary arteriography will confirm the diagnosis.

Pulmonary Infarction

Small emboli cause pulmonary infarction. There is frequently pleuritic pain and pleural effusion may develop; about 50% of patients have haemoptysis. Dyspnoea is variable and linked with the degree of pleuritic pain; there may be a varying degree of pyrexia present and tachycardia of over 100 per minute is found in the majority of cases. Symptoms are frequently slight and it is the most commonly overlooked serious respiratory lesion. It should be remembered that repeated small pulmonary emboli may seriously obstruct the pulmonary vascular bed and lead to pulmonary hypertension and right ventricular failure.

TREATMENT

Treatment is primarily prophylactic and is directed towards those patients at greatest risk – the old and obese, the patient with cardiac disease, the post-partum and postoperative patient. Acceleration of the venous return by means of exercise and early ambulation is important. Patients confined to bed should be examined frequently for the development of evidence of phlebothrombosis. If there is any suspicion of deep venous thrombosis, anticoagulant therapy should be started immediately unless there are strong contra-indications.

Massive pulmonary embolism requires urgent treatment and intravenous anticoagulants may prevent extension of the clot. Oxygen should be given freely and the usual measures for acute circulatory failure employed. Morphine or pethidine may be given for relief of pain and apprehension. Methods of treatment include the use of anticoagulants, fibrinolytic agents and emergency pulmonary embolectomy.

Treatment of pulmonary infarction will be by means of anticoagulant therapy, oxygen and bed rest. Morphine may be required for the associated pain.

PHYSIOTHERAPY

Treatment is mainly prophylactic and all patients at risk should be given active leg exercises and breathing exercises in order to assist the venous return. These patients should be encouraged to carry out active foot and leg movements at frequent intervals during the day.

If a pulmonary embolus should occur, physiotherapy should be discontinued until anticoagulant therapy has been established when treatment will be re-ordered by the physician or surgeon. At this stage some patients may cough up a certain amount of old blood and clot and chest movements may be limited due to pleuritic pain. Localised breathing over the affected area should be encouraged and it may be necessary to give postural drainage. Leg exercises should be continued until the patient is ambulant.

If a pulmonary embolectomy is performed, physiotherapy will be carried out on the same lines as for other patients undergoing cardiopulmonary bypass (see Chapter 10).

TUMOURS OF THE LUNG

Carcinoma of the Bronchus

This is the commonest tumour of the lung and its incidence has greatly increased over the past thirty years. All the available evidence attributes the great rise in mortality from this disease to the smoking of tobacco, particularly cigarettes.

The majority of these tumours arise centrally either in, or proximal to, a segmental bronchus. A few are peripheral.

Histologically 56% are found to be squamous cell carcinomas, 37% are anaplastic (oat cell carcinomas), 6% adenocarcinoma and 1% alveolar cell carcinomas.

SYMPTOMS

A dry cough or a change in the nature of the cough is often an early symptom; haemoptysis may also occur. A persistent wheeze and dull, deep-seated pain are common symptoms.

As the growth increases in size it may cause progressive bronchial obstruction with mucopurulent sputum and eventual collapse of the segment.

In some patients the disease is discovered by means of mass X-ray. Others may remain symptom-free until complications occur.

COMPLICATIONS

Inflammatory complications may present as pneumonia or lung abscess. Any patient with a segmental pneumonia which fails to resolve, or recurs repeatedly in the same area, should be investigated for a bronchial carcinoma.

Pressure by the tumour may cause collapse of a lung segment or obstruct the superior vena cava.

Tumour cells may directly invade the pleura and cause pleural effusion or this may be the result of spread of inflammation. Again, the cells may infiltrate the pericardium or heart muscle causing atrial fibrillation or pericardial effusion.

Distal metastases may occur in any part of the body and endocrine and metabolic disorders occasionally occur.

Neurological complications are not uncommon. There may be involvement of the brachial plexus together with pain and weakness in the arm (Pancoast's tumour), or of sympathetic ganglia (producing Horner's syndrome). The recurrent laryngeal and phrenic nerves may be affected with resultant hoarseness and hiccough respectively.

Finger clubbing with pulmonary pseudo-hypertrophic osteo-arthropathy may sometimes be present. This causes pain and swelling in the joints, particularly the fingers, wrists and ankles. The X-ray will show typical subperiosteal reaction leading to new bone formation.

Any patient presenting with the above features should have a chest X-ray which may confirm the presence of bronchial carcinoma. The sputum should be examined for carcinoma cells which can be found in two cases out of three (Oswald et al., 1971). If there is any doubt as to the diagnosis, bronchoscopy is carried out. It is always done if surgery is being contemplated in order to decide whether the tumour is operable.

TREATMENT

Apart from anaplastic (oat cell) carcinoma when radiotherapy may be the treatment of choice, the main hope of a cure lies in the surgical removal of the affected lobe or lung. Unfortunately many patients are not suitable for this type of treatment either because of the extent of the growth or because of poor respiratory function.

Radical radiotherapy may be considered but not all patients are suitable for this. If the disease is too advanced malaise produced by irradiation sickness may outweigh the benefit gained.

Palliative radiotherapy is more commonly used, in order to relieve symptoms and make the patient more comfortable, particularly for those with obstruction of the superior vena cava, pain, haemoptysis, distressing cough or obstruction of a large bronchus.

Cytotoxic drugs may be used in the treatment of malignant pleural effusion and antibiotics may be used for secondary infection.

In many cases only symptomatic measures are possible and with each individual the physician will have to consider carefully what he will tell the patient and his relatives. All possible measures should be taken to relieve physical and mental suffering.

PHYSIOTHERAPY

Physiotherapy is most often required for the pre-operative or pre-bronchoscopy preparation of the patient and in the postoperative treatment and is carried out on the lines indicated in Chapter 9.

If the patient is being treated by means of radiotherapy and if there is infection beyond the bronchial obstruction, as the tumour reduces in size and the obstruction is relieved, the patient will start to expectorate purulent sputum. This can be considerably facilitated by means of postural drainage. Gentle vibrations may be given but it is wiser not to give percussion and vigorous shaking in view of the possibility of haemoptysis or the presence of metastases in the spine or ribs.

A physiotherapist may be asked to help patients in the terminal stages of the disease if they are troubled by excessive secretions and are having difficulty in expectoration. It may be possible to help in the removal of secretions by means of postural drainage and gentle vibrations. Very occasionally nasopharyngeal suction may be contemplated, but this should only be done if the patient is alert and in extreme distress. This procedure should not be carried out in comatose patients in the terminal stages of the disease.

Some patients may develop pulmonary fibrosis as a result of radiotherapy. They will be short of breath and it may be helpful to teach them controlled breathing, particularly when walking (see Chapter 11).

Adenoma of the Bronchus

This is a benign tumour which rarely undergoes malignant change. It is less common than carcinoma of the bronchus and may present as haemoptysis or as bronchial obstruction with infection. Diagnosis is confirmed by bronchoscopy. The tumour is surgically removed.

Hamartoma

This is a benign tumour of the lung and it is composed of a mixture of tissues found in the lung, particularly cartilage.

Patients are often symptom-free and a hamartoma is usually discovered on chest X-ray. It is frequently surgically removed as it is difficult to distinguish it from peripheral bronchial carcinoma or tuberculoma.

DISEASES OF THE PLEURA

Pleurisy

Inflammation of the pleura may be dry or associated with effusion, the former often proceeding to the latter.

Dry Pleurisy

Dry pleurisy may be caused by: tuberculosis which rapidly progresses to pleurisy with effusion; pneumonia or lung abscess; pulmonary infarct; injury to lungs or pleura; rarely in the terminal stages of uraemia. Occasionally primary pleurisy may occur without underlying disease.

CLINICAL FEATURES

The main symptom is a sharp and stabbing pain over the affected area, aggravated by coughing and deep breathing. The respirations may be short and grunting and chest movement limited on the affected side. The diagnosis is confirmed by the presence of a pleural rub. The pain diminishes as an effusion forms.

The chest X-ray may reveal underlying disease, if present, but otherwise shows no specific sign of dry pleurisy.

TREATMENT

Bed rest and treatment of the underlying condition will be required. Analgesics and local heat may be of help in relieving pain, but due regard must be paid to the underlying condition. The patient should be nursed in a position that is most comfortable for his breathing and may choose to lie on the affected side.

Pleural Effusion

An accumulation of fluid in the pleural cavity may represent a transudate or an exudate.

TRANSUDATES

These occur when the venous pressure is high or the osmotic pressure of the plasma is reduced. The fluid is usually clear and of low specific gravity and contains less than 2·0g protein per 100ml.

Causes of pleural transudates are cardiac failure, the nephrotic syndrome and cirrhosis of the liver.

EXUDATES

These occur in the presence of inflammation or neoplasm. The fluid is of high specific gravity and contains more than 2·0g protein per 100ml. Exudates may be clear or cloudy; they will be clear in tuberculous or neoplastic disease but cloudiness may be due to the presence of blood as in neoplasm or pulmonary infarct, or pus cells as in pneumonia or lung abscess.

Causes of pleural exudates are: bacterial pneumonias; pulmonary infarction; secondary pleural malignancy or rarely, a primary tumour such as diffuse malignant mesothelioma; tuberculosis; subphrenic abscess and other complicating inflammatory lesions; collagen disorders; fungal infections. There are also very rare causes such as the postmyocardial syndrome, acute pancreatitis, Meig's syndrome.

TYPICAL SIGNS OF PLEURAL EFFUSION

There is diminished movement on the affected side. If the effusion is large, there may be mediastinal shift to the opposite side. Tactile vocal fremitus is diminished over the fluid. On percussion there is stony dullness over the fluid, the line tending to rise in the axilla with moderate effusions. On auscultation there are absent breath sounds and voice sounds over the fluid. Sometimes bronchial breathing occurs above the upper level of the fluid.

TREATMENT

The pleural reaction which is frequently associated with bacterial pneumonias may progress to pleural effusion and should always be suspected if fever persists despite appropriate antibiotics. These effusions should always be aspirated to dryness at once. The fluid is amber or straw-coloured.

Pleural involvement in pulmonary infarction is almost invariable and pleural pain is a constant clinical feature. Pleural effusion commonly develops, small to moderate in size. Aspiration is seldom required, but if performed the fluid may be blood-stained but is more commonly clear and straw-coloured.

Primary pleural neoplasm is rare but secondary pleural malignancy is common. They have two characteristics, the fluid is often bloodstained and it recurs promptly after aspiration. The patient must be kept comfortable by repeated aspiration; it is sometimes possible to slow down the re-accumulation of fluid by radiotherapy or chemotherapy, but on the whole results are disappointing.

Pleural effusion is commonly associated with primary tuberculosis. The onset is variable, sometimes it is acute with fever, malaise, sweating and severe pleuritic pain as in pleurisy. Other patients may have little pain but complain of vague ill-health and dyspnoea on effort. Treatment will be by means of aspiration and the use of antituberculous drugs. It is important to prevent the development of pleural fibrosis.

Pleural effusion associated with subphrenic abscess should be promptly aspirated and appropriate antibiotic therapy instituted. Surgery may be necessary.

Pleural effusion may occur in association with collagen disorders, fungal infections and other rare disease. Management will consist of treatment of the underlying condition.

PHYSIOTHERAPY

Physiotherapy has no part to play in the treatment of dry pleurisy, transudates or malignant pleural effusion.

Following aspiration of other types of pleural effusion, breathing exercises should be started in order to prevent chest deformity and loss of respiratory function due to thickening of the pleura.

The patient should be given localised expansion exercises to all areas of the affected side; attention should be paid to the apical area even though the effusion is usually in the posterior basal area. Belt exercises are often helpful and the patient should be encouraged to practise several times a day.

If chest movement does not improve, the patient should lie on his unaffected side with two pillows under his thorax in order to open out the ribs on the affected side. He should take up this position for half an hour at a time at least four times a day and should be encouraged to practise intermittent expansion exercises whilst in this position.

Treatment should be continued until chest expansion is equal and the X-ray has improved.

EMPYEMA

This is a localised collection of pus in the pleural cavity. It is most commonly a complication of lobar pneumonia but it may also be associated with bronchiectasis or due to spread of infection from a lung abscess, subphrenic abscess, mediastinal sepsis, a chest wound or a complication of thoracic surgery. It may also result from a tuberculous infection of the pleural cavity.

CLINICAL FEATURES

Empyema most commonly occurs one to two weeks after the start of a pneumococcal pneumonia. Instead of the normal process of recovery, the patient remains ill, the temperature begins to rise again and is of a remittent character accompanied by drenching sweats; there is general malaise and anorexia.

Examination of the chest reveals signs of fluid, i.e. dullness to percussion and absent or diminished breath sounds over the area; in children there may be bronchial breathing over the area which may lead to the erroneous diagnosis of unresolved pneumonia.

Postero-anterior and lateral X-rays will reveal the locality of the fluid and diagnosis will be confirmed by aspiration. In the early stages of empyema the fluid is thin and serous but in the later stages it becomes thick and purulent. The aspirated fluid should be cultured for organisms. Fluid may become loculated and difficult to aspirate.

PROGNOSIS

With correct treatment, the prognosis for empyema is good.

TREATMENT

The aims of treatment are control of infection, removal of pus and obliteration of the empyema space.

In the early stages of empyema, the infected pleural effusion must be aspirated daily and an appropriate antibiotic should be injected into the pleural cavity. An antibiotic should also be given orally or parenterally. These measures will usually result in a cure. In the case of tuberculous empyema, antituberculous drugs will be given.

If this treatment is not effective, the aspirated fluid will become thick and purulent and a chronic empyema will develop. In this case, surgical intervention will be necessary by means of a decortication or drainage by rib resection (see p. 158).

Physiotherapy will be on the same lines as for pleural effusion, although chest deformity is more likely to occur and recovery will be slower.

Pre- and postoperative treatment may be required.

HAEMOTHORAX

Haemothorax usually follows trauma to the chest wall, but it may also be associated with pneumothorax, when it is known as haemopneumothorax. Occasionally an aneurysm may rupture into the pleural cavity and cause a haemothorax.

Blood in the pleural cavity clots rapidly and fibrin will be deposited on the pleural surfaces. Pleural reaction will occur with further outpouring of fluid. If blood is left in the pleural cavity, pleural fibrosis occurs which will result in serious interference with lung function.

CLINICAL FEATURES

If pleural bleeding is excessive, the patient will be shocked and collapsed, with rapid pulse and respiration. There may not be external evidence of trauma but there will be signs of fluid in the chest. Diagnosis will be confirmed by aspiration of blood from the pleural cavity. It is important to distinguish between the presence of haemorrhage and blood-stained pleural effusion.

TREATMENT

General treatment for internal haemorrhage should be given. The effusion should be aspirated daily in order to keep the pleural space as dry as possible. Antibiotics should be given at this stage as there is danger of secondary infection.

Surgical intervention may be necessary in cases of severe bleeding or damage to the chest wall, or if the blood cannot be evacuated by aspiration.

Physiotherapy will be as for pleural effusion once the haemorrhage has been controlled.

SPONTANEOUS PNEUMOTHORAX

A collection of air in the pleural cavity as a result of a pathological process is known as a spontaneous pneumothorax.

Spontaneous pneumothorax most commonly occurs in young males and is caused by the rupture of a bleb under the visceral pleura. It is thought these blebs are caused by a congenital defect in the alveolar wall.

It may also complicate lung disease such as asthma, emphysema, pulmonary tuberculosis, congenital cysts, cystic fibrosis, lung abscess and pneumoconiosis. Air in the pleural cavity may also be caused by wounds, perforation of the oesophagus or trachea, or following thoracic surgery.

When a spontaneous pneumothorax occurs as the result of a ruptured bleb, the leak usually seals off rapidly and air in the pleural cavity absorbs in a week or so. Occasionally a valve-like leak occurs and air will enter the pleural cavity on inspiration but is unable to escape on expiration; this leads to an accumulation of air and is known as a tension pneumothorax.

CLINICAL FEATURES

Onset is usually sudden and is associated with pain on the affected side of the chest and dyspnoea. It is occasionally precipitated by a sudden movement. The degree of distress suffered varies according to the size of the pneumothorax and the condition of the lungs.

On examination, the chest movement will be diminished on the affected side. There will be mediastinal displacement away from the affected side, the degree varying according to the size of the pneumothorax. The percussion note is either normal or hyper-resonant. There will be diminished breath sounds over the site of the pneumothorax.

The development of a tension pneumothorax will be indicated by increasing dyspnoea, cyanosis and distress. There will be signs of a pneumothorax with considerable mediastinal displacement. Measures to relieve the tension must be taken immediately, otherwise death may occur.

The chest X-ray will show air in the pleural cavity with a varying amount of lung collapse.

TREATMENT

When a spontaneous pneumothorax has been diagnosed shortly after onset, it is wiser to admit the patient to hospital as there is always a risk of tension pneumothorax or haemopneumothorax developing.

If there is a large pneumothorax or if the patient is in great distress, a needle should be inserted into the pleural space and the pressure recorded; if a tension pneumothorax has occurred the pressure will become positive instead of negative. It is often necessary to insert a pleural drain connected to an underwater seal, then expansion of the lung will usually take place within a day or so. If expansion fails to take place, or if the pneumothorax recurs, it may be necessary to consider pleurodesis (the induction of chemical pleurisy), abrasion pleurodesis or pleurectomy.

If the pneumothorax is very small, the patient should rest in bed for a few days and re-expansion will probably occur without further measures being taken.

Physiotherapy is contra-indicated in the early treatment of spontaneous pneumothorax. Once a drainage tube has been inserted, breathing exercises may be ordered to obtain full re-expansion of the lung and expansion exercises should be given to all areas of the affected side. Full range arm movements should also be given.

If pleurodesis is carried out the patient will have a severe pleural reaction and breathing exercises should be started the day after introduction of the irritant substance into the pleural cavity. Treatment will be on the same lines as for pleural effusion but the patient is often in a great deal of pain and it is helpful to administer an analgesic before treatment is attempted. A drainage tube is often inserted and arm exercises should also be given.

If pleurectomy is to be carried out, pre- and postoperative physiotherapy will be necessary (see p. 157).

REFERENCE

Oswald, N. C., Hinson, K. F. W., Canti, G. and Miller, A. A. (1971). 'The Diagnosis of Primary Lung Cancer with Special Reference to Sputum Cytology.' *Thorax*, 26, 623.

BIBLIOGRAPHY

Anderson, C. M. and Goodchild, M. C. (1976). *Cystic Fibrosis. Manual of Diagnosis and Management*. Blackwell Scientific Publications.
Basmajian, J. M. (1971). *Grant's Method of Anatomy*, 8th ed. The Williams and Wilkins Co., Baltimore.
Bates, D. V., Macklem, P. T. and Christie, R. V. (1971). *Respiratory Function in Disease*. W. B. Saunders Co., Philadelphia, London, Toronto.
Chest and Heart Association (1964). *Cystic Fibrosis*.
Houston, J. C., Joiner, C. L. and Trounce, J. R. (1975). *A Short Textbook of Medicine*. English Universities Press.
Last, R. J. (1972). *Anatomy — Regional and Applied*, 5th ed. Churchill-Livingstone.
Miller, G. A. H. and Sutton, G. C. (1970). 'Massive pulmonary embolism.' *British Journal of Hospital Medicine*, June.
Reid, Lynne (1967). *The Pathology of Emphysema*. Lloyd-Luke (Medical Books) Ltd.
Thacker, E. W. (1971). *Postural Drainage and Respiratory Control*. Lloyd-Luke (Medical Books) Ltd.
West, J. B. (1976). *Respiratory Physiology — the Essentials*. The Williams and Wilkins Co., Baltimore.

ACKNOWLEDGEMENT

The author expresses her thanks to Dr. J. V. Collins, M.D., M.R.C.P. for his help in the revision of these chapters.

Chapter 15

Common Diseases of Blood Vessels and their Investigations

by J. PICKERING, M.C.S.P. and R. BOURNE, F.R.C.S.

The number of people affected by vascular diseases is increasing yearly, and more are dying from either these disorders or their complications.

As yet there is no definite known cause for atherosclerosis, but many factors appear to have some effect on the course of the disease. These are mainly wrong diet, obesity and hypertension. A raised serum cholesterol level and a soft water supply are believed by some schools of thought to increase the risk of disease. Cigarette smoking is believed by many people to be an important factor because some diseases, e.g. Buerger's disease, seem to be arrested when the patient gives up smoking. Smokers, according to some surveys, run twice the risk of myocardial infarction as do non-smokers. The risk lessens on giving up smoking. Peripheral arterial disease occurs in only 1% of non-smokers compared with up to 30% of the average population. Men who smoke and have a raised serum cholesterol level and hypertension have ten times the risk of coronary disease as men in whom all three factors are absent (Framlingham study). Men and women in the 30 to 60 age group with a raised systolic pressure show a high rate of coronary disease and morbidity. 'Strokes' and abdominal aneurysms are also more common in hypertensive patients according to post-mortem evidence.

ATHEROSCLEROSIS

Obliterative arterial disease is the commonest cause of death in middle and later life. Men are affected more often than women, and those in the 60 to 70 age group are more at risk (though the incidence in younger people is increasing). The nature of the disease is still uncertain; in fact there is not even agreement on the meaning of the name itself. Crawford in 1960 defined atherosclerosis as the 'widely prevalent arterial lesion characterised by patchy thickening comprising accumulations of fat and layers of collagen-like fibres, both being present in widely varying proportions'.

Suggestions have been made that the aortic intima may buckle due to the shearing action of the pulse wave, but this is not universally accepted. The thickening of the intima leads to narrowing of the lumen and eventually to complete occlusion.

The disease is generalised, thus if it is present in one limb it is likely that the coronary and cerebral arteries and the vessels of the other limbs are also involved.

As the lumen of the vessels becomes diminished, the blood flow decreases. Many people may not notice this because their normal activities are low, but the more active person will feel the effects of ischaemia during exercise. Eventually, as flow continues to decrease, a level may be reached when the area becomes ischaemic even at rest, and at this stage nutrition may be inadequate to maintain life of the tissues and gangrene may develop.

INTERMITTENT CLAUDICATION

The symptom which usually causes a patient to seek advice is pain. This is initially pain on exercise though later it becomes rest pain. Pain occurs in the region supplied by the affected artery after a regular amount of work of a given group of muscles, and is relieved by rest. It develops again on repetition of that amount of work. As the disease progresses so pain develops on decreased amounts of exercise. Thus a patient may be able to walk 100 yards before the onset of pain in the calf. This forces him to stand still until the pain has subsided, then he can repeat the distance. Gradually the distance he can walk before pain forces him to stop decreases. The pain is usually described as cramp-like or as a tight feeling in the calf which causes him to limp.

The most common site for block is at the femoro-popliteal junction, but changes may occur at other sites (see Fig. 15/1), when the symptoms produced are not so immediately obvious and may lead to confusion in diagnosis. Thus an aorto-iliac block may appear as backache and anterior tibial compartment syndrome as a foot problem.

The explanation of intermittent claudication lies in the fact that in walking, the gastrocnemius and soleus muscles need extra blood; if the vessels are normal the arterial bed in the muscles becomes wide open to supply the need and avoid ischaemia. The pressure in the normal vessels maintains the bed open during the phase in which the

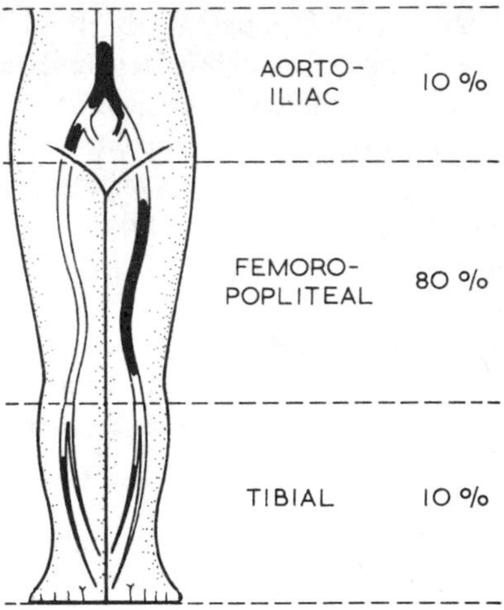

Fig. 15/1 The sites where blocks most commonly occur in the lower limbs

AORTO-ILIAC	10 %
FEMORO-POPLITEAL	80 %
TIBIAL	10 %

muscles relax. If the vessels are diseased and the blood supply therefore deficient the pressure will not be adequate to perfuse the muscles. Hyperaemia and post-exercise inflow are smaller and slower than in normal vessels.

Almost all people who present with intermittent claudication have at least one absent pulse.

From follow-ups on patients suffering from this disease, it has been found that they are more likely to die or become seriously disabled from atherosclerosis of the coronary or cerebral arteries than from increased severity of the disease in the peripheral vessels or from loss of a limb. Over 50% of the patients die from myocardial infarcts, the next highest group being 14% from cerebrovascular accidents.

REST PAIN

Rest pain develops when the resting blood level is lower than is needed for adequate perfusion. During sleep there is widespread vasodilation of the whole body, with gradual shunting of the blood away from the affected limb. The pain threshold is eventually reached, the patient wakes up in pain and hangs the leg over the side of the bed to refill the blood vessels. At this stage skin changes begin to appear and nail growth slows down. These symptoms may be relieved by sympathectomy or by reconstructive surgery where possible.

As the disease progresses, muscle wasting and gangrene may occur.

GANGRENE

This implies death with putrefaction of the involved parts. The distal part of a limb is usually affected. It can be due to atheroma directly occluding the vessel, infection from boils or gas-gangrene (*Clostridium welchii*), trauma or physical means such as burns, frostbite and electrical damage. Gangrene can be either dry or wet.

Dry gangrene occurs when there is gradual slowing of the blood supply as in atherosclerosis. The area demarcates and separation occurs. Quite often no surgery is needed other than tidying up of the distal portion.

Wet gangrene occurs when the area is suddenly deprived of blood. Infection is usually present and there is a surrounding area of inflammation extending higher than the line of demarcation.

ULCERATION

The legs are the sites of many types of ulcers. Venous ulcers are discussed in Chapter 19. Arterial ulcers may result from thrombosis of diseased arteries though gangrene of the most distal area, e.g. the toes, is most common. Patches of gangrene due to trauma, pressure or mild infection may occur anywhere. The patches of necrosed tissue may develop into deep sloughing ulcers, leaving deep structures, such as tendon and bone exposed. Unlike venous ulcers these are usually painful.

Treatment includes warmth, relief of pressure and rest. Sympathectomy may help by improving blood flow and so warmth. If the oxygen-carrying capacity of the blood is increased e.g. by hyperbaric oxygen (see references), tissues may survive when under normal situations they would not. Hyperbaric oxygen can be given either locally or generally in a hyperbaric chamber. Oxygen is given at 2 to 3 atmospheres of pressure for a given period of time. The patient is then decompressed and rested. This treatment may be administered twice a day for several days. This is still not widely available and there is considerable controversy as to whether it does have a beneficial effect on arterial disease. The ulcer however will not heal unless the circulation improves and an adequate amount of blood reaches the ischaemic area. Many patients come to amputation because the pain is so severe and there is little chance of the healing of the ulcer.

ARTERIAL THROMBOSIS AND EMBOLISM

A thrombosis is a solid body forming within a blood vessel where there is some irregularity in the vessel wall. The lumen of the vessel may be widened or narrowed or there may be an atheromatous plaque. The thrombus consists of platelets and leucocytes with fibrin and red cells. It may occlude the whole artery so that the only blood flow in that part is through the collaterals, and these vessels may themselves eventually be affected by atherosclerosis.

Should a part or the whole of the thrombus become detached before it completely blocks the vessel, it becomes an embolus and may lodge at the bifurcation of, or block, a smaller artery.

It has been stated that there are no differences in the symptomology of embolic and thrombotic obstruction of an artery. With few exceptions the manifestations and symptoms of both forms of obstruction are the direct or indirect results of limb ischaemia. Usually there is a feeling of numbness followed by the onset of pain on movement. The limb is pale, cold and the superficial veins are collapsed showing as thin blue lines. With a few exceptions the pulses will be absent. Often hyperaesthesia is present with muscle weakness. An operation is often essential as the distal point will die from lack of nutrition and accumulation of metabolites. As this is a sudden advance there is not usually time for a collateral circulation to develop.

Survival of the limb depends therefore on the rate at which blood flow is returned to the limb. If embolectomy (see p. 289) is considered then it should be performed within 6 to 10 hours from onset for a good result.

ANEURYSMS

An aneurysm is defined as a localised swelling of a pulsating vessel. Aneurysms were first recognised as long ago as the second century,

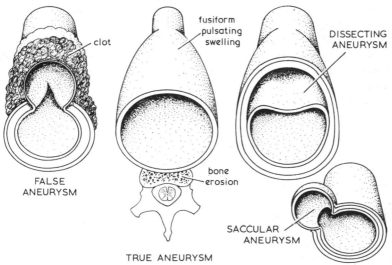

Fig. 15/2   Types of aneurysms

but it was only in the latter half of this century that replacement grafts began to be undertaken (see p. 294) and since that time treatment by such surgery has become more common practice.

FALSE ANEURYSMS (see Fig. 15/2)

These are due to damage to the artery either in surgery or by direct injury. Bleeding occurs and continues until the pressure of blood in the haematoma equals that of the artery. The haematoma organises and gradually a central cavity communicating with the lumen of the artery develops. This cavity becomes lined with endothelium continuous with that of the damaged vessel.

TRUE ANEURYSMS (see Fig. 15/2)

These are mainly the result of vascular disease, most commonly atherosclerosis. The weakened arterial wall gradually dilates with consequent thinning of all its coats. This dilatation may be saccular or fusiform in shape (see Fig. 15/2). It can occur in any artery but those most usually affected are the aorta and popliteal arteries.

Symptoms

Some aneurysms give rise to negligible symptoms. The artery concerned may widen over a long distance so that the upper and lower limits are often difficult to assess prior to surgery. This type of aneurysm is more common in the older patient in whom activity is gradually lessening and consequently it may remain undetected.

When symptoms do occur they are usually the result of pressure. The aneurysm may actually press on the branches, obstructing the blood flow. This is often observed when the popliteal artery is involved, and it may result in ischaemia and gangrene in the foot. Adjacent veins may be compressed giving rise to venous stasis, oedema and thrombosis. A pulsating sac pressing on bone may cause erosion, thus a thoracic or abdominal aortic aneurysm may destroy a vertebra and paraplegia may result. Pressure on neighbouring nerves will cause pain and muscular weakness.

Many patients however do not present until the aneurysm is in danger of rupturing.

Diagnosis

There is usually a pulsating mass which can be painless or may give rise to symptoms due to pressure.

Plain X-rays may show in a lateral view erosion of bone if the aneurysm is long-standing. The shadowy outline of the aneurysm may show up, as would calcification if this has occurred in the aneurysmal sac.

Aortograms are carried out if possible to give the surgeon a more definite picture of what he will find. A water-soluble contrast medium is injected into the aorta to define the limits of the aneurysm.

Dissecting aneurysms occur when there is a tear in the tunica intima (see Fig. 15/2). Blood passes into the media and tracks up and down in the artery. This may be treated by drastically lowering the blood pressure and putting the patient on complete bed rest. Careful monitoring of size is necessary to make sure it is no longer increasing. Once stable then replacement of the affected segment can be more safely undertaken or a re-entry operation performed (see p. 298).

BUERGER'S DISEASE

There is some doubt as to whether this disease does exist as a separate entity. Certainly a disease in which the distal vessels become inflamed, thrombosed and eventually obliterated does exist. This is a disease in which cigarette smoking is thought to be one of the main causes. If the patient can be persuaded to stop smoking, the progress of the disease is slowed down and may practically stop.

Both arms and legs may be affected, although usually the disease starts in the vessels of one limb. Even with incipient gangrene, the pulses are usually present but rest pain is a feature and is often acute. The distal areas of the limbs are red and the nails deformed. As the disease becomes chronic, the skin appears thin and the toes become blue.

Reconstruction is not always possible because it is a distal vessel disease so there are no decent vessels on to which a graft may be attached. Smoking must definitely be stopped with, hopefully, recession of the disease. Vasodilators can be used and Buerger's exercises practised (see p. 286). Great care is needed to keep the toes and fingers healthy as once infection develops the wounds will fail to heal.

RAYNAUD'S DISEASE

This disease is characterised by spasm of the digital arterioles. Raynaud himself did not actually describe a disease as such but rather a syndrome of intermittent claudication which occurs after subjection to cold. The cause of primary disease is not fully known but it may be hereditary. The incidence is greater in females and in cool damp climates.

The spasm of the digital arterioles causes capillary flow to cease so that the fingers or toes go white and numb. As the spasm disappears there is a reactive hyperaemia, the colour of the fingers changes from blue to red, they throb, and the patient experiences 'pins and needles'. In some patients, as the disease advances, the spasm fails to relax completely and in the course of time actual necrosis of the finger-tips may develop.

Similar phenomena may occur in diseases such as arteriosclerosis, embolism, cervical rib, and in connective tissue and blood diseases and may be known as secondary phenomena.

Whether the disease is primary or secondary, the main feature is the intermittent appearance of the symptoms with progressive ischaemia leading to necrosis.

DIABETES

In diabetics the small distal vessels become involved and ulcerated areas develop. As there is often associated neuropathy these can occur from badly fitting footwear. It is important that the diabetes is adequately controlled otherwise there will be failure to heal and infection will just increase. This condition may present on its own or may be present with atherosclerosis.

INVESTIGATIONS

General examination

As we have seen, most patients with arterial disease have generalised atherosclerosis and may have had or are at risk from coronary or cerebral thrombosis so that a chest X-ray and E.C.G. are mandatory. Other disease such as peptic ulceration, diabetes, anaemia or polycythaemia are often present and should be excluded by the relevant investigations.

Local examination

The colour varies from dead white to mottled purple with a shiny atrophic skin and loss of normal hair distribution. In the pre-gangrenous state swelling and small haemorrhages are often present, the skin being withered and dry with loss of sweating. The limb is cold unless infection has become evident when it may feel warmer. A secondary fungal infection is often found in skin folds e.g. between the toes. Loss of sensation and reduced movement are signs of

A Summary of How to Recognise Sites of Obstruction

SIGNS AND SYMPTOMS	BIFURCATION OF AORTA	BIFURCATION OF ILIAC ARTERY	BIFURCATION OF COMMON FEMORAL ARTERY	TRIFURCATION OF POPLITEAL ARTERY
Pain	Mainly whole of lower extremities	Mainly whole of lower extremities	Foot and leg below knee	Foot, calf, ankle
Numbness	Legs, thighs	Leg, thigh	Foot, ankle	Foot, ankle, lower $\frac{1}{3}$ of leg
Cold as symptom	Entire lower extremity (Bil.)	Entire lower extremity	Leg, lower part of thigh	Leg
Paraesthesia	Legs	Leg	Foot, ankle	Foot, ankle, calf
Pulses	None below aorta	None below aorta on affected side	None below common femoral artery	None below femoral artery
Mottling Pallor	Both extremities, lower abdomen, trunk	Lower extremity to groin	Lower extremity to upper $\frac{1}{3}$ of thigh	Foot, ankle, leg
Cold as sign	Groins	To groin	Nearly to knee	Knee
Hyperaesthesia	Legs	Leg	Foot and sometimes ankle	Foot, ankle, lower $\frac{1}{3}$ of leg
Weakness	Hips, lower extremities	Lower extremity	Foot, ankle	Foot, ankle, knee
Paralysis	Thighs, legs, feet	Leg and foot	Toes, sometimes foot or ankle	Toes and foot

ischaemia and in the pre-gangrenous state the limb should be handled carefully as hyperaesthesia is also often present.

The detection of arterial pulsation as an indicator of flow either by palpation or auscultation over the course of the main arteries is essential in all patients. An increased pulsation with an audible bruit (or murmur) on listening indicates aneurysmal dilatation and therefore disease; a murmur without dilatation suggests narrowing of the vessel. The sounds heard are due to abnormal turbulence of blood within the lumen of the vessel. The lack of venous refilling also supports the diagnosis of poor arterial flow.

Physiological Measurements

The volume of flow to the tissues such as skin and muscle determines the oxygen supply and removal of waste products; this is a factor of the pressure difference between two points divided by the resistance.

$$\text{Flow} = \frac{\text{pressure difference}}{\text{resistance}}$$

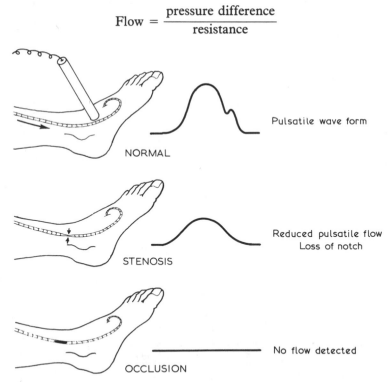

Pulsatile wave form

NORMAL

Reduced pulsatile flow
Loss of notch

STENOSIS

No flow detected

OCCLUSION

Fig. 15/3   Diagram of the wave form using a Doppler flow probe on the dorsalis pedis artery

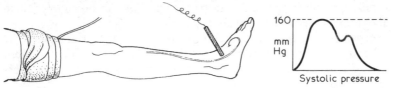

Fig. 15/4   Diagram to show technique and the pressure trace at the ankle following exercise in a patient with peripheral vascular disease, using the flow probe

Flow can either be measured directly, indirectly or by predicting its volume from the pressure and resistance.

Pressure can be measured directly by inserting a needle into the vessel and reading the level from a manometer or by transducing the pressure into an electrical signal. Direct pressure is thus commonly measured in the central vein and less commonly in the peripheral vein, portal vein system or from a peripheral artery.

Flow can be measured by detection of marker dilution; directly applied flow meters such as the electromagnetic flow probe which requires to be placed around the vessel and can only be used at operation, or the ultrasound 'Doppler' flow probe where ultrasound is beamed at a moving wave front of blood, producing a frequency shift which is a function of the rate of blood flow. By applying the probe over the skin a semi-qualitative measurement is obtained and flow patterns varying with the degree of obstruction recorded (see Fig. 15/3).

The flow is absent in a total occlusion with no collateral flow. This is an extremely useful instrument which in addition to indicating changes in flow can be used to measure pressure in an indirect way when flow is present but the peripheral pulse by palpation is absent. Readings are taken before exercise, immediately after and two to five minutes later. In a normal person the resting systolic pressure in the limb concerned does not alter significantly after exercise; in peripheral vascular disease, however, there is a drop in the pressure at the calf (see Fig. 15/4).

Tissue clearance of a local marker, such as ^{133}Xe, a radio-isotope that can be detected by counting the gamma emission with a Geiger counter, can be used to measure skin or muscle blood flow.

Plethysmography (venous occlusion) can be used to measure skin (hand or foot) and muscle (forearm, calf) flow.

Thermography, *skin temperature*, and *oscillometry* only indicate qualitative changes.

Treadmill: By walking the patient under controlled conditions on a moving platform at a standard incline repeated measurements of a patient's exercise tolerance can be made. This can be coupled with flow measurements as indicated above.

Arteriography: By injecting contrast medium into the arteries to be studied, e.g. the aorta and lower limb vessels, the course, size, stenoses, dilatations and state of collaterals can be seen. Then catheters can be introduced in a retrograde fashion e.g. transfemoral arteriography or by direct puncture e.g. lumbar aortogram. By skilled manipulation of the catheter tip most organs in the body can be studied in this way e.g. kidney, liver, gut, cerebral circulation.

Biochemical and Haematological Studies

We have seen how changes in the patient's fat metabolism can predispose to atherosclerosis and how diabetics suffer from small blood vessel changes. It is therefore obvious that other conditions are important when considering the pathological changes in arterial disease. Conditions which are known to increase the viscosity and hence reduce the flow of blood must be detected if patients are to be relieved of their symptoms or surgical operations are to succeed. The following tests are some of the important ones included in the screening of patients with vascular disease.

BIOCHEMICAL

By measuring fasting serum cholesterol, lipoprotein and triglyceride levels, patients' fat abnormalities can be classified and thus treated. Fibrinogen when elevated can be reduced and so reduce blood viscosity. Diabetes must always be detected by urine analysis and blood sugar estimations.

HAEMATOLOGY

Blood is examined for evidence of polycythaemia, platelet abnormalities and clotting changes.

OTHER FACTORS

Blood is screened for serological evidence of rheumatoid arthritis, polyarthritis and syphilis which are all known to predispose to various pathological changes in blood vessels from small vessel disease to aneurysm formation. Other collagen diseases such as scleroderma and systemic lupus erythematosus must also be considered.

These are only some of the main factors which are studied in patients with proven or suspected arterial disease and which have been shown to be important both aetiologically and with an increased morbidity. As our knowledge increases patients will benefit from these more accurate screening methods and eventually it is hoped that many conditions will be prevented or reversed by correct treatment of the underlying abnormalities.

REFERENCES

Crawford, T. (1960). 'Some Aspects of the Pathology of Atherosclerosis.' *Proceedings of the Royal Society of Medicine.*
Framingham (1962). 'Enquiry.' *Proceedings of the Royal Society of Medicine.*
Proceedings of the 2nd International Congress of Hyperbaric Oxygenation. (1964). Churchill Livingstone.

BIBLIOGRAPHY

See end of Chapter 18.

Chapter 16

Veins and Lymphatics

by R. BOURNE, F.R.C.S.

In this chapter we look at the more common disorders of the venous system, a knowledge of which is essential when caring for patients on both the medical and surgical wards. Also included is a brief review of the lymphatic system as diseases of the system are often looked after by general and arterial surgeons as well as general physicians and general practitioners. Figure 16/1 shows the basic anatomy of the veins of the lower limb.

VARICOSE VEINS

A vein is varicose when it is dilated and tortuous; many sites are affected e.g. oesophageal, haemorrhoidal and spermatic but the veins of the leg are most commonly involved. They are usually thought of as a minor condition but as many as 10% of all admissions are patients with varicose vein disease and its complications.

Primary Varicose Veins

Saccular dilatation develops spontaneously and often the veins are tortuous. There seems to be no simple explanation of their development, though several factors may precipitate varicosity.

Inherited structural weakness may be present in the walls of the vein e.g. defective collagen. Some authorities believe that this alone would not cause varicosities but that it may be one factor among many. The erect posture of the human body must therefore play some part in the development of varicosity. Occupations which involve prolonged standing have a higher incidence of the disease, as do labouring and other heavy jobs.

Obesity leads to large deposits of fatty tissue around the larger vessels and so increases the pressure in the veins.

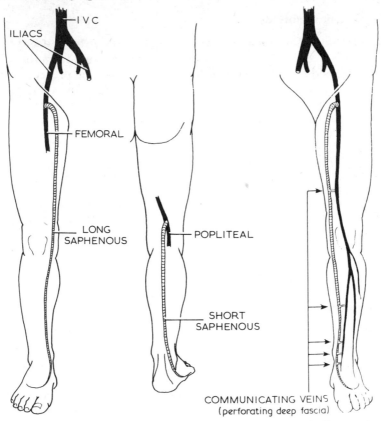

Fig. 16/1 The basic anatomy of the veins of the lower limb (Deep veins black)

During pregnancy minor varicose veins may become worse due to the increased abdominal pressure on the iliac veins.

Secondary Varicose Veins

In these cases the veins become varicose distal to venous obstruction. This may be due to obstruction to free, deep venous flow by outside pressure on the veins such as benign or malignant intra-pelvic tumours or even tight-fitting abdominal garments. Deep vein thrombosis in the lower extremities may destroy the valves which normally prevent flow from deep to superficial veins. Two rare causes are arteriovenous fistulae, which raise the venous pressure, and venous angiomata. These will be discussed in Chapter 18.

Signs and Symptoms

Venous blood flows forwards from the superficial vein to the deep vein and back to the right side of the heart under pressure from the left ventricle and the calf muscle pump, reverse flow being prevented by competent valves. When the valves in the communicating veins from the superficial to the deep system become incompetent the pressure in the superficial veins rises and symptoms are produced:

Ugly tortuous veins
Aching pain due to high venous pressure
Oedema due to reduced absorption of tissue fluid
Brown pigmentation due to blood leaking from capillaries
Fat necrosis, eczema and ischaemia of the skin with ulceration
Complications include thrombophlebitis with hard tender cord like
  veins, haemorrhage which follows spontaneous rupture of thin
  walled veins, and periostitis in underlying bone and talipes equinus
  due to long standing ulceration.

Investigation

This is designed to localise the sites of communication between the deep and superficial venous systems and the incompetent perforators, as treatment is to stop these leaks. Clinical methods by palpating the veins while the patient is coughing often detects the incompetent sites and the use of tourniquets localises these levels further. Other more scientific methods such as thermography, ultrasound and phlebography can also help.

Treatment

This is aimed at reducing or abolishing the leakage of blood from the deep to superficial systems at the site of incompetent communicating veins and may be conservative, by injections or surgery.

CONSERVATIVE TREATMENT

This aims at supporting varicose veins and preventing flow from deep to superficial vessels, so keeping the dilatations empty. This is achieved by firm elastic support by the use of one-way stretch bandages or elastic stockings (see Fig. 16/2). The patient is advised on how to apply the bandages and how to care for them. He is told to rest with the legs elevated and to avoid prolonged standing. Foot bending and stretching will stimulate the soleal pump and aid venous return.

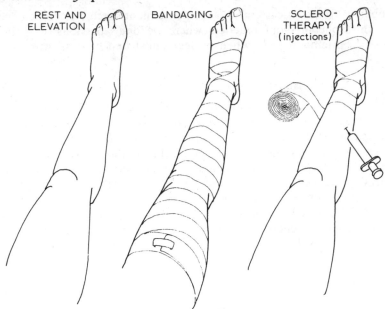

Fig. 16/2 Diagram to illustrate 3 conservative methods of treatment for varicose veins

He is also warned to avoid damage to the skin and instructed on what to do if the vein should rupture.

These measures are not curative but are suitable for elderly patients, those suffering from debilitating illness and those unsuitable for or unwilling to undergo surgery.

Physiotherapy is not usually ordered but many patients being treated for other conditions suffer also from varicosities and it is essential in this case for the physiotherapist to take precautions to avoid minor damage to the area.

INJECTIONS

A sclerosing fluid is injected into the affected vein to damage the intima of the vessel and thrombosis occurs obliterating the lumen and preventing blood flow through the vessel. The limb is bandaged to help the adhesion of the damaged intimal surfaces and the patient is encouraged to walk once the bandages are applied (see Fig. 16/2). This relatively simple method deals with the superficial veins and if injected at the site of incompetent perforators can be very effective; it does carry a risk of thrombosis spreading to the deep veins and occasional sensitivity reactions are encountered. It is becoming obvious from clinical trials that for permanent success incompetence at the saphenofemoral junction (where the long saphenous vein joins the deep femoral vein) when present, must first be dealt with surgically.

SURGERY (see Fig. 16/3)

This consists of ligating the incompetent perforators from above down starting at the point where the long saphenous joins the femoral vein. This can be achieved by stripping the veins from the ankle to the groin although many surgeons avoid doing this as the vein can often be useful in later life for reconstructive arterial surgery. This leg is then firmly bandaged and after 12 hours of elevation of the leg the patient is encouraged to get up and walk. The bandage is kept on for three to six weeks. The physiotherapist can often help with the early mobilisation and encouragement of the patient. Early and active movement lessens the potentially dangerous extension of thrombosis into the deep veins and possible pulmonary embolus.

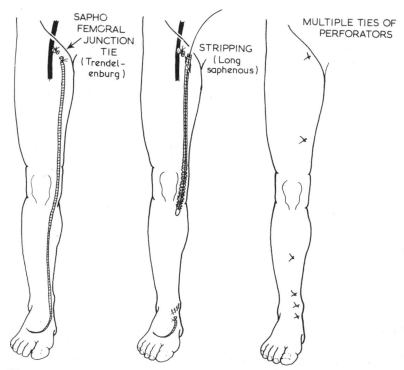

Fig. 16/3   Diagram to illustrate some surgical methods of treatment for varicose veins

Treatment of the Complications

Thrombophlebitis: early ambulation with elastic support.

Eczema: prevention of itching and secondary infection. Lanolin is often used to soften the skin and topical steroids are often employed.

Venous ulcers: (see Chapter 19).

Haemorrhage: local pressure and elevation. A tourniquet should not be applied as the pressure is often inappropriate.

Talipes equinus: here the physiotherapist can help with remedial exercises.

DEEP VEIN THROMBOSIS

Deep vein thrombosis (D.V.T.), and often fatal pulmonary embolism are very important complications of routine surgery, medical illness and following childbirth. When possible these complications should be prevented or at least adequately treated. The aetiology of thrombosis has been discussed in an earlier chapter and can be due to changes in the vessel wall and damaged endothelium; reduced blood flow as seen during operation, periods of inactivity, debilitating disease and compression of the pelvic veins by tumour or pregnancy; and hypercoagulability of the blood.

The results are seen locally as occlusion with late calcification and occasionally localised abscess formation. Oedema then occurs with later development of superficial vein varicosities. When the clot extends or propagates, more major veins such as the iliacs may be occluded; if the clot becomes detached pulmonary embolus occurs.

Diagnosis

It is important to establish the site and extent of the disease in order to institute adequate treatment. When gross, the clinical signs of oedema and swelling, dilatation of the superficial veins and increased skin temperature enable the diagnosis to be made.

The fibrinogen uptake test: This utilises fibrinogen labelled with the radio-isotope I^{125} and which when injected is taken up either by pre-existing thrombus or is laid down in new clot formation, thus enabling early detection of thrombus. This test has revealed that 30% of all patients undergoing surgical operations have thrombosis present in the deep veins.

Further information can be obtained by using the ultrasound flow detector and by phlebography. The latter, a technique of injecting contrast medium into a vein in the foot and taking X-rays of the venous system which is then outlined enables the extent of the thrombus to be seen and estimation of its age to be made. This is important in predicting whether the clot might detach itself from the circulation and so cause a pulmonary embolus. Chest X-rays, E.C.G., isotope lung scans and arteriography are all important in investigating the possibility of a pulmonary embolus.

Treatment of Deep Vein Thrombosis

A variety of treatments are available, the indications varying with each individual patient. Medical opinion also varies as to the best methods used.

NON-SURGICAL

Supporting crêpe bandage with an anticoagulant given either intravenously as heparin or orally as warfarin form the mainstay of treatment. Sometimes the patient is kept in bed with the leg elevated; at the other extreme the patient is kept ambulatory. Physicians and surgeons vary as to their use of long- or short-term anticoagulants. Clot can also be dissolved (lysed) by the judicious use of streptokinase or urokinase, but they cannot be used immediately after surgery or trauma as bleeding is a major complication.

Surgery

Thrombectomy – the surgical removal of the clot – has a part to play although thrombosis can occur rapidly unless anticoagulation is also employed. It is often combined with vein ligation.

In recurrent pulmonary emboli veins are often tied off or partially interrupted e.g. plication of the vena cava. An 'umbrella' device is also available which can be introduced into the vena cava from a large peripheral vein and when 'opened' acts as a filter to prevent large clots reaching the lungs.

LATE COMPLICATIONS

Swelling due to oedema of the limbs and varicose veins has been discussed earlier. Recannulation of the thrombosed system does occur and this prevents many of the serious consequences of the so-called post-phlebotomy syndrome.

Prevention of Deep Vein Thrombosis

This is a very important but still controversial subject as to the best methods currently available although all surgeons and physicians agree that some method should be instituted at least with high risk patients. The high risk group included all patients over 40 years and those with malignant disease, vein obstruction, previous history of D.V.T. and women on the contraceptive pill. The methods can be summarised under the following headings.

REDUCTION IN STASIS AND PREVENTION OF VENOUS FLOW

The main methods are elevation of the legs, elastic stockings, passive movement of the foot, intermittent compression of the calf with pneumatic stockings and the stimulation of the muscle contraction with an electric current. Pre- and postoperative encouragement of active movement of the leg is an important function of the physio-therapist.

REDUCTION IN BLOOD HYPERCOAGULABILITY

Small doses of heparin, when given subcutaneously, reduce the inci-dence of thrombosis and possibly pulmonary embolus although this has still to be proven by clinical trials. Low molecular weight dextran given intravenously has the same beneficial effect. Much research is still being carried out in this important field of preventive medicine.

PORTAL VENOUS SYSTEM

Although this is usually discussed when considering diseases of the liver, a short note is included here as both general and vascular surgeons are often called upon to operate when portal hypertension has occurred and diversion from the portal to the systemic venous system is required.

The portal veins carry blood from the intestine, pancreas and spleen to the liver; 60–80% of the blood to the liver is carried in this way. Obstruction of this system occurs in the portal vein itself, within the liver or in the extremely rare post-hepatic vein obstruction. Clinically patients with high pressure in the portal system have varices develop-ing in the oesophagus, rectum or around the umbilicus, viz at sites where the portal and venous systems meet. When patients bleed from these sites, the most serious bleeding from the oesophagus, operations are often performed in the portal system. Different methods are available e.g. porto-caval, spleno-renal, mesenterico-caval; the prin-ciple of treatment being to bypass the area of obstruction and there-fore to reduce the pressure and prevent the complications of bleeding.

LYMPHATIC SYSTEM

This consists of dermal capillaries which drain via plexuses into main connecting trunks that follow the course of superficial veins. Thus, in the leg they run with the long and short saphenous veins into deep trunks in the groin and popliteal fossa and thence into the inguinal, iliac and eventually via the cisterna chyli into the subclavian veins. Flow is achieved by contraction of skeletal muscle, numerous valves preventing back flow. The circulation of lymph from its formation as interstitial fluid to its reintroduction into the blood system at the termination of the thoracic duct removes large protein molecules from the tissue and this prevents oedema.

Signs, Symptoms, Investigations

Incomplete formation of lymphatic channels, acquired blockage or valvular incompetence are the three main aetiological factors in lymphatic disease. The result is lymphoedema. Abnormalities are investigated by lymphangiography. Lymphatic vessels are cannulated after first delineated with the subcutaneous injection of patent blue violet; ultrafluid lipiodil is then injected into the small lymphatics. This shows the main channels and concentrates in the lymph nodes.

The commonest causes of lymphoedema are primary (congenital, *praecox* in early life, or *tarda*, onset after age 35) and secondary to either surgical excision or radiotherapy of lymph nodes, malignant disease or filiriasis.

Treatment

CONSERVATIVE MEASURES

Well-fitting elastic stockings, elevation of the legs and massaging before sleep are the most important factors; the use of diuretics also has a small part to play in the management. All methods may need to be continued after surgery.

OPERATIVE SURGERY

Excision of the diseased skin and oedematous subcutaneous tissue with skin grafting is the traditional method. Dilated incompetent lymphatics can also be ligated or direct lympho-venous anastomosis performed. Either lymph nodes are anastomosed direct to vein or by utilising magnifying techniques, such as the operating microscope, dilated channels are anastomosed direct to the adjacent veins. In the future many cases of lymphoedema following surgical procedures, such as block dissection of lymph nodes, mastectomy or peripheral tumours, might be helped in this way.

Primary tumours although rare, do occur, and are either capillary or cavernous lymphangiomata, cystic hygromas or lymphangio-sarcomas. The two former are treated by excision, the latter often accompanied by radiotherapy and amputation if necessary. All these conditions are rare. They are encountered in busy vascular units although treatment is often carried out at specialised centres. The physiotherapy is concentrated on measures to reduce swelling and this is accompanied by passive and active exercise with elevation and support as outlined above.

BIBLIOGRAPHY

See end of Chapter 18.

Chapter 17

Treatment of Peripheral Vascular Disorders

by J. PICKERING, M.C.S.P.

The treatment of peripheral vascular disease may be medical, surgical or a combination of both. There is an increase in the awareness of the importance of preventive treatment.

PREVENTIVE TREATMENT

Diet

Many people may be living a sedentary life and may be overweight. These patients will benefit from a reducing diet. The fat intake is limited and this is due to the fact that a high cholesterol level is thought to affect the course of the disease. There is strong evidence that the elevation of the plasma fat concentration, i.e. primarily triglycerides and cholesterol, contributes to the formation of atherosclerosis (Stanbury, Wyngarden and Fredrickson, 1972). Therefore patients should reduce animal fat intake and when plasma concentration levels are elevated drug treatment can be instituted.

Smoking

It cannot be emphasised too strongly that there is a far greater risk of myocardial infarcts and actual death in smokers than in non-smokers. Just over 10% of patients suffering from intermittent claudication are non-smokers, while up to 30% of the general population do not smoke. Vasoconstriction of the terminal vessels occurs during smoking. It is therefore clear that in vascular disease smoking should be avoided since a limb surviving on a limited blood supply would be at an even greater risk in a patient who smokes. This means he can almost choose between his legs and his smoking!

Hygiene

Gangrene can start very easily in an ischaemic limb through only minor trauma. Home chiropody is one of the most common causes of this. Many patients, whether diabetic or not, will try to treat their own corns and cut their nails and in doing so may damage the surrounding skin and introduce infection. Again, new or badly fitting shoes can cause blistering which could be severe if sensation in the feet is poor.

Hot water bottles should not be allowed near ischaemic limbs but the bed should be warmed before the patient gets into it. If any abrasion does occur it must be kept very clean and dry and all pressure on it relieved. This is all much more important with diabetic patients as their ability to heal is poor.

Activity

Exercise within the limit of producing claudication, and normal activities, as far as possible, must be encouraged. Most patients are told to walk to the limit of the pain-free distance at regular intervals, and to try to increase this distance slightly. This helps to build up the collateral circulation and to keep as much blood as possible flowing through the affected arteries. Lying in bed or prolonged standing leads to venous stasis and therefore lack of oxygen to the already deprived tissues.

Drugs

Vasodilators and anticoagulants have both been tried with varying success. If vasodilators are given orally, their effect is general, over the whole body, with the normal vessels dilating more easily than those diseased, and stealing blood from the areas where it is most needed.

If large arteries are blocked there is little benefit to be obtained from dilating a distal vessel. The blood will not flow through in an increased amount however much the arterial bed is opened up. Injecting vaso-dilators directly into an affected artery is too dangerous a procedure to be carried out regularly. If these drugs could give relief then a sym-pathectomy would be preferable to avoid the regular use of drugs.

Anticoagulants may help prevent deep vein thrombosis and pul-monary emboli. It is still unproven that they prevent the formation of arterial thrombi. There is also the risk that if the patient is on long-term therapy then even minor surgery such as dental extractions, and trauma such as cuts and bruises, could become serious when the clotting time is lengthened.

Physiotherapy

Some patients may be referred for physiotherapy, although the treatments offered have very little specific benefit. In fact many may even be contra-indicated.

HEAT OR COLD THERAPY

Infra-red or any form of heat is usually contra-indicated in peripheral arterial disease. At one time heating of a proximal area such as the trunk for an involved foot was considered beneficial, but in the majority of patients suffering from atheroma the disease is so widespread that it would be impossible to find an unaffected area without total body arteriograms. Quite often skin sensation is impaired so both heat and cold could lead to a burn which would be difficult to heal.

EXERCISE

Exercises to build up muscle power in the unaffected limb when possible are of value, especially if the patient has to rely on this limb after amputation of the other one.

Buerger's exercises are sometimes ordered, especially if the patient has to be in bed for some time. Unfortunately there is little evidence to prove that there is any real success from this regime. These exercises consist of three changes in position of the limbs:

1. In lying, with the limbs well supported and elevated at an angle of 45° to the horizontal, until the feet or hands blanch completely. This should then be maintained for a further two minutes.

2. In sitting, with the limbs dependent until full filling of the veins occurs, and then for a further three minutes.

3. The patient lies completely flat for at least five minutes. This sequence is then repeated several times in each session of treatment and the patient told to continue this routine at home.

When giving exercises the physiotherapist has to be especially careful in handling the ischaemic limb and in avoiding minor injury such as might occur if the patient knocked against a piece of equipment. Not only is an ischaemic area less sensitive but even minor trauma causing slight swelling or infection, will further reduce the blood flow and increase the metabolites and may thus precipitate gangrene.

Patients with venous ulcers will benefit from physiotherapy.

SURGICAL TREATMENT

The most common operations performed for arterial disease are sympathectomy, endarterectomy, bypass and replacement grafts.

SYMPATHECTOMY

This involves destruction of the ganglia reducing vasomotor control and therefore causing vasodilation. The limbs involved will be dry, warmer, and the incidence of infection, e.g. web-space, is decreased.

If chemical sympathectomy is to be performed then phenol solution is injected into the ganglia under X-ray control. A patient who would be at risk from general anaesthesia can be treated by this method as Valium is often used, with the area of injection numbed by lignocaine.

Open surgery is preferred in some centres and then of course a general anaesthetic is needed.

Cervical Sympathectomy

Raynaud's disease, affecting the hands, will benefit from this. The effect is greatest during the first few months so therefore this should be performed at the start of the colder weather rather than during the summer months. Patients suffering from hyperhydrosis may also benefit from this operation as their hands will no longer sweat so profusely. Some surgeons believe that a cervical sympathectomy is not complete unless the stellate ganglia is removed, but this is not such a common fact nowadays. Side-effects may be drooping of the eyelid, dilated pupils and a sunken eye (delayed).

Lumbar Sympathectomy

Again hyperhydrosis affecting the feet to such an extent that the shoes will actually rot may be helped by this, as will Raynaud's sufferers. Old people and those where the disease is too widespread for reconstruction may benefit from sympathectomy. Sexual function may be impaired if the first lumbar ganglion is not preserved.

PHYSIOTHERAPY

There is no need for treatment when the patient has a chemical sympathectomy as he is on bed rest for 24 hours and is then at least as mobile as before. With operative treatment pre- and postoperative breathing exercises and effective coughing should be taught. As with all lower abdominal surgery there is a risk of thrombosis so leg exercises until mobile should be encouraged. Postoperatively all cervical sympathectomy patients will have had check chest X-rays to exclude pneumothorax and some may have chest drains in situ. Expansion of the apical segments is therefore important and there are no real contra-indications to any form of treatment for this, only the usual precautions of moving a patient with a chest drain (Chapter 8). Many lumbar sympathectomy patients may already have impaired sensation or movement and therefore mobilisation is difficult, but must be performed, even if a frame or crutches have to be used.

ENDARTERECTOMY

This operation was introduced over 30 years ago and still is frequently used in many centres.

Open Endarterectomy

The artery is opened directly over the obstruction and the plaques of atheroma, together with the tunica intima are removed (see Fig. 17/1). This operation is most suitable for short blocks and at arterial bifurcations.

Closed Endarterectomy

In this method a small incision is made at a suitable site and then an instrument such as a ring stripper is passed along the artery to beyond

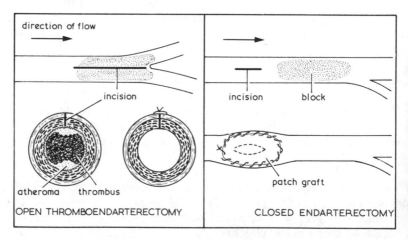

Fig. 17/1   Diagram illustrating open and closed methods of endarterectomy

the block (see Fig. 17/1). This is then pulled back. If it is thought that suturing the arteriotomy may cause constriction of the lumen then a patch graft will be used. This may be of vein or man-made fibre. The patch is sutured round to increase the size of the lumen.

PHYSIOTHERAPY

As the physical treatment is very similar in both grafting and endarterectomies they will be discussed together later on. The only difference is in slightly earlier mobilisation with an endarterectomy.

EMBOLECTOMY

This type of surgery to the affected vessel should be performed as soon as possible after the onset as viability of the limb decreases with time loss. As the methods of detecting the site of embolus improve so that

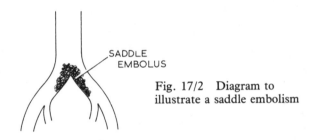

SADDLE
EMBOLUS

Fig. 17/2   Diagram to illustrate a saddle embolism

operations become less extensive, some emboli in the limbs can be removed under a local anaesthetic. Pulmonary emboli are discussed in Chapter 14.

If a large embolus passes down the aorta it may lodge at the bifurcation and so block both limbs of the distal vessel. Any embolus lodging at any bifurcation is called a saddle embolus (see Fig. 17/2). This can break up and block the distal vessels individually needing separate incisions for removal, i.e. both radial and ulnar arteries from brachial, and both iliac arteries from the aorta. If the embolus does fragment like this then several incisions may be needed. A catheter such as the Fogarty balloon catheter is introduced into the vessel and the obstruction cleared, making sure that there is distal flow and, hopefully, pulses at the end of the operation.

PHYSIOTHERAPY

Usually these are emergency operations so the patients are not seen pre-operatively. If by chance they are already in-patients then exercises to the affected part must *not* be done as further breaking up of the embolus could occur.

Postoperatively general exercises can be performed to the legs and breathing exercises where necessary. If viability of the limb may still be doubtful, advice from the surgeon must be sought before active exercises are begun. Sometimes only passive stretching of the tendo Achilles may be done. This is important because the nutrition of the nerves may have been affected by the interruption of blood flow through the limb and foot-drop may occur. It is not much use having a viable leg if the patient cannot walk on it.

GRAFTS

A long incision over the site of the affected vessel or several small incisions are made with the graft tunnelled under the overlying tissues from the exposed ends of the blocked area.

The following materials are used.

MAN-MADE FIBRES

These are usually of woven or knitted Dacron. The most suitable sites for these are in fast flowing arteries such as the aorta. As the diameter lessens so the success of this material decreases. However it may be used in conjunction with a vein graft if sufficient length of vein cannot be found. (Hitch hike graft.)

VEIN GRAFTS

The most common vein used is the long saphenous vein. It is very carefully removed and the tributaries tied off so that the wall is as smooth as possible. The vein is then anastomosed in reverse so that the valves offer no impediment to flow. The cephalic vein may also be used. In some patients the saphenous vein may not be suitable due to venous disease or may already have been used for surgery (coronary artery grafting, previous leg or arm surgery, varicosities). As the cephalic vein is not very long a length of Dacron may be used as well, the vein being used over the joint as it is more capable of accommodating the movements of the joint without kinking.

XENO-GRAFTS

Intensive investigations are being carried out on de-natured animal vessels to assess their suitability. It seems that as they are already in use in heart surgery it will not be long before they are in more common use in peripheral sites.

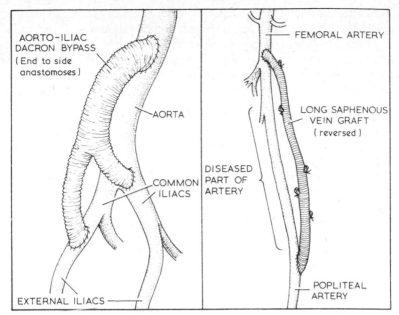

Fig. 17/3   Diagram to illustrate methods of bypass grafts

Methods of Grafting

BYPASS GRAFTS

With these operations the diseased portions of the vessel are not removed but left in situ and it does therefore have some blood flow through it. The graft is usually anastomosed end to side (see Fig. 17/3).

REPLACEMENT GRAFTS

The affected artery is completely replaced by the graft. Some aneurysms are treated by this method. An area of healthy material is exposed above and below the site of disease. The affected part is removed and the graft anastomosed between, making sure all three coats of artery are sewn to the graft. If this is not done blood will leak between the layers causing dissection.

SURGERY OF THE AORTA

The graft will usually be from below the renal vessels and on to either the iliac or femoral vessels. As the supply to the internal iliacs is still often poor, claudication in the buttocks and disturbance of sexual function may still be present. Patients may not complain of impotence until after the operation but it is part of the disease process and not the result of operation. However if the internal vessels are by-passed then circulation to them is not increased. For this reason in younger patients an endarterectomy to these vessels may be performed. Often the patients are elderly and because of the length of anaesthesia chest complications are quite common.

PRE-OPERATIVE PHYSIOTHERAPY

Breathing exercises and leg exercises are taught, if possible.

POSTOPERATIVE PHYSIOTHERAPY

Adequate analgesia should be given regularly for the first few days and physiotherapy can then be done in conjunction with this and with bed bathing. Breathing exercises in alternate side lying on the first day are usually permitted unless there has been great trouble in securing the graft. Co-operation with the nursing staff means that the patient is not disturbed unnecessarily. Postural drainage involving tipping should *not* be done unless absolutely essential as the supply to the legs may still only be adequate in lying. The surgeon's permission should always be obtained before this is carried out. As the colon has been handled quite a lot a paralytic ileus will probably be present and again may make tipping uncomfortable.

Leg exercises are done routinely until the patient is mobile. No definite rule can be made for this as surgeons differ greatly. It may be as soon as the second day or as late as the tenth. When an end-arterectomy has been done, rather than a graft, there is no problem with security of the arterial incision so chest care can be much more vigorous if needed.

SURGERY OF THE LIMBS

For a good result the 'run off' must be good or the graft will shut down. The femoro-popliteal section may be replaced quite easily with a vein graft but unless the trifurcation of the peroneal, anterior and posterior tibial arteries is patent then the graft will block off. However much blood is pumped down the vessel the limb will not remain healthy unless the terminal vessels are able to cope with the flow.

PRE-OPERATIVE PHYSIOTHERAPY

As there is no incision into the abdomen there is less of a problem with coughing. Breathing exercises should however be taught so that the patient is as fit as possible for a probable long anaesthetic. Leg exercises with great emphasis on quadriceps contractions must be done.

POSTOPERATIVE PHYSIOTHERAPY

The patient can be rolled from side to side for treatment without harm but once again tipping is not encouraged but is possible for short periods. Weight-bearing exercises in the form of 'lilting' (alternate heel raising) is begun very early, sometimes on the first day, at the surgeon's discretion – usually with endarterectomies. No patient should be allowed to walk any distance unless he has good quadriceps control and can fully lock the knee when walking. In fact the physiotherapy very closely follows that used after a meniscectomy, apart from the early mobilisation.

If the surgery has been a combination of both limb and aortic grafting then special care must be taken. Hips and knees can be bent for coughing but the position should not be maintained for too long so that the graft does not become kinked in the groin or compressed in the iliac fossa. With a long popliteal incision the patient tends to lie with a pillow under the knee and the knee in a slightly flexed and rotated position. The pillow should be removed immediately and encouragement to keep the knee straight given. As many of the patients have associated arterial disease in other places it is often difficult to gain their full co-operation so many visits have to be made to check that the position is maintained. It is amazing how many things can be used to keep the knee flexed, towels, newspapers and spare blankets are often to be found hiding in the bed.

SURGERY OF THE CAROTID ARTERIES

Carotid surgery may be either preventive or done as an emergency. This is an area where a large number of endarterectomies are done. Many of the patients will have had transient ischaemic attacks and therefore a good pre-operative assessment must be made. Sometimes this includes a psychological assessment. Hypothermia may be used if the operation is thought to be extensive. If there has already been a major cerebral incident on one side then preventive surgery may be done on the other side in the hope of preventing another episode. The internal carotid artery is difficult to operate on at its upper limit and the method of overcoming blocks at this level is discussed later under new procedures.

PRE-OPERATIVE PHYSIOTHERAPY

The usual routine of breathing exercises is carried out whenever possible. A general test of voluntary muscle strength should be charted before surgery and again immediately afterwards. This need not involve more than a comparison of large muscle groups on each side (see Table 17/1).

		RIGHT		LEFT	
		pre	post	pre	post
Fingers	bend				
	stretch				
Wrist	bend				
	stretch				
Elbow	flexion				
	extension				
Shoulder	abduction				
	adduction				
	flexion				
Hip	abduction				
	adduction				
	flexion				
	extension				
Knee	flexion				
	extension				
Ankle	dorsiflexion				
	plantar flexion				

Table 17/1   A Chart to show voluntary muscle strength pre- and postoperatively

POSTOPERATIVE PHYSIOTHERAPY

Most patients are able to be up and walking the following day providing there are no side-effects. The chart should be filled in and any differences reported to the surgeon if they are not immediately apparent – some changes would of course have already been reported, i.e. hemiplegia, lack of awareness, speech loss.

There is no special treatment to be carried out for this operation if the result is good but if any complication has developed, such as hemiparesis, then the specific physiotherapy for this must be done. Some people are reluctant to move their necks but this does not last long.

SURGERY OF ANEURYSMS

Replacement grafts are the most usual form of treatment. The aneurysm is dissected out, clamps are applied proximally and distal to it, and the contents of the sac removed. The graft is sewn into place and whenever possible the sac is sewn round the graft. This applies to most aneurysms and physiotherapy follows that stated above for the limb vessels and 'cold' aneurysms.

Wiring is used if the aneurysm is considered inoperable, because too many arterial trunks are involved, or the tissue at either end is too friable, or the patient is a bad risk for surgery owing to any other condition. About 100 metres of narrow gauge stainless steel wire is inserted into the sac which then slowly becomes obliterated and the nutrition of the lower limbs becomes dependent on collateral vessels.

PRE-OPERATIVE PHYSIOTHERAPY

If the patient is admitted from the waiting list for cold surgery, physiotherapy is started as soon as possible. Patients admitted with either leaking or dissecting aneurysms and as emergencies should not be treated unless specific instructions to do so are given since the danger of the aneurysm rupturing is very great. If treatment is ordered then breathing and leg exercises should be demonstrated rather than performed vigorously. Any sudden increase in symptoms while treating the patient must be taken seriously as an increase in size makes surgery a far greater risk.

POSTOPERATIVE PHYSIOTHERAPY

The larger the extent of surgery the less the patient is permitted to do immediately afterwards. If the aneurysm had ruptured then the patient will have been in shock beforehand and will be very frightened at the thought of moving. Some patients may have been rushed miles by ambulance to a specialist centre and will have added worries about this. The physiotherapist is often the one to whom the patient will confide these worries – there may be an unattended dog at home or some other problem and the patient may not want to worry the nurse and so tells the physiotherapist. Many patients feel that the 'physio' belongs to the patient rather than to the ward as the nurse does, so it is very important that any problems, whether real or imaginary, are reported to the right people, i.e. social workers, making sure that the nursing staff are also informed.

Breathing exercises with good support to the abdomen during coughing are performed. Leg exercises with a lot of foot movements are essential as although anticoagulants such as heparin are injected into the femoral vessels the blood supply to the legs may have been stopped temporarily and the risk of deep vein thrombosis is therefore increased. From the second day onwards breathing and leg exercises are continued until the patient is up and about. This may mean sitting out in a chair and progressing to walking a short distance from the third day onwards, but often much later. The greater the surgery the later the ambulation.

REFERENCE

Fredrickson, D. S. and Levy, R. I. (1972). 'Diseases characterised by evidence of abnormal lipid metabolism.' Chapter in *The metabolic basis of inherited disease*, (Ed. Stanbury, Wyngarden and Fredrickson). McGraw-Hill.

BIBLIOGRAPHY

See end of Chapter 18.

Chapter 18

Less Common Procedures and Recent Advances

by J. PICKERING, M.C.S.P.

Axillary-Femoral Subcutaneous Grafts

This is a fairly new operation which has so far been performed on only a few patients in recent years. The patient may originally have had a graft for an aneurysm which has failed in some way, so that the nutrition of the lower limbs is inadequate. If there is widespread arterial disease, a graft may be used to aid nutrition to the proximal part of the leg when the distal part is to be amputated.

The grafts, usually of Dacron, are passed from the axillary artery beneath the skin, but outside the ribs, to be anastomosed with the femoral artery (see Fig. 18/1). As neither the chest nor the abdominal cavity are opened, the patient's chest is usually unaffected so the operation is suitable for a patient who otherwise might be a bad risk for reconstructive surgery because of his chest.

PHYSIOTHERAPY

Since the operation is often a salvage procedure and may be done as an emergency, physiotherapy is not usually started pre-operatively but if the patient is in the ward for a time prior to surgery he can be given breathing exercises.

The first day postoperatively breathing exercises must be done with care because it is easy to compress the graft. This can usually be seen by the bruising that occurred when the tunnelling was done, and with light pressure pulsation in the graft may be felt. If the patient rolls into side lying then he should only roll far enough to keep the graft free from the bed.

Leg exercises are done routinely. Treatment continues as needed with early ambulation. When the patient is mobile care should be taken to see that the pyjama cord is not pulled tightly over the graft. The physiotherapist should explain this to the patient and suggest help with everyday clothing, e.g. braces, not a belt.

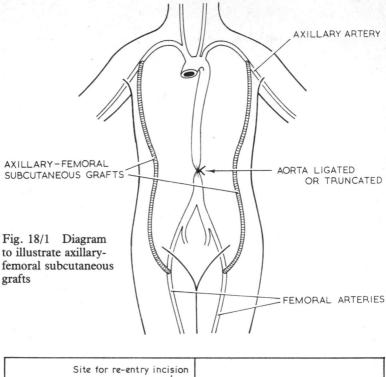

AXILLARY ARTERY

AXILLARY—FEMORAL
SUBCUTANEOUS GRAFTS

AORTA LIGATED
OR TRUNCATED

Fig. 18/1 Diagram
to illustrate axillary-
femoral subcutaneous
grafts

FEMORAL ARTERIES

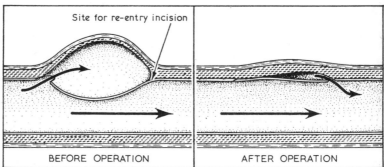

Site for re-entry incision

BEFORE OPERATION

AFTER OPERATION

Fig. 18/2   Diagram to show re-entry operative procedure

Re-Entry Procedures

Sometimes surgery is carried out for acutely dissecting aneurysms to
prevent further dissection. A small incision is made in the artery wall
through the tunica intima to allow re-entry of blood (see Fig. 18/2). As
the blood flows back into the stream dissection stops and the layers
adhere to each other again.

Arterial Injuries

These are often part of a complicated injury. The artery may be damaged by either open or closed injury and the result is one of acute ischaemia of the distal part. Therefore the presentation and the investigations are similar as for arterial obstruction as mentioned in the previous chapters.

The treatment is one of haemostasis and the restoration of circulation to the affected part. This may include removal of the obstruction, i.e. bone fragment, dislocated joint or crush injury. The surgery to the damaged artery follows the basic reconstruction, i.e. direct resuture vein grafting or Dacron replacement of the damaged section.

PHYSIOTHERAPY

This will depend on any associated injury. If the initial injury was directly to the artery then the treatment will be the same as for any arterial procedure. Fractures may mean immobilisation of the limb so treatment will be modified accordingly.

Renal Atheroma

Atheroma can affect these vessels as any others. The patients usually present with hypertension and other associated renal complaints. No special physiotherapy is needed other than routine care. Dialysis may be necessary if both arteries have been involved.

Mesenteric Surgery

These vessels become occluded with thrombus and necrosis of the gut follows. Until recently this was not easily recognised and many patients died from it. At laparotomy the unhealthy segment of bowel will be removed if gangrenous. This may or may not include colostomy depending on the extent of necrosis. It may be possible to carry out an endarterectomy on the vessel; if not, bypass surgery will be required. When the flow is re-established it is obvious which parts will survive.

Embolism or thrombosis can involve the mesenteric vessels to produce acute massive necrosis of the gut. Subsequent ischaemia and stricture formation may cause symptoms of pain after meals ('gut claudication').

Once the diagnosis of acute ischaemia has been established medical measures are instituted to replace fluid loss and to lessen the extension of thrombus and tissue destruction. After a few hours, surgery is undertaken to restore flow to the devitalised tissue or to excise those areas of irreversible bowel ischaemia.

The mortality from treated cases is 80–90% but those that survive become a difficult or complex nutritional problem often requiring extensive intravenous feeding on either a long or short term basis.

Chronic ischaemia can be investigated by arteriography and reconstructive vascular surgery performed where indicated.

Tumours of Blood Vessels

These are congenital malformations of vessels which occur as a result of defective development of blood vessels from the diffuse mesenchymatous plexuses that are the beginnings of the definitive endothelial tubes. The resulting haemangiomata are present at birth and are capillary or cavernous in nature. Treatment after an adequate period of waiting as a majority regress as growth of the patient occurs, is by surgical excision. As well as on cosmetic grounds excision is performed because they often bleed. Haemangiopericytomas are found in deeper soft tissues of the limbs and often in the uterus.

Carotid Body Tumours

These arise from paraganglia adjacent to vessels commonly at the carotid bifurcation and aortic arch and present as a swelling in the neck or in deep areas such as the thorax. They are treated by careful excision with facilities for vessel replacement and blood transfusion.

Glomus Tumour

This painful red or blue dermal or subcutaneous nodule can be found throughout the body but commonly at the finger-tip. Again these are excised surgically for the relief of symptoms.

Some vascular tumours can become malignant by developing sarcomatous changes (angiosarcoma). The other rare tumour is the Kaposi sarcoma, being more prevalent in Equatorial Africa.

Microvascular Surgery

Surgeons in many fields of surgery are becoming skilled in the use of magnifying aids to perform surgery on delicate tissues. These techniques using an operating microscope are in common use by ophthalmological and E.N.T. surgeons. The vascular surgeons can use these refined optical instruments and precision tools to perform anastomoses on small vessels as small as 0·8mm in diameter and obtain a high patency rate. As many as 10 sutures are accurately placed around the vessel to perform the anastomosis.

CLINICAL APPLICATIONS

Since re-implantation of an amputated thumb was performed in 1966, many successful cases of digital re-implantation have been performed. The plastic and traumatic surgeons have further developed their skill to include free tissue transfer such as full thickness skin pedicle grafts, omentum, muscle and rib cartilage. In 1961 these techniques were pioneered in vascular surgery as applied to operations in neurosurgery on the cerebral vessels and techniques of revascularising the brain from the extracerebral superficial temporal artery by anastomosing it to the middle cerebral artery are being used more and more.

It can be seen therefore that as surgeons become more adept at these fundamental techniques the practising physiotherapist will be called on to help rehabilitate patients who have undergone this intricate and delicate surgery.

Arteriovenous Fistulae

These are abnormal communications between an artery and vein varying in size from being little larger than a capillary, to a connection between the aorta and vena cava. The large fistulae are often traumatic in origin whereas the small multiple ones are congenital and represent an arrest in development of the blood vessels. They can be found in all regions and organs of the body and appear as characteristic port wine or strawberry birth marks. They either involve the skin as part of vascular tumour formation, or present as abnormal growth of a limb with compensating heart enlargement and high output heart failure. When present in internal organs such as the stomach, intestines or liver they can present with blood loss from bleeding or abnormal enlargement.

TREATMENT

The unsightly congenital multiple arteriovenous fistulae can be excised and efforts made to prevent regrowth of the area; stapling of the epiphysis of long bones to reduce growth is often performed. Multiple ligation of bleeding arteries can produce a degree of palliation. Selective embolisation, viz the injection of particles into the circulation in order to occlude the fistulae has some advocates but has not gained world wide acceptance due to the difficult techniques and uncertainty of the results. It may become acceptable for areas such as the pelvis where excision or amputation is not feasible.

Localised congenital fistulae: Here an attempt can be made to ligate the feeding arteries and veins and to excise the fistulous tissue.

Acquired arteriovenous fistulae: The extent can be obtained from arteriography then ligation performed.

Shunts: Arterial venous fistulae are becoming commonly performed for easy access to patients' vessels requiring repeated haemodialysis.

COMPLICATIONS OF SURGERY

Respiratory Failure

Deep anaesthesia for a lengthy period is required during extensive reconstruction. Chest complications, therefore, do develop. Aneurysms are usually found in the older patient who perhaps has less respiratory reserve and who has smoked all his life. Postoperative shock can also be a complication. If these factors are taken into consideration it is not surprising that after prolonged surgery it is a long time before the patient breathes spontaneously.

Treatment of a patient on a ventilator following arterial surgery is the same as for anyone being ventilated (see Chapter 6). Tipping may be carried out if essential but not for any length of time, as circulation may only be adequate in the supine position.

Paralytic Ileus

Due to handling of the colon during the exploratory laparotomy there is often spasm of the muscular wall of the intestine. If the reconstruction involves either of the mesenteric vessels then the condition may last longer.

Embolism

When the artery is clamped for any length of time during reconstruction there is stasis of blood in the distal vessels. Should a thrombosis start to form in these vessels when the artery is unclamped the thrombus may be pushed on to block a smaller artery. There is also pressure on veins during surgery and this may lead to stasis and pulmonary emboli may occur. For these reasons pulses are carefully charted every 15 minutes after surgery for a certain length of time to make sure the vessels remain patent. The blood pressure should not be allowed to drop either as this will cause the flow to be reduced through the graft.

False Aneurysm

This can occur round the suture line in any reconstruction.

Failed Graft

The graft may fail for several reasons.

a) There may be deposits of atheroma laid down in the graft after surgery.

b) The vessel may collapse due to pressure on it from the surrounding structures or from leakage of blood flowing through at the suture line.

c) If the blood pressure is not maintained at a good level then the graft may slowly clot in the first few hours after operation.

d) An infection may develop round the graft and as a result the suture line may break down. If Dacron or some other foreign body is present then antibiotics are necessary. The theatre dressing should be left intact for as long as possible as this helps prevent the introduction of infection. Obesity can almost be considered a complication in its own right – where the skin overlaps as in the groin, there is an ideal breeding ground for bacteria.

Deep Vein Thrombosis

The less able the patient is to keep mobile the higher the risk of thrombosis. There are many reasons why the patient does not move after the operation. Respiratory failure requiring ventilation means that the patient is often deeply sedated and so is unable to move his own limbs. Confusion is quite common in elderly patients or those who have had massive surgery involving the carotid or innominate arteries. A confused patient may move but will damage himself so he may require sedation for this reason.

For these and other reasons it may be necessary to move the patient's limbs regularly until he can do it himself. Anti-embolic stockings should be worn to theatre and afterwards if the patient is known to be at risk.

Acute Renal Failure

The shock of a leaking aneurysm with the sudden drop in blood pressure and the subsequent surgery may be sufficient to cause renal failure. This may mean reduced output or complete failure. If the blood urea rises significantly the patient may become confused and difficult. Usually either peritoneal dialysis or haemodialysis is started to bring the level down, and is continued until kidney function is adequate. If surgery has been on the renal vessels or on the associated portion of the aorta then the incidence of renal failure is greater. Sometimes the damage may be permanent and then a shunt is necessary (see p. 302).

In this chapter we have looked at the more complex recent advances and the less common procedures. It is important to stress that many of the developments have only been made possible by improved para-medical and surgical techniques in the fields of anaesthesia, monitoring instrumentation and laboratory support. The careful investigation by the laboratory with a supply of cross-matched blood and the availability of autotransfusion techniques is also essential.

Autotransfusion: The patient's own blood is collected at operation or after trauma, filtered and retransfused and enables the surgeon to perform emergency surgery on patients who would otherwise have died.

Skills have increased to keep pace with these advances and the knowledgeable physiotherapist, in addition to providing the essential day to day care of the respiratory and cardiovascular systems, can contribute to the complex management of the more specialised problems as outlined in this chapter.

BIBLIOGRAPHY

Atkins, P. and Hawkins, L. A. (1965). 'Detection of venous thrombosis in the legs.' *Lancet*, ii, 1217.
Attinger, E. O. (Ed.) (1964). *Pulsatile Blood Flow*. McGraw-Hill, New York.
Birnstingl, Martin (Ed.) (1973). *Peripheral Vascular Surgery*. William Heinemann Medical Books Ltd.
    Particularly the following chapters:
        Browne, N. L. – The Vein
        Marston, A. – Surgery of the Mesenteric Arteries
        Negus, D. – The Lymphatic System
Donaghy, R. M. P. and Yasargil, M. S. (Eds.) (1967). *The Development of Microsurgical Technique in Microvascular Surgery*. C. V. Mosby Company, St. Louis and Georg Thieme Verlag, Stuttgart.
Eastcott, H. H. G. (1973). *Arterial Surgery*. Pitman Medical Press.
Holford, C. P. (1976). 'Graded compression for preventing deep venous thrombosis.' *British Medical Journal*, ii, 969–970.
Mavor, G. E. (1971). 'Surgery of deep vein thrombosis', *British Journal of Hospital Medicine*, 1, 755.
Moore, J. M. and Frew, I. D. O. (1965). 'Peripheral vascular lesions in diabetes mellitus.' *British Medical Journal*, ii, 19.

Richards, Robert L. (1970). *Peripheral Arterial Disease — a Physician's Approach*. Churchill Livingstone.

Wheelock, F. C. and Filtzer, H. S. (1969). 'Femoral grafts in diabetics. Resulting conservative amputation.' *Archives of Surgery*, **99**, 776.

Yao, S. T. (1970). 'Haemodynamic studies in peripheral arterial disease'. *British Journal of Surgery*, **57**, 761.

ACKNOWLEDGEMENTS

The author would like to express her sincere thanks to Mr. H. H. G. Eastcott, M.S., F.R.C.S., who taught her so much when she was working for him at St. Mary's Hospital, London. She thanks also Mr. R. Greenhalgh, M. CHIR, F.R.C.S., at Charing Cross Hospital, London, for his advice. She is grateful to Miss M. Wigham, M.C.S.P., and the staff of the physiotherapy department of Charing Cross Hospital, London, for their help and tolerance while she was revising these chapters.

Chapter 19

Leg Ulcers

by C. R. BANNISTER, M.C.S.P.

Definition

Leg ulcers are chronic lesions of the skin and connective tissues, although deeper structures may be involved. Caused by abnormalities of the circulatory system, ulcers rarely occur upon a normal limb.

They are designated venous or arterial types according to the vessels at fault. The first presents the problem of impaired venous return, the second that of diminished arterial supply. Signs, symptoms and treatment fundamentally differ. About 95% of leg ulcers seen in our departments are venous in origin, the remainder being arterial, although cases involving both systems are seen.

BASIC ANATOMY OF LOWER LIMB CIRCULATION

The following simple description concentrates upon the practical needs of our study. Anatomy cannot be fully discussed in such a brief chapter and reference should be made to a standard textbook.

The Arterial System

Leaving the heart at the left ventricle the aorta passes through the thorax and abdomen where mesenteric, coeliac, renal and other visceral branches form. At the level of the fourth lumbar vertebra it divides to form the right and left common iliac arteries. Opposite the lumbosacral articulation the common iliac arteries divide into the internal and external iliac arteries. The external iliac runs downwards along the medial border of psoas major muscle and enters the thigh beneath the centre of the inguinal ligament, becoming the femoral artery. Four centimetres below the ligament the arteria profunda femoris branches. The main vessel proceeds along the adductor canal to pass through the opening in adductor magnus muscle where it becomes the popliteal artery.

THE POPLITEAL ARTERY

This distributes the geniculate branches which form part of the anastomosis round the knee, and at the lower border of popliteus muscle divides into anterior and posterior tibial arteries.

THE ANTERIOR TIBIAL ARTERY

This passes between the tibia and fibula, through the upper part of the interosseous membrane, on the anterior surface of which it then runs to the front of the ankle. Proceeding to the dorsum of the foot it becomes the dorsalis pedis artery. It then continues along the medial side of the dorsum of the foot to pass through the proximal end of the first intermetatarsal space to complete the plantar arch. Branches are given off to the muscles on the antero-lateral side of the leg, to the bones and ankle joint as well as to the foot and toes.

THE POSTERIOR TIBIAL ARTERY

This descends from the lower border of popliteus, at which level the peroneal artery emanates, then courses along the back of the leg, lying on the deep muscles and being covered by gastrocnemius and soleus. Becoming superficial, it is palpable below the medial malleolus. Branches are disposed to the muscles on the back of the leg, the peronei, and to the foot and toes.

The Venous System

This consists of superficial and deep groups of vessels, connected to each other directly and by the perforating veins.

The Superficial Veins

These lie within the layers of the superficial fascia and comprise the long and short saphenii and their tributaries.

LONG SAPHENOUS VEIN

This courses upwards along the medial aspect of the leg. From the small veins of the toes and metatarsal region, the dorsal venous arch, and the medial marginal vein, it passes along the inner aspect of the foot to the front of the medial malleolus, along the medial border of the tibia, then postero-medially behind the knee and antero-medially along the inner aspect of the thigh, passing through the saphenous opening in the deep fascia to join the femoral vein approximately three centimetres below the inguinal ligament. It receives tributaries from the superficial veins of the thigh and from the lower part of the abdominal wall. In addition it drains the superficial tissues of the greater part of the leg with the exception of the lateral side of the leg and foot. A small area on the medial side between the tibia and the tendo Achilles drains directly into the deep veins. *Thus interference with flow in the deep veins of the calf is particularly liable to affect the venous drainage of the lower third of the medial side of the leg – the area where venous ulceration occurs most frequently* (see p. 314).

SHORT SAPHENOUS VEIN

From the lateral marginal veins of the foot, it passes postero-laterally behind the lateral malleolus, along the back of the calf and, piercing the deep fascia, joins the popliteal vein at the back of the knee.

The superficial vessels are connected to each other by a complicated network of small veins.

PERFORATING OR COMMUNICATING VEINS

These are very important vessels connecting the two parts of the venous mechanism and normally allow blood to flow only from superficial to deep veins. They are mainly located in the lower third of the leg, though important vessels are found above and below the knee.

The Deep Veins

The deep system consists of the anterior and posterior tibial, popliteal and femoral veins and their tributaries. They lie beneath the fibrous inextensible deep fascia and the muscles immediately below this.

ANTERIOR TIBIAL VEINS

These arise from the vena comitantes of the dorsalis pedis artery. Lying deep to the anterior tibial muscle group, they ascend the leg, pass between the tibia and fibula through the upper part of the interosseous membrane and join the posterior tibial vein to form the popliteal vein.

POSTERIOR TIBIAL VEINS

These accompany the artery. In the lower part of their course they are covered only by skin and fascia. Ascending, they lie upon the deep muscles and beneath soleus and gastrocnemius, joining the anterior tibial veins to form the popliteal vein. Perforators are received from the long and short saphenii.

THE POPLITEAL VEIN

This commences at the lower border of the popliteus muscle, ascends behind the knee to the opening in adductor magnus through which it passes to become the femoral vein. The popliteal receives the short saphenous and geniculate veins.

THE FEMORAL VEIN

This progresses upwards in the adductor canal to pass beneath the inguinal ligament near its centre. Its principal tributaries are the vena profunda femoris, one perforator just above the knee, and the long saphenous vein. At the inguinal ligament it becomes the external iliac vein.

EXTERNAL ILIAC VEIN

This passes along the brim of the lesser pelvis and at the level of the sacro-iliac joint receives the internal iliac vein to form the common iliac vein. At the level of the fifth lumbar vertebral body, the common iliac veins unite to form the inferior vena cava which, passing through the diaphragm, enters the right atrium of the heart. In the abdomen the inferior vena cava receives tributaries from the abdominal viscera.

Valves

These are bicuspid structures, placed at intervals along the veins. Their function is to prevent venous back-flow. They are especially numerous in the veins of the lower extremities, particularly in the deep veins.

It should be noted that whilst the superficial veins are supported solely by the partially extensible superficial fascia, the deep veins are sustained by both muscle and the inextensible deep fascia. The deep system assists blood return of the weakly supported superficial group by means of musculo-venous pumps.

The principal musculo-venous pump is composed of the following structures: posterior tibial muscles, deep fascia, deep veins of the lower leg, and perforating veins. On contraction of the calf muscles, the posterior tibial veins are closed and emptied, the blood being propelled upwards. On relaxation, the veins are refilled, not only from the deep veins of the foot, but also from the lower part of the long saphenous vein via the perforating veins and directly from the tissues of the lower part of the medial side of the leg between the tibia and the tendo Achilles. Thus venous return from the superficial veins is assisted.

AETIOLOGY AND TREATMENT

Normally blood supply and return are in balance. If either is chronically disturbed, tissues may degenerate and the leg become predisposed to ulceration.

THE ISCHAEMIC ULCER

SITE

The ischaemic ulcer is usually found on or below the malleolus (see Fig. 19/1).

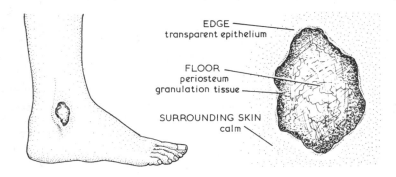

Fig. 19/1   A typical ischaemic ulcer

PAIN

This is often intense, possible causes being infection or anoxia.

The *surrounding skin* is usually calm unless the lesion is infected. The *edge* of the ulcer is of transparent epithelial tissue or, if infected, possibly serpiginous in form. The *floor* often consists only of periosteum with a narrow circumference of granulation tissue.

In such a lesion, the periosteum has little protection and should infection intervene there is a risk of osteomyelitis occurring. Granulation tissue must be stimulated in order to protect the periosteum and initiate healing. Sub-erythema doses of ultraviolet light are indicated, followed by a dressing such as Lassar's paste or paraffin Tulle Gras. In general, a greasy dressing will stimulate granulation tissue growth, but a saline dressing will tend to control this.

Utmost care must be taken in the selection and application of the bandage for compression is harmful because the arteries are already damaged. A crêpe bandage may be all that is required.

Briefly, as far as physiotherapists are concerned, all that can be done for these patients is to make the most of such circulation as remains.

THE VENOUS ULCER

If preventive measures are not, or cannot be, pursued, the limb slowly regresses and ulcers can easily result.

Types

They occur spontaneously or have traumatic origin, and assume one of the following forms:

SPECIFIC INFECTION

The *edge* of the ulcer may be serpiginous and possibly undermined. The *floor* of the ulcer may present a thick yellow or black slough or be itself discoloured. It is deep and often uneven and dark. The *base* may or may not be present according to the duration of the ulcer. The *surrounding skin* may be inflamed, an indication of acute infection or even the beginning of cellulitis (see Fig. 19/2).

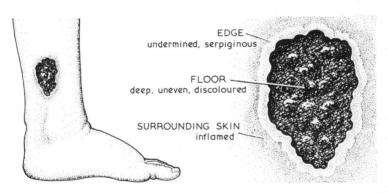

EDGE
undermined, serpiginous

FLOOR
deep, uneven, discoloured

SURROUNDING SKIN
inflamed

Fig. 19/2   An infected venous ulcer

A swab for culture and sensitivity would probably be taken and the dressing prescription based upon this.

Rest is an essential part of treatment.

When inflammation has subsided, a fourth degree (E_4) or a double fourth degree ($2E_4$) erythema dose of ultraviolet light may be given, this being bactericidal; the skin is protected, usually by sterile paraffin Tulle Gras.

In order to prevent cross-infection of other ulcers, strict pre-cautions must be observed in dealing with this type.

HEALING

The *edge* of the ulcer is of transparent epithelium, even and calm. The *floor* is clean granulation tissue level with the skin. It is shining and a healthy pink in colour. The *base* is probably non-existent and the *skin* calm (see Fig. 19/3).

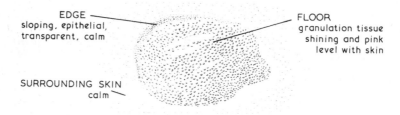

EDGE
sloping, epithelial,
transparent, calm

FLOOR
granulation tissue
shining and pink
level with skin

SURROUNDING SKIN
calm

Fig. 19/3   A healing venous ulcer

This stage of ulceration needs only sub-erythema ultraviolet light, a bland dressing and a suitable support.

HYPERGRANULATING

The *edge* of the ulcer is epithelial and even in form. The *floor* is clean granulation tissue growing above the level of the surrounding skin. The *base* is probably non-existent and the *skin* calm (see Fig. 19/4).

In this type the exuberant tissue must be controlled, for epithelium will not grow over hypergranulation. A pressure pad over the ulcer dressing is often sufficient but it may be necessary to precede this with a $2E_4$ dose of ultraviolet light, the skin and non-hypergranulating areas being protected by sterile paraffin Tulle Gras.

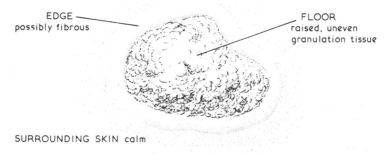

EDGE
possibly fibrous

FLOOR
raised, uneven
granulation tissue

SURROUNDING SKIN calm

Fig. 19/4   A hypergranulating ulcer

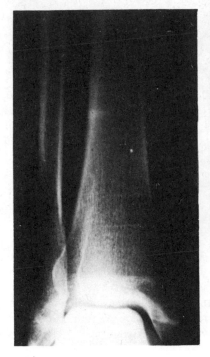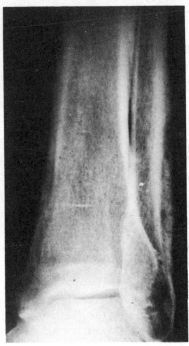

Plate 19/1   Radiographs showing the effect of fibrous base of ulcer of 15 years' duration. Compare the tibia and fibula of the same patient: (*left*) the normal right limb; (*right*) the ulcerated left limb

CHRONIC

The *edge* of the ulcer is fibrous, thick and vertical. The *floor* is pallid, and deeply set below the skin level. Sometimes low-grade infection is evident. The *base* is a thick, fibrous and almost avascular mass beneath and somewhat larger than the ulcer. It may be mobile but is probably closely enmeshed in the bone below (see Plate 19/1). The base delays healing and its effect must be removed before an ulcer can heal. The *skin* is calm, but possibly thick and indurated (see Fig. 19/5).

All parts of a chronic ulcer need to be stimulated and mobilised, using massage, ultraviolet light, ultrasound and exercises.

This type is the one most frequently seen in physiotherapy departments.

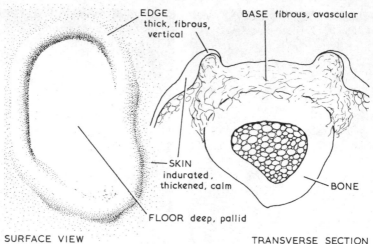

Fig. 19/5   A chronic ulcer

Site

Venous ulcers occur in the lower third of the limb excluding the foot, more often on the left than on the right leg. There are four commonly seen positions, each with their own characteristics.

MEDIAL LOWER THIRD

This is the most frequent site. Probably a late result of deep vein thrombosis and the consequent incompetent perforators.

LATERAL AND MEDIAL LOWER THIRD

This most often results from varicose veins, the ulcer lying at the lower end of the inefficient vessel distal to the above.

ANTERIOR

This site is frequently at the junction of middle and lower thirds. Always traumatic and infected, the injury usually damages the periosteum and its minute blood vessels. Stumbling when climbing on to a chair or boarding a bus is the usual cause.

POSTERIOR ANKLE

This is a very painful site, often traumatic.

Type of Patient Affected

Patients aged from 20 to 93 years have been treated, the greater number being in the 50–70 age-group. Approximately 66% of the patients are women and 34% men. Venous ulcers occur on people of all physiques, but mostly on those of heavier build.

TREATMENT

All regimes are subject to modification according to the general condition of the patient. Many of these patients have chest, heart or other diseases. Allergic reaction contra-indicates the substance causing it.

In general terms the objects are to re-establish as nearly as possible normal circulation in the limb and to the ulcer site. *Only when efficient blood metabolism is restored can infection be controlled and healing initiated.*

Treatment is based upon the study of predisposing and maintaining causes and changes in structure such as the fibrous base or induration of connective tissue and skin (see Plate 19/2). It is also dependent upon the patient, particularly in regard to the selection of the bandage, i.e. the ability to remove and re-apply this and the extent of activity.

EXAMINATION OF PATIENT

Ascertain the history. Closely examine the limbs and the lesion; compare the size and shape of the legs and the tension and extent of oedema; note areas of induration; determine the range of movements and the reasons for limitation, e.g. contractures. Examine for varicose veins, signs of phlebitis or thrombosis and incompetent perforators. Note the dorsalis pedis and posterior tibial pulses. Pay particular regard to the incidence of pain and try to elicit the cause. Allergies must be noted.

A tracing of the ulcer may be taken, as follows. A piece of cellophane is sterilised and laid on the ulcer. This should be covered by a second piece on which is traced the ulcer outline. The first piece of cellophane is discarded and the tracing is transferred onto the patient's record card with carbon. Fortnightly comparisons may be made and recorded.

Close observation of tissue changes is essential. Although tracings afford useful edge comparisons, the visible progression or regression in all parts actually guides our treatment. Cleansing of the lesion, proliferation of granulation tissue, the filling in of the floor and the formation of a healing edge, are all to be noted.

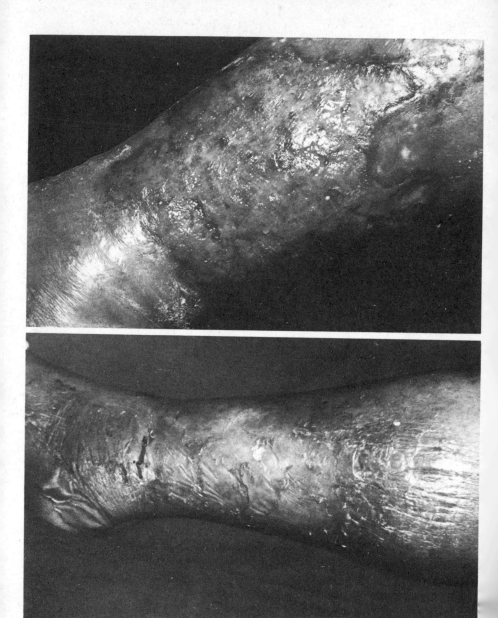

Plate 19/2   *Upper*: A chronic gravitational ulcer complicated by congestive cardiac failure, bronchitis and natural obesity. *Lower*: The same limb after healing by hospitalisation, medical care and physiotherapy to the ulcer

Objects of Treatment

REDUCTION OF OEDEMA

Oedema inhibits circulation, healing and phagocytosis. It is itself trauma and will, according to its tension, thrombose minute blood vessels to the skin, connective tissue and fat, causing degeneration of these parts. Oedema limits movement, will become organised, is a culture medium for bacteria, and is a source of pain.

CONTROL OF INFECTION

Infection maintains the lesion and in some specific invasions such as *Proteus, Pseudomonas pyocyanea* or *Staphylococcus aureus* will actually enlarge the ulcer by destroying tissue. Infection is also a source of pain. *These pathogenic conditions contra-indicate all physiotherapy*, with the possible exception of ultraviolet light.

MOBILISATION OF ALL STRUCTURES and STIMULATION OF ULCER FLOOR AND EDGES

This is to increase vascularity.

ALLEVIATION OF PAIN and INITIATION OF THE HEALING PROCESS

This results from the realisation of the above aims of treatment.

Physiotherapy (Regimes of Treatment)

Make the patient comfortable; in elevation if the general condition allows.
Prepare the trolley:
Sterilise the trolley top. Drop onto this the dressing pack from its envelope. Place two pairs of sterile forceps on trolley top, with which the sterile dressing pack will later be opened. Place a pair of disposable plastic gloves in wrappers, and a spare paper sterile towel.
On lower shelf place: cleansing solution; dressing solution; cream; skin barrier; bandages; plastic foam.
Wearing disposable plastic gloves, remove bandages and discard, remove gloves and discard. Place sterile paper towel under limb. Open dressing pack with spare forceps.
Pour out solution (Savlon 1%, Eusol, or sterile normal saline). Thoroughly wash the hands. Using 'no touch' technique clean surrounding skin. Clean ulcer and dry with sterile gauze.
Cover lesion with antiseptic pack (toilet solution), and retain this where practicable throughout physiotherapy. Now commence physiotherapy.

Reduction of Oedema

The most suitable treatment may be selected from the following.

COMPRESSION FARADISM

In effect, this is the formation of an artificial musculo-venous pump. Pressure localising pads of plastic foam should be placed on the malleolar hollows, over the ulcer and possibly along the course of varicose veins. Electrodes are placed on the plantar surface of the foot, the antero-lateral tibial muscle group, and possibly the femoral triangle, and the whole held in place by a simple bandage. Pressure is by the blue line, or Bisgaard bandage, applied firmly from toes to knee or above. Comfortable stimulation, enough to elicit a definite contraction, is given for two periods of about 10 minutes each with a rest between. Faradism is also useful if given without compression.

EXERCISES IN THE BISGAARD BANDAGE

Remedial exercises can be performed whilst the legs are in elevation and firmly bandaged as above.

AIR COMPRESSION

The development of intermittent pulsating instruments such as the 'Auto-pulse' gives another means by which the swollen leg may be controlled. The limb is placed into a double-skinned plastic tube which is alternately filled and emptied of air, both compression and relaxation being sensitively controlled and giving a possible maximum of 100mm Hg; the usual being 60 to 80mm Hg for 10 minutes. The treatment mechanically reduces the oedema. Simple and quick to apply, this apparatus appears to be a most effective method. It is also indicated for the treatment of contractures of joints, such as the knee.

HIGH ELEVATION

This is a home exercise. For a period of 20 minutes twice daily, the patient lies on the floor with the legs vertical, supported by the wall.

Control of Infection

Except in the acute and sub-acute infective stages, all techniques that aid the restoration of the normal blood metabolism assist this aim. Without adequate blood supply, infection cannot be contained. Provided there is no inflammation, the specific physiotherapy treatment for this object is a *bactericidal dose of ultraviolet light*. This is sometimes as high as a $2E_4$ depending upon the state of the ulcer floor. With a third degree (E₃) erythema dose or stronger application it is essential to protect the surround of the ulcer, and this is most easily done by applying sterile paraffin Tulle Gras right up to the edges. Ultraviolet light of this intensity is usually given once, or at the most, twice per week.

Mobilisation of Skin and Connective Tissue

Gained primarily by massage, the technique is the rolling of these structures between lightly held fingers and thumb. This can be extremely painful and should not be continued for more than two or three minutes at any one site. This movement should be alternated with kneading. These manipulations may with advantage be preceded by a short treatment of ultrasound, of the order of $1 \cdot 5$ Wcm² pulsed 1:1 for 10 minutes.

Massage to ulcer edges is essential in order to regain mobility here and to retain flexibility as the ulcer heals in order to give a free, well vascularised scar. Cover the lesion with dry sterile gauze. Wearing sterile disposable gloves, feel the ulcer edge and give finger kneading along it, flattening and moving the fibrous wall. Painful areas should be avoided.

Stimulation of Ulcer Floor and Edges

Ultraviolet light is the treatment of choice for this specific object.

At the chronic ulcerative stage using the Kromayer lamp a second degree (E₂) erythema dose is suggested to the floor and surrounding skin. As the ulcer becomes cleaner and acquires a better colour, the dose should be reduced because intensive ultraviolet light deepens a granulating area. At that stage a sub-erythema dose is indicated. *Ultrasonics* may also be used. This treatment is given to the surrounding area and stimulates and mobilises by increasing the vascularity of a part. It is contra-indicated when an ulcer is maintained by an incompetent vein as this may bleed into the ulcer floor.

Ice is a very convenient method of improving the local circulation.

Alleviation of Pain

Pain in a gravitational ulcer is caused by oedema, infection, thrombosis, phlebitis, a varix, or adherent dressings. Relief should follow the treatments indicated, coupled with a thoughtful and carefully applied dressing and support.

THE DRESSING

On completion of physiotherapy, it is necessary to take a fresh dressing pack, and possibly to re-lay the dressing trolley.

Remove the antiseptic pack with which the ulcer has been covered throughout treatment and dry the ulcer. The skin will have to be treated if eczema or maceration are present. A skin barrier such as titanium dioxide paste or zinc and menthol ointment may be used for protection.

The ulcer dressing plays a very important part in infection control and in the healing of an ulcer. This may take the form of a base of tulle, cream, ointment, powder, paste or a solution in which the medication is suspended, or one of the proprietary non-adherent types. The effect of the base on skin and ulcer must be noted.

The simplest effective dressing should always be used. When using tulles or ointment, it must be applied so that the skin is not attacked. The doctor will often prescribe a specific lotion or ointment; if he does not then Lassar's paste, paraffin Tulle Gras, Eusol, lotio rubra, aluminium subacetate are all suitable. Modern proprietary applications are legion. All are effective in various circumstances and it behoves the physiotherapist engaged in this work to study their properties and effects.

Two recently introduced dressings are Debrisan and Lyophilised Porcine Skin. The former acts by absorbing the debris and bacteria, the latter acts by the application of almost pure collagen in the form of reconstituted freeze dried pigskin, and cleanses the ulcer and stimulates healing.

If a culture and sensitivity swab indicates a specific infection requiring an antibiotic, the doctor will prescribe or must be consulted. These should be used only under medical instructions, the dangers being allergic reaction in the patient or the raising of a resistant bacterial strain.

The dressing for a painful ulcer or one crossing a joint should be non-adherent, divided horizontally and put on as separate pieces. This may relieve the pain caused by an adherent dressing. An absorbent pad, also divided, is placed over the dressing and the support applied.

THE SUPPORT

This is the most important single factor in the treatment of venous ulcers. By it we can reduce oedema, simulate the venous pump, and ease pain by giving relief to pendulous and distended veins. Reaction to any support must be watched for.

Where local pressure is required, thin pads of plastic foam or folded gauze may be placed in the malleolar hollows, over the ulcer and along the course of obvious varicose veins. The bandage must be carefully selected according to the needs and abilities of the patient. If the Bisgaard method is chosen, the dressing and pads are held in place by toes-to-knee crêpe bandage, this being retained at night, the Bisgaard bandage being removed and then re-applied in the morning before rising. This is a very efficient support, but those most likely to benefit from it are the younger and more active patients. The Bisgaard bandage should not be placed directly on the skin as the sensitive areas could be abraded by its edges.

The most frequently used alternative is the medicated type such as Viscopaste, Calaband, Coltapaste etc., supported by an outer elastic bandage such as crêpe, Elastocrêpe, Lestreflex, Elastoplast, or Poroplast.

The medicated bandage is non-extensible and must be carefully applied without tension and cut where necessary to conform to the limb. The outer bandage is applied firmly, but never tightly, to the foot and lower third of the leg and eased somewhat as the bandage is progressed upwards. The bandage must extend from the bases of the toes to just below the knee (Fig. 19/6). (If needed the support may be continued above the knee by Tubigrip.) Alternatively, crêpe, double-crêpe, Tubigrip, Lastonet, Elastocrêpe, Elastoplast and Poroplast may be used without a medicated under-bandage.

As the course of treatment progresses, it is necessary frequently to re-assess tension, for blood vessels protected by oedema in the early stages become vulnerable to constriction as that oedema is reduced.

REMEDIAL EXERCISES

To complete the treatment, simple foot exercises are taught. These must be regularly and frequently repeated at home. They are essential in order to prevent contracture and to maintain the strength of the foot muscles, the long-continued wearing of a bandage being weakening. They will actively assist in the reduction of oedema; when the leg is correctly supported, the musculo-venous pump is simulated and the excess fluid slowly expelled.

Excision and graft

The object of this surgical procedure is to remove the avascular, fibrous base on which the ulcer lies in order to graft the skin on to normally vascularised tissue. Physiotherapists are sometimes asked to provide pre- and postoperative care.

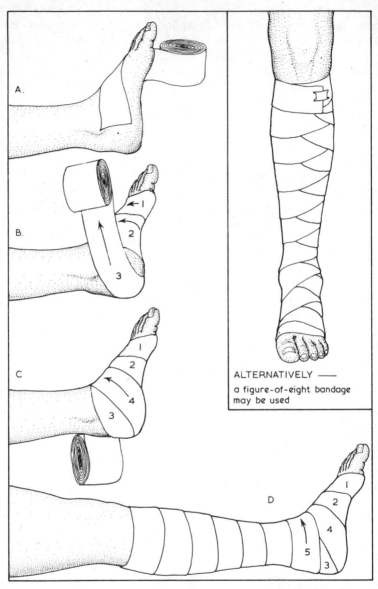

A.

B.

C.

D.

ALTERNATIVELY ——
a figure-of-eight bandage
may be used

Fig. 19/6   The application of the support bandage

PRE-OPERATIVE CARE

Conservative treatment is given to clean the wound, mobilise joints and stimulate epithelisation.

POSTOPERATIVE CARE

The aims at this stage are to aid circulation to the graft and to strengthen, thicken and mobilise it. Surgeons vary in their instructions but the following is a successful postoperative regime.

Ten to fourteen days after the graft, daily sub-erythema doses of ultraviolet light are given. The author believes that five seconds at two inches (5cm) with the Kromayer lamp is the most effective starting dose. Two or three more treatments are given without progression and then minimal increases are made. This treatment appears to stimulate epithelisation, improve the colour and strengthen the grafts.

Wearing sterile gloves, massage may be given above and below the lesion as the graft improves in colour and stability. This is to mobilise soft tissue, particularly near the excised border for this area tends to become fibrous. Mobility is essential, for circulation to the graft would otherwise be impaired.

Progression is made to finger kneading to the excised border and when it is stable, gradually introduce this movement across the graft. Still later, ultrasonics may be given to the area around the graft. Remedial exercises are introduced as soon as possible. Continue in this way until a mobile, well-vascularised graft results.

Physiotherapists should only be called in for the problem cases of leg ulcers – particularly for the extensive but inoperable lesions. Modern medical treatment should be given at the earliest pre-ulcerative stage and is therefore prophylactic. The extensive ulceration that we now see is largely the result of public ignorance of the treatment available. But the work of the great pioneers is being recognised and their methods used. Just as the effects of so many other conditions have been eliminated or minimised, so in the future will the worst of leg ulceration be controlled.

Leg ulceration appears to be a particularly useful study for physiotherapy students because other facets of their work are introduced, viz.:

The behaviour and control of oedema whatever its cause.

Recognition of the fact that swelling is itself traumatic and that wherever it occurs reduction needs to be achieved as quickly as possible.

The care of infected lesions.
The principle of infectious precautions.
The care of skin grafts.
The prevention and treatment of contractures.
The care of unique chronic conditions such as the balance and walking re-education of a patient who has not stood for ten years.

Most important of all is the emphasis on teamwork, for in dealing with the worst of these lesions all disciplines may be called in at one stage or another because, not infrequently, such an ulcer is only a sign of a deeper and much more serious condition requiring the most thorough examination, diagnosis and treatment.

BIBLIOGRAPHY

Bremner, D. N., Moffat, L. E. F., Lee, D. (1977). 'Porcine Dermis as a Temporary Ulcer Dressing'. *The Practitioner*, May.
Dodd, Harold and Cockett, F. B. (1976). *Varicose Veins and the Pathology and Surgery of the Veins of the Lower Limb*, 2nd ed. Churchill Livingstone.
Fegan, W. G. (1967). *Varicose Veins, Compression Sclerotherapy*. William Heinemann Medical Books Ltd.
Fegan, W. G. (1974). 'Varicose Feet.' *Nursing Mirror*, August 30.

ACKNOWLEDGEMENT

The author wishes to express his gratitude to Mr. J. L. Stephen, M.A., M.CH., F.R.C.S. for the benefit of his knowledge and advice for many years, and permission to use photographs of his patients.

Chapter 20

Cardiac Pathology

by E. A. BEAZLEY, M.C.S.P., DIP.T.P.

DISTURBANCES OF CARDIAC RATE AND RHYTHM

Disturbances of cardiac rate and rhythm are due either to disturbances in forming an electrical impulse or failure to conduct electrical impulses correctly.

IMPULSE FORMATION

The normal heart rate varies but has an average rate of 70 rhythmical cycles per minute at rest. The electrical impulse is initiated at the sinuatrial node (pacemaker) and spreads out over the atria; it is picked up by the atrioventricular node and conducted by the atrioventricular bundle to the apex of the ventricles.

FACTORS INFLUENCING IMPULSE FORMATION

All factors which affect the heart rate will affect impulse formation:

COMMON FACTORS	HEART RATE INCREASED	HEART RATE DECREASED
Nervous	Sympathetic	Parasympathetic (vagus)
Chemical	Noradrenaline Thyroxine	
Temperature Emotion	Increased	Decrease

Pain may alter heart rate. Coronary vascular disease may deprive the sinuatrial node of adequate nutrition for normal function.

IMPULSE DISORDERS

Sinus tachycardia occurs when impulses are initiated at a faster rate than normal. Sinus bradycardia occurs when impulses are at a slower rate than normal. Sinus arrhythmia occurs when the heart rate is arrhythmic. Ectopic foci are heart beats initiated in either the atria or the ventricles. They are premature beats which interrupt the normal heart rhythm, and may be found in association with atrial tachycardia, atrial flutter or fibrillation; ventricular tachycardia or ventricular fibrillation.

Atrial or Ventricular Tachycardia

This is nearly always paroxysmal and consists of a succession of rapid rhythmical premature beats. The attacks usually pass off suddenly. In each case there may be no underlying heart disease but anoxia of the ventricular muscle, or an overdose of digitalis, may be the cause of ventricular tachycardia, e.g. following myocardial infarction. The attack is accompanied by palpitations, anxiety and weakness.

TREATMENT

D.C. electroversion may be used in both instances to re-establish a normal rhythm (see ventricular fibrillation).

Atrial tachycardia may be treated by drugs, e.g. digitalis, providing this has not been the cause of the tachycardia.

Ventricular tachycardia may be treated by a myocardial depressant such as propranolol to try to re-establish normal rhythm.

Atrial Flutter

Atrial flutter is due to a rapid regular stimulus formation in an ectopic form producing contraction waves at the rate of about 300 per minute. The functional tissue is unable to respond at this rate, due to the natural refractoriness of the atrioventricular conducting tissue, and will induce ventricular contractions at a rate of 2:1, 3:1 or 4:1 (partial atrioventricular block). If this rate continues for some days or longer, congestive failure is likely to develop.

Atrial Fibrillation

This differs from atrial flutter in its speed. The stimulus formation is more rapid (450 per minute or more), and irregular. The atria appear to be 'twitching' rather than contracting and they no longer eject blood into the ventricles. The danger of this is the possible formation of clots in the atria, particularly in the left auricular appendage. Clots may be dislodged from the left side causing cerebral or systemic arterial emboli, or from the right side causing pulmonary emboli.

The effect on the ventricles depends on how many contraction waves spread to the ventricles. If a high proportion reach the ventricles cardiac failure is likely to ensue.

In both atrial flutter and fibrillation there is usually underlying heart disease, which is most commonly mitral stenosis.

The object of treatment is to restore sinus rhythm, and lower the rate of conductivity so that fewer stimuli reach the ventricles. This can usually be achieved by the use of digitalis.

Ventricular Fibrillation

This type of fibrillation is characterised by rapid irregular ineffectual twitchings of the ventricles. They do not produce an adequate cardiac output, and so this condition is likely to be rapidly fatal. It is usually the cause of death following coronary thrombosis. Sometimes it can be arrested by the use of the defibrillating machine. In this method an electric shock depolarises the myocardium and when the heart begins to beat again it is hoped that the normal rhythm will be re-established.

Interference in Conduction

This is known as heart-block. The interference may be in any part of the conducting system, but the commonest sites are the atrioventricular node and the atrioventricular bundle. The lesion is usually calcification or fibrosis of the conducting system which occurs in coronary artery disease or chronic rheumatic carditis; or it may be a congenital defect.

The passage of the impulse is either delayed (partial heart-block) or prevented (complete heart-block). The atria and ventricles beat independently and if no impulse reaches the ventricles they beat at their inherent rate of about 40 per minute. This ventricular rate cannot change to meet the varying needs of the body.

The danger of this condition is the occurrence of Stokes-Adams attacks which may prove fatal. Occasionally in heart-block the slow ventricular rate changes to ventricular tachycardia or fibrillation; or as a partial heart-block changes to a complete heart-block the ventricles stop contracting; in each case the patient becomes unconscious and pulseless. Convulsions develop due to cerebral anoxia, breathing becomes stertorous and the sufferer becomes deeply cyanosed. After about half a minute the ventricle starts to beat again, which may be due to anoxia; convulsions cease and the patient's colour and pulse return.

TREATMENT

Treatment of acquired heart-block is usually by the administration of drugs which quicken the heart rate, but if these are ineffective and there are frequent Stokes-Adams attacks the rate of ventricular contraction may be controlled by an artificial pacemaker (see p. 172).

CARDIAC FAILURE

The heart, a muscular pump, supplies the metabolic needs of the tissues. The needs vary, the tissues demanding more on exercise and less at total rest. They are met by a rapid response which alters the force, or the rate of contraction of the heart, or both.

The heart responds like voluntary muscle, and can increase its output on severe exertion; or if necessary, providing there is an adequate oxygen supply to the myocardium, it will hypertrophy, as for example in athletes.

The cardiac reserve and ability to hypertrophy enable the myocardium to cope with damage or disease, i.e. to compensate, so that an individual may have a heart lesion for years but be totally unaware of it.

When the oxygen supply becomes inadequate for the increased needs of the now hypertrophied myocardium, the heart muscle ceases to hypertrophy and the strength of contraction gradually fails to maintain an adequate cardiac output. The cavity dilates and back pressure causes a rise in venous pressure. Signs and symptoms of heart involvement appear and the heart is said to be decompensating or failing.

Compensation is the ability of the myocardium to respond to more work, by hypertrophy. The area of hypertrophy depends on the site of the lesion. At first there will be an increased volume of blood in a chamber, e.g. the left ventricle with aortic stenosis. The ventricle dilates slightly, which stimulates a stronger contraction to overcome the resistance and maintain a normal output volume. This will occur over a long period but eventually the limit of hypertrophy will be reached. Decompensation then follows. Output begins to fall and the ventricle dilates. This decompensation is made more likely as the nutrition of the subendocardial muscle is impaired by the high ventricular pressure, and ischaemic fibrosis gradually develops.

There are no symptoms of impending failure while the heart's chambers are responding by hypertrophy. As compensation fails, symptoms appear on severe exertion, so that the patient decreases his activity. Fatigue and breathlessness gradually appear on mild exercise such as walking, and eventually symptoms appear at rest. This is cardiac failure.

The whole heart, all four chambers, may fail together, but frequently the clinical picture is one of failure of one side more than the other.

Left ventricular failure usually occurs in association with hypertension when the peripheral resistance is high. Disease of the aortic valve, either stenosis or incompetence, or both together, force the left ventricle to work harder, to hypertrophy and eventually to fail. Coronary artery disease and myocardial infarction may cause left ventricular failure. The disease of the coronary vessels deprives the heart muscle of adequate oxygen, and ischaemic fibrosis develops.

Left atrial failure occurs where there is an obstruction to the flow of blood into the left ventricle as in mitral stenosis, and there is a reservoir of blood left in the atrium following each phase of emptying.

Left-sided heart failure is the failure to maintain an adequate circulation of the systemic flow of blood, and so the needs of the tissues are not met, and the patient feels weak and lethargic.

Right ventricular failure may follow left ventricular failure, as there is back pressure exerted through the pulmonary circulation to the right ventricle. When pulmonary hypertension becomes too great, the right ventricle fails. Pulmonary hypertension will occur in the presence of hypoxia, a condition associated with many of the chronic respiratory diseases and in association with the pathology of the pulmonary vessels, e.g. pulmonary emboli.

Right-sided failure in which there is an inadequate return of blood to the heart, results in peripheral oedema seen in the lower limbs, and in recumbent patients in the sacral area. Congenital heart disease, e.g. septal defects, or stenosis of the pulmonary valve, and any condition which interferes with the return of blood to the heart or to the right ventricle, e.g. tricuspid valvular disease, will result in right-sided failure.

Thyrotoxicosis which may be associated with heart failure, is a precipitating factor, not a cause of heart failure.

Congestive Cardiac Failure

This is a term which is usually applied when the left side of the heart fails and the lungs become congested. Ultimately there is congestion of the peripheral circulation, but this may not be in evidence at first.

The congestion may be in the pulmonary system, or in the systemic system, or in both systems. It is usually due to the retention of sodium and water by the kidneys resulting in a larger blood volume.

In left-sided congestive failure the left side of the heart fails to provide an adequate pump and pulmonary congestion develops. The pulmonary vessels constrict, increasing the work of the right ventricle. While the right side of the heart continues to pump adequately, pulmonary congestion gradually increases. There will be oedema of the lung parenchyma and, as it increases and the congestion becomes chronic, there is thickening of the interstitial tissue and the lungs become 'stiff'. There is an increasing resistance to airflow and breathing becomes more difficult.

CLINICAL SIGNS OF LEFT-SIDED HEART FAILURE

Dyspnoea on exertion progressing to dyspnoea at rest.
Shallow and an increasingly rapid rate of breathing.
Orthopnoea.
Paroxysmal nocturnal dyspnoea which occurs when a patient sleeping in a sitting position slips down the bed during sleep.
Cardiac asthma in advanced cases associated with pulmonary oedema.

CLINICAL SIGNS AND SYMPTOMS OF RIGHT-SIDED CARDIAC FAILURE

These are the signs of systemic venous congestion:
Pulsating veins at the root of the neck above the medial third of the clavicle.
Distension of the external jugular vein.
Liver palpable below the right costal margin.
Pain in the right hypochondrium due to the stretched capsule of the swollen liver.
Loss of appetite and nausea with vomiting due to portal congestion.
Ascites if there is outpouring of a serous fluid into the peritoneal cavity.
Peripheral oedema which usually has a low protein content, and gravitates to the most dependent parts of the body. If the pad of a thumb or finger is pressed into the oedema, and on release the impression made is retained for a short while, it is known as pitting oedema.
Peripheral cyanosis if the right-sided failure is associated with a left-sided cardiac failure. This may disappear when the limbs are warmed.
Central cyanosis if lung disease is present.

CHANGES OF RIGHT AND LEFT-SIDED CARDIAC FAILURE

There will be changes in the:

Electrocardiogram
P_{CO_2} and P_{O_2} levels
X-ray projection of the heart and pulmonary vessels
Heart sounds
Kidney function which may occur secondary to fluid control.

COMPLICATIONS OF CONGESTIVE CARDIAC FAILURE

These are the complications associated with bed rest:

Chest infection (e.g. hypostatic pneumonia)
Deep venous thrombosis
Pressure sores associated with lack of nutrition and excess oedema in
    the tissues, where body weight is supported
Muscular weakness which is generalised
Postural tone of the antigravity muscles and small muscles of the feet
    diminishes with prolonged immobility; and the tendo Achilles may
    shorten.

TREATMENT OF CARDIAC FAILURE

The treatment of this condition is medical. Physiotherapy may be used to prevent the complications mentioned above once the pulmonary oedema is being controlled by the use of diuretics.

The lungs are kept free from infection through the use of breathing exercises and effective coughing which may need to be achieved using reinforcement of the abdominal muscles. Where indicated, postural drainage may be used or modified.

Circulation in the legs is improved with breathing exercises and exercises for the feet, knees, and hips as appropriate to the cardiac condition.

Pressure sores should be prevented by adequate turning of the patient; if a reddened area appears prevention of deterioration to a sore may be achieved either by the careful use of infra-red rays, or ice massage to the area and its surrounds. Should pressure sores develop, they may be treated with infra-red rays, ultraviolet rays or ice massage to the surrounding area.

Progressive schemes of exercises which may be used to increase the tolerance of the heart once the heart failure is controlled will also help strengthen weakened muscles. They will only be given on the direct request of the consultant in charge of the patient.

Pain in the forefoot on ambulation can be prevented by exercising the lumbricals and interossei during the recovery period; exercises of the ankle into dorsiflexion with the knee straight will help prevent shortening of the tendo Achilles.

Tension often seen in patients with cardiac conditions may be relieved with relaxation. The state of the heart must be considered when choosing the method of teaching relaxation.

Chapter 21

Some Cardiac Disorders

by E. A. BEAZLEY, M.C.S.P., DIP.T.P.

RHEUMATIC FEVER (ACUTE RHEUMATISM)

Rheumatic fever is an inflammatory condition affecting connective tissues; particularly those of the heart in the young, and the joints in adults. It has a tendency to recur.

CAUSE

The cause is frequently an upper respiratory tract infection by group A haemolytic *Streptococcus*. The cardiac symptoms may appear two to four weeks later. Some authorities think there may be an auto-antifactor present, which reacts with the antigen found in the myocardium.

CHANGES

The changes which occur in the heart are primarily in the myocardium. There is a myocarditis which spreads to involve the endocardium and may spread to involve the pericardium in an inflammatory process.

The *myocardium* develops numerous Aschoff nodes: small necrotic areas of collagen tissue surrounded by histiocytes and leucocytes, which will heal by fibrosis and contraction, and interfere with myocardial function so that it may fail. Many of these nodes form beneath and adjacent to the endocardium, which frequently becomes inflamed in acute rheumatism.

The *endocardium* of the heart chambers, valves, chordae tendinae and papillary muscles become inflamed and the changes which occur are similar to those of the myocardium, except for the valves. The valves develop tiny wart-like vegetations along the margins of the cusps.

Pericardial inflammation gives rise to a sero-fibrinous exudate which may, but often does not, impede the function of the heart. It does not lead to a constrictive pericarditis.

TREATMENT

This is by drugs to combat the infection, and bed rest with oxygen to relieve all strain on the myocardium. If there is joint involvement these are rested in a pain-free neutral position.

Physiotherapy is not used in the acute phase. If there is joint involvement this is treated as an acute rheumatoid arthritic joint once the patient's myocardial condition allows.

CHRONIC RHEUMATIC HEART DISEASE

This commonly follows an acute attack of rheumatism.

CHANGES

The changes are mainly those of chronic endocarditis, in which there is an overgrowth of connective tissue followed by contraction, which gives rise to valvular deformities.

The myocardium shows Aschoff nodes, and small areas of myocardial fibrosis where Aschoff nodes have healed.

There may be pericardial adhesions which are unimportant unless the pericardium becomes attached to mediastinal structures or there is severe fibrosis which impedes cardiac function.

The endocardial structures affected by acute rheumatism – the papillary muscles, chordae tendinae and walls of the chambers – thicken and contract slowly as part of the continuing healing process.

The valvular cusps fuse along their edges as organisation of the warty vegetations occurs (stenosis). Contraction and thickening of the valvular cusps and fibrous rings leads to incompetence.

The mitral valve is the valve most frequently damaged by rheumatic heart disease, while the pulmonary valve seldom seems to be affected.

While the chronic changes take place there may be a recurrent attack of the original infection with more vegetations forming on the cusps, and more Aschoff nodes in the myocardium.

TREATMENT

This is medical, though the valvular diseases may require surgery (see Chapter 10).

COMPLICATIONS

Cardiac failure is a common occurrence due to the stenosis and/or incompetence of one or more valves.

Angina pectoris occurs when the coronary blood flow to the hypertrophied myocardium becomes inadequate because of poor cardiac output.

Atrial fibrillation is a common result of myocardial and endocardial scar tissue.

Thrombi often form in the atrial appendages of patients with mitral or tricuspid stenosis and atrial fibrillation. These may circulate as emboli in the arterial network or pulmonary veins.

Subacute bacterial endocarditis is a common development following disease of valves in chronic rheumatic heart disease.

SUBACUTE BACTERIAL ENDOCARDITIS

Subacute bacterial endocarditis is an infection of the endocardium. There is formation of large vegetations on the cusps of valves, which usually have pre-existing cardiac lesions.

CAUSE

There is probably an infective focus in the mouth or upper respiratory tract. The infection often appears following minor surgery, e.g. tooth extraction.

The infective bacteria, often classified as *Streptococcus viridans*, are usually of low virulence.

The changes of rheumatic heart disease or congenital valvular defects are often present, and the bacteria cause further damage to the diseased valves.

The circulating bacteria and any other matter circulating in the blood become attached to platelets. The platelets are attracted to, and deposited on, the edges of the valvular cusps, which may have been deformed previously. These vegetations, formed of a small area of calcification surrounded by a soft crumbly mass of bacteria, platelets, fibrin and white blood cells, are larger than those of rheumatic heart disease, and tend to spread to the endocardial walls, particularly the atrial wall behind the mitral valve.

Signs and symptoms of subacute bacterial endocarditis are often a low grade, fluctuating fever with an enlarged spleen and haematuria in a person who has a congenital defect, e.g. a persistent ductus arteriosus or valvular defect, or in one who has had rheumatic heart disease.

Blood cultures, which may have to be taken frequently to establish a diagnosis, usually confirm it, if taken during an active phase of the condition when there are circulating emboli containing bacteria.

Cardiac failure is not an early feature of this condition.

TREATMENT

Treatment of this condition is medical. When the patient is well enough, surgery to correct any underlying cardiac abnormality may be considered.

VALVULAR HEART DISEASE

The valves are continuous with the endocardium which lines the chambers of the heart.

The tricuspid and mitral valves, which lie in the atrioventricular fibrous ring, shut when the pressure in the ventricles is rising so that the blood does not regurgitate into the atria.

The pulmonary valve between the right ventricle and the pulmonary artery, and the aortic valve between the left ventricle and the aorta, remain shut until the ventricular pressures exceed the pressures on the arterial side of the valves.

CAUSES OF VALVULAR DISEASE

Valvular disease may be acquired or congenital.

Rheumatic endocarditis often precedes valvular disease and is the most frequent cause of mitral valve pathology. It may also affect the aortic and tricuspid valves.

Subacute bacterial endocarditis may add to the damage already caused by rheumatic endocarditis, or its effect may be superimposed on congenital lesions.

Syphilis may affect the aortic valve.

Congenital lesions usually affect the pulmonary valve, and also may affect the aortic and tricuspid valves.

Trauma will occasionally rupture a cusp of a valve.

PATHOLOGY OF VALVULAR DISEASE

Rheumatic endocarditis involves the endocardium and the valves – ring, cusps and chordae tendinae – to a greater or lesser extent. It causes inflammatory changes and the structures involved will fibrose and shrink. Wart-like vegetations of platelets and fibrin form along the edges of the valvular cusps. These warts gradually become part of the valve and add to its structural distortion. The repair process may take place over a period of years.

Subacute bacterial endocarditis usually attacks previously diseased or congenitally defective valves. There is an endocarditis and further inflammation of the valves, but this time the warty vegetation is formed by septic foci containing the organism which has caused the infection.

The inflammatory disease process may lead to stenosis or incompetence or a combination of the two. The other coats of the heart may be affected also.

Stenosis is the thickening and fusion of the valve's cusps leading to an overall reduction in the cross-sectional area of its open orifice. The chamber behind the stenosis will dilate and then hypertrophy in response to a greater volume of blood.

Incompetence is the ineffective closure of a valve due to distortion, contraction, and fusion of the valves and in disease of rheumatic origin the chordae tendinae will also contract and fibrose. During systole, blood regurgitates through the unclosed valve. There will be an initial dilatation, and hypertrophy of the chambers behind the incompetent valve. As the volume of blood passing through the valve increases, the same sequence of events occurs distally – first dilatation followed by hypertrophy of the muscular wall, and eventually failure.

Disease of the Mitral Valve

CAUSE

Rheumatic endocarditis is the usual cause of mitral valve disease. The affected cusps will be thicker and stiffer than normal and may be calcified. The orifice will be narrower (stenosis), and may not shut (incompetence). If the ring and the chordae tendinae are contracted this will increase the incompetence.

Mitral stenosis leads to dilatation and hypertrophy of the left atrium due to the increased volume of blood in the atrial chamber. The back pressure caused by the stenosis will eventually cause pulmonary congestion and hypertension and then an increased volume of blood in the right ventricle. The right ventricle responds by dilating, and then hypertrophies until eventually there is right-sided heart failure. Atrial fibrillation is often present with this condition.

Mitral incompetence is where the mitral valve fails to close during ventricular systole, and allows regurgitation of blood to the left atrium. This will dilate and hypertrophy forcing more blood through to the left ventricle, which will respond by dilating, then hypertrophying and eventually going into failure.

SYMPTOMS OF MITRAL VALVE DISEASE

Mitral stenosis produces dyspnoea on exertion due to pulmonary congestion. This becomes worse, and occasional attacks of acute pulmonary oedema occur.

Palpitations and a persistent cough are present, and there is a gradual increase in dyspnoea until it occurs at rest. Eventually orthopnoea develops.

Symptoms of congestive cardiac failure also occur.

Mitral incompetence produces no symptoms until the left ventricle can no longer compensate. Then as failure begins there is an increased back pressure causing pulmonary hypertension, and the symptoms become the same as those for mitral stenosis.

TREATMENT

This is surgical for both mitral stenosis and mitral incompetence (see Chapter 10).

Disease of the Aortic Valve

CAUSES

Rheumatic endocarditis may cause aortic stenosis in association with other valvular lesions, or aortic incompetence. Incompetence may also be due to a syphilitic infection of the aorta, subacute bacterial endocarditis, or trauma.

A congenital bicuspid valve is sometimes associated with calcification and may give rise to an aortic stenosis in an elderly person.

SYMPTOMS OF AORTIC STENOSIS

These are absent until the hypertrophied left ventricle can compensate no longer. Then there will be progressive dyspnoea on exercise which progresses until there is dyspnoea at rest. Finally there is orthopnoea and congestive cardiac failure.

In addition, probably due to cerebral anaemia resulting from low pressure in the arch of the aorta, there are symptoms such as dizziness, faintness, and transient loss of consciousness (syncope) and, due to low pressure in the coronary arteries, myocardial ischaemia may result in angina, heart-block and sudden death.

SYMPTOMS OF AORTIC INCOMPETENCE

The left ventricle may dilate and hypertrophy over a period of years. Eventually failure of the left ventricle becomes apparent, and there is progressive dyspnoea on exercise. This progresses until it occurs at rest, and then becomes orthopnoea, and there is congestive cardiac failure.

TREATMENT

This is surgical for both aortic stenosis and aortic incompetence (see Chapter 10).

Disease of Pulmonary Valves

CAUSE

Pulmonary stenosis is usually a congenital deformity. It may be an isolated lesion, but is more commonly found in association with a ventricular septal defect (see page 182).

Pulmonary incompetence is usually associated with pulmonary hypertension in which the pulmonary artery dilates. This is followed by dilatation of the right ventricle leading to an enlarging of the orifice from the right ventricle to the pulmonary artery, e.g. as with mitral stenosis.

SYMPTOMS OF PULMONARY CONGESTION AND OEDEMA

The patient is dyspnoeic and becomes cyanosed; there is a productive cough with expectoration of copious frothy sputum which is white, pink or streaked with blood; there are coarse bubbling sounds over the lung fields with secretions in the larynx, trachea and main stem bronchi. These make an audible rattle.

TREATMENT

This is directed to the primary cause of the hypertension.

Tricuspid Valve Disease

CAUSE

Rheumatic endocarditis may affect the tricuspid valve at the same time as the mitral valve, and frequently the aortic valve.

SYMPTOMS

Symptoms of tricuspid stenosis are overshadowed by symptoms from other valvular disease. There is, however, little dyspnoea or orthopnoea if there is associated mitral stenosis; the output of the right ventricle is lower than normal, and so there is not much pulmonary congestion.

Incompetence occurs in dilatation of the heart in association with right ventricular failure.

TREATMENT

This is surgical for tricuspid stenosis. The treatment of incompetence will be directed towards the cause.

Treatment of Valvular Heart Disease

The presence of one or more defective valves throws a strain on the myocardium which must work harder to maintain an adequate output. This extra load can be reduced by surgery in some patients. Contracted and deformed valves can be repaired; adhered cusps and fibrosed valve rings can be dealt with by valvotomy; or valves can be completely replaced by a prosthesis. These operations often have spectacular results, but they are serious procedures and are accompanied by particular risks (see Chapter 10).

Conservative treatment, which will vary with the age and state of the patient, is used when surgery is not suitable or is refused.

The young patient known to have a valvular lesion may be advised in the choice of a suitable career, i.e. avoiding heavy manual work.

Pregnancy may have to be terminated, or special precautions taken; this will possibly involve a period of bed rest.

Cardiac arrhythmias are treated by suitable drugs.

Lung infections must be avoided, and if signs of infection appear rapid and effective treatment is essential.

If failure has occurred, rest, diet, drugs and oxygen will relieve the work of the heart. As the heart recovers the patient has to learn to live within the limits imposed by the defective heart without becoming a chronic cardiac invalid.

The complications of valvular disease require treatment and involve such methods as anticoagulant therapy for arterial embolism, antibiotics for lung infections, drugs for atrial fibrillation and congestive failure.

PHYSIOTHERAPY

This has a part to play in helping to prevent or treat the complications of cardiac surgery (see Chapter 10) and in recovery from congestive cardiac failure. The physiotherapist will be called in to treat such complications as hemiplegia, or paralysis resulting from cerebral anaemia or a cerebral embolism.

ISCHAEMIC HEART DISEASE

The coronary arteries anastomose, and there is usually a good anastomosis between the smaller vessels, which branch from the main

SUMMARY OF TREATMENT OF VALVE DISEASE

VALVE	CAUSE	CONDITION	SIGNS AND SYMPTOMS	TREATMENT
Mitral	Rheumatic endocarditis	Stenosis	palpitations; persistent cough; dyspnoea on exertion, later at rest; pulmonary oedema; orthopnoea	Medical and/or Surgical
		Incompetence	no symptoms until left ventricular failure occurs, then pulmonary hypertension and changes as for stenosis	
Tricuspid	Rheumatic endocarditis	Stenosis	likely to be those of either associated mitral valve disease or aortic valve disease	Surgical
		Incompetence		
Aortic	Rheumatic endocarditis Acute bacterial endocarditis Syphilis Trauma Congenital	Stenosis	dyspnoea on exercise, later at rest; orthopnoea; dizziness and syncope; angina	Surgical
		Incompetence	left ventricular failure; progressive dyspnoea; orthopnoea; congestive cardiac failure	
Pulmonary	Congenital + Ventricular septal defect Pulmonary hypertension	Stenosis		Surgical
		Incompetence	pulmonary hypertension	Medical and/or Surgical

branches of the coronary vessels, but not with the larger arteries. If the lumen of the coronary vessels gradually becomes smaller, the myocardium will show ischaemic changes (fibrosis).

Sudden occlusion of the blood supply to a part of the myocardium will lead to necrosis of the area supplied exclusively by the blocked vessel. If this occurs in the proximal 2 or 3cm of a coronary artery there will be a large infarct, but if the occlusion occurs distally and the area of heart muscle affected receives nutrition from anastomotic vessels, few changes occur in the myocardium.

CAUSES OF ISCHAEMIC HEART CONDITION

Atherosclerosis of the coronary vessels is the commonest cause in Western civilisation
Aortic valvular incompetence
Mitral stenosis of a severe nature
Syphilitic aortitis if the entrances to the coronary arteries are restricted

INCIDENCE OF CARDIAC ISCHAEMIA

Men of middle age in the professional and administrative occupations have a higher incidence of atherosclerosis than their peers. Recent research seems to indicate that people who have a high calorie intake, a high energy output and incorporate a large amount of cereal fibre in their diet have a lower incidence of coronary heart disease (Morris, 1977).

COMPLICATIONS OF CARDIAC ISCHAEMIA

Angina pectoris
Coronary occlusion
Arrhythmias

Angina Pectoris

This condition is characterised by sudden retrosternal pain, probably due to the inadequate removal of the waste products of cardiac muscle contraction.

Angina of effort occurs on activity and may be intense.

CLINICAL SIGNS AND SYMPTOMS

Pain of varying intensity starts behind the sternum from which it radiates up into the neck and spreads into one or both arms, and the jaw if it is very intense. Breathing may become shallow and laboured.

PRECIPITATING FACTORS

Intense emotion	Hypertension
Atherosclerosis	Anaemia
Cardiac ischaemia	Thyrotoxicosis

TREATMENT

Medical treatment will include prescribing a vasodilator drug to be taken as necessary. There are both short and long-acting dilators. It is the short acting one, glycerine trinitrate, which the patient should have with him, and use, if necessary, before or during physiotherapy.

Surgical treatment to improve the blood supply to the myocardium may be suitable in some cases (see p. 170).

Physiotherapy may involve the use of progressive exercises, whereby it is hoped to hypertrophy the heart, decrease the heart rate, and improve the nutrition to the heart (see Chapter 22).

Coronary Occlusion

This is the blocking of a coronary vessel due to a thrombus or embolus which may be secondary to coronary atherosclerosis and leads to a myocardial infarct.

Myocardial Infarction

This is the death of muscle cells of the myocardium. The affected area varies in size and the severity depends on the site of the coronary occlusion and any previous occlusions.

Changes of inflammation occur, organisation and healing with fibrous tissue taking from four to six weeks. Small necrotic areas form firm fibrous scars; large areas of necrosis may destroy the efficiency of the cardiac pump. The scar tissue may then become stretched with diffuse bulging of the wall from the pressure of the blood inside the heart chamber, or a saccular aneurysm may develop (see p. 265).

CLINICAL SIGNS AND SYMPTOMS

The pain is retrosternal, spreading up to the jaw and neck. It starts lower with less intensity and lasts longer than that of angina pectoris and is not relieved by vasodilator drugs.

Breathlessness, shock, pallor, sweating, coldness, giddiness, syncope and vomiting may all be present.

The blood pressure will fall after one or two days. The pulse is rapid with a low pressure and the temperature up slightly because of inflammatory changes.

COMPLICATIONS

These are primarily due to alteration in the conductivity of heart muscle, and alteration in the mechanical function of the heart.

Disorders due to electrical conductivity include:
Rhythmic disorders
Fibrillation of the atria or ventricles
Ectopic beats which may be atrial or ventricular
Cardiac arrest.

Disorders due to mechanical malfunction include:
Thrombi forming in the affected heart chamber
Emboli which may circulate from any thrombotic site in the cardiovascular system
Hemiplegia from an embolus circulating from the left ventricle
Frozen shoulder usually on the left side, three to four weeks after the occlusion

TREATMENT

The treatment of this condition is medical, although surgery may be tried to improve the blood supply to the heart or to correct a cardiac aneurysm (see Chapter 10).

Physiotherapy in the acute stage may be required to prevent any respiratory complications. Deep breathing exercises with effective coughing affects the respiratory and cardiovascular system. There is usually no contra-indication to the patient lying down for treatment if required, but this should be checked with the doctor first if in doubt. Active leg exercises within the patient's tolerance, and not causing breathlessness, are encouraged to help prevent deep venous thrombosis in the early stages.

Following the acute stage, physiotherapy may not be required as the patient's activity may be increased adequately without formal exercise. Physiotherapy during the recovery phase may be used to help increase cardiac efficiency with the use of progressive exercises. This may continue on an out-patient basis following discharge. The design of the exercise regime will depend on the degree of damage to the heart and the patient's progress, and what the doctor in charge of the case considers to be suitable in terms of work for the heart. This may be linked to each patient's pulse rate. Patients may be advised to continue exercises long after they have returned to work, and many big companies have gymnasia where people working for them may go and exercise during the day (see Chapter 22).

REFERENCE

Morris, J. M., Marr, Jean W. and Clayton, D. G. (1977). 'Diet and heart: a postscript.' *British Medical Journal*, 2, 1307.

BIBLIOGRAPHY

Conybeare's Textbook of Medicine (Ed. W. N. Mann and M. H. Lessoff, 1975). 16th ed. Churchill Livingstone.

Davidson, Sir Stanley and MacLeod, J. (Eds.) (1974). *The Principles and Practice of Medicine*. 11th ed. Churchill Livingstone.

Muir's Textbook of Pathology (Ed. J. R. Anderson, 1971). 10th ed. Edward Arnold.

Price's Textbook of the Practice of Medicine (Ed. R. B. Scott, 1973). 11th ed. Churchill Livingstone.

ACKNOWLEDGEMENTS

The author thanks the Principal, Staff and Students of the School of Physiotherapy, St. Mary's Hospital, London for their help and advice in the revision of these chapters.

Chapter 22

Rehabilitation following Coronary Thrombosis

by P. McCOY, m.c.s.p.

INTRODUCTION

Rehabilitation following coronary thrombosis should start from the beginning of the patient's illness and should continue until the patient has reached his maximum physical potential commensurate with his clinical condition. Thus the aim of the coronary care team will be to have the patient return to work or normal circumstances as soon as the patient's clinical state allows. Inevitably some patients will not be able to resume work or participate in any physical activity because of the severity of the cardiac muscle damage following the coronary thrombosis.

Generally the policy of three weeks bed rest followed by very restricted physical activity has been replaced in most units by a programme of more rapid mobilisation and earlier discharge from hospital. The time scale of mobilisation and level of physical activity will vary widely in different hospitals. The physiotherapist must always follow the policy of the consultant cardiologist responsible for the patient.

INTENSIVE CORONARY CARE – FIRST 48 HOURS

The patient will probably be admitted to an intensive care bed in a coronary care ward. He will be nursed there for the initial 48 hours which is the crucial period following a coronary thrombosis. During this time the patient's electrocardiograph (E.C.G.) is monitored continuously so that potentially dangerous arrhythmias can be treated as they arise thereby minimising the risk of sudden arrhythmic death. Other observations which will be recorded frequently include blood pressure, heart rate, respiratory rate, temperature and fluid intake and output. This information will be used in the patient's regular medical assessment.

During the intensive care stage the patient will be nursed in the semi-recumbent position in bed. Patients in cardiogenic shock or with low blood pressure will probably be nursed lying flat or in the head down position to assist blood flow to the brain. Some doctors will permit the patient to sit up in a chair by the bedside for an hour in the later part of the first day if the patient's condition is stable. This will be extended to two hours in the second day if clinical stability is maintained. Some patients may be permitted to have short walks around the bed while still attached to the electrocardiograph monitor.

Factors which would prevent early mobilisation include tachycardia, ventricular arrhythmias, persistent chest pain and congestive heart failure.

Physiotherapy in the First 48 Hours

The main aim of physiotherapy during this early period is preventive. It is important to prevent accumulation of secretions in the lungs which may predispose to chest infection and its possible complications. Stasis in the deep veins of the legs should be prevented and so lessen the danger of deep venous thrombosis and its possible complications.

Deep breathing exercises should be taught and the patient should be asked to repeat them at least every hour. Patients, who have a history of respiratory disease such as chronic bronchitis, or present with chest infection may need other physiotherapy measures such as postural drainage. Foot and ankle exercises should be repeated regularly by the patient to increase blood flow in the legs.

THIRD DAY UNTIL DISCHARGE FROM HOSPITAL

If the patient's condition has remained stable during the first 48 hours he is moved out of the acute monitoring area. He will now be allowed to be more active and will probably be encouraged to have frequent short walks within the ward. The practice of including supervised exercises in the mobilisation programme is becoming more widespread. This enables staff to monitor progress by recording the duration and type of activity and recording the patient's response. Speed of mobilisation may be modified if the patient develops symptoms. Occasionally clinical deterioration will require return to acute monitoring.

Recording of Information

In order to record patients' response to activity it will be necessary to divide the mobilisation programme into stages. An example of a possible mobilisation programme is set out below.

Stage I	Monitoring; bed rest; patient washed and fed if necessary.
	Physiotherapy: breathing exercises. Foot and ankle exercises.
Stage II	Monitoring; sit up in chair for one hour; patient feeds and washes himself; may use commode.
	Physiotherapy: as Stage I.
Stage III	Monitoring; sit up in chair for two hours, morning and afternoon.
	Physiotherapy: as Stage I.
Stage IV	Off monitor; walk to toilet and bathroom.
	Physiotherapy: Bed End exercises. 5 repeats of each exercise.
Stage V	As Stage IV, plus 6 repeats of Bed End Exercises.
Stage VI	As Stage IV, plus 7 repeats of Bed End Exercises.
Stage VII	As Stage IV, plus 8 repeats of Bed End Exercises.
Stage VIII	As Stage IV, plus walk up and down 1 flight of stairs.

Bed End Exercises

Starting Position. Patient stands facing the end of his bed.
1. Double knee bending.
2. Arm abduction to shoulder level.
3. Alternate leg swinging.
4. Finger tips on shoulders, arm circling.

Figure 22/1 illustrates a chart which could be used to record the patient's response to the various stages of mobilisation. This chart may be kept at the patient's bed so that it is readily available to physiotherapy, nursing and medical staff. The post-infarct day and the date are recorded on the horizontal axis, and the various stages are displayed along the vertical axis. The appropriate line can be ticked to indicate the Stage the patient is at. The pre-exercise heart rate and the maximum and post-exercise heart rate can be recorded. Symptoms which arise during exercise should be noted in the remarks column.

Indications for stopping exercise are shortness of breath, chest pain, irregularities of the pulse, and tachycardia (heart rate above 100 beats per minute).

The patient should be accompanied on the flight of stairs and if

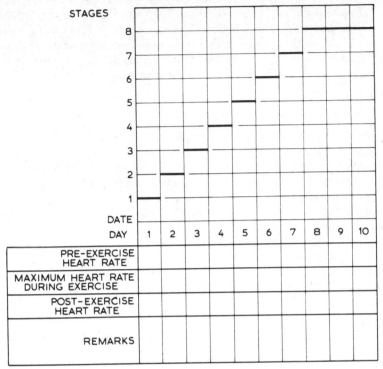

Fig. 22/1 A chart to record the patient's response to mobilisation following coronary thrombosis (ward use)

facilities are available the electrocardiograph should be monitored by telemetry.

The length of time patients spend in hospital following coronary thrombosis will vary between six days and four weeks depending on the policy of the cardiologist.

Physiotherapy in Some Early Complications which may follow Coronary Thrombosis

Chest infections. Physiotherapy and antibiotic therapy are usually prescribed. Postural drainage may be carried out but it will often be necessary to modify the postural drainage position.

Cerebral embolism. The signs and symptoms will vary with the size and site of the blocked vessel. If the patient develops a hemiplegia then physiotherapy treatment should be undertaken in the usual way. It will be necessary to modify the treatment in the early days so as not to overtire the patient.

Limitation of movement in left shoulder girdle. If the patient has had his left arm immobilised because a temporary pacing catheter has been in situ he may have some limitation of shoulder movements. Shoulder movement should be checked after removal of the catheter and mobilising exercises can be taught if necessary.

Convalescence following Discharge from Hospital

On discharge from hospital most patients are able to return home but some will spend a few weeks at a convalescent unit for social or other reasons. The first week at home is spent indoors. The patient is advised to have eight to ten hours rest at night and one or two hours rest in the afternoon. Most patients will be able to climb stairs once or twice daily. Inevitably some patients with extensive cardiac damage and severe heart failure will not be able to climb stairs. Their exercise tolerance will be low and their activity will be limited by shortness of breath and fatigue. By the second week at home the patient will be able to have short walks out of doors in the garden. After the third week the daily walk can be gradually extended so that by the sixth week following discharge the patient is walking three or four miles daily.

Driving a car is usually forbidden for at least six weeks following a coronary thrombosis. Air travel is usually not advised for about three months.

Clinical Review

Patients are usually reviewed at the hospital out-patient department within a month or two of discharge from the ward. The doctor can then assess the patient's ability to return to work, normal life, or embark on an exercise programme. Most patients will be medically fit to return to their former employment within three months of their illness. Some patients may have to take a lighter job because of the inability to do heavy work. Government regulations will debar those who need Heavy Goods Vehicle or Public Service Vehicle licences from their former employment because of coronary thrombosis. These patients will need advice from the social worker as early as possible in their illness so that suitable alternative employment can be found. There are wide variations in medical practice with regard to length of time off work and level of physical activity advised after coronary thrombosis.

REHABILITATION EXERCISE PROGRAMME

Many hospitals now offer facilities for selected patients to attend exercise courses in the physiotherapy department. Not all post-coronary thrombosis sufferers will be clinically fit to attend so it will be necessary to have criteria for selection. The criteria may vary in different centres and the ultimate decision will be the responsibility of the physician.

AIMS OF REHABILITATION PROGRAMME

1. Reduce frequency and severity of myocardial infarction.
2. Provide psychological benefits of exercise.
3. Increase exercise tolerance.
4. Return the patient to work and normal activity as early as possible after the infarction.
5. Restore the patient's confidence in his ability to lead a normal life.

Criteria for Selection for Exercise Class

1. Age up to sixty.
2. Reasonable cardiovascular function based on heart size, X-ray evidence of heart failure and previous history.
3. No serious locomotor disability or concurrent disease.
4. Acceptance of concept by the patient.

Testing Exercise Tolerance

Exercise testing before training provides guidelines for exercise prescription. The exercise tolerance can be tested on a static bicycle ergometer in the physiotherapy gymnasium. If monitoring facilities are available the patient should have his electrocardiograph monitored throughout the test. The blood pressure and resting heart rate are recorded before the test. The heart rate can be observed continuously throughout the test by means of a finger pulsometer. The resistance on the ergometer is increased by increments at each completed minute provided the patient does not show signs of distress. The precise length of time of an exercise test will depend on the physician. The test should always be stopped if any of the following symptoms occur:

Chest pain
Severe shortness of breath

Fatigue
Premature ventricular beats
Dizziness
Muscle cramp
Heart rate in excess of the maximum recommended for the patient.
(See Table below.)

TABLE TO SHOW MAXIMAL HEART RATE RELATED TO AGE
(Astrand et al. 1977)

20–29 years	170 beats per minute
30–39 years	160 beats per minute
40–49 years	150 beats per minute
50–59 years	140 beats per minute
60–69 years	130 beats per minute

There are a great variety of exercise training programmes in operation. To some extent the actual choice of exercises and equipment will depend on the available resources. Many centres, particularly in Scandinavia and the United States of America, have sophisticated gymnasium facilities available for rehabilitation. In the United Kingdom many hospitals offer an exercise programme supervised by a physiotherapist. The hospital-based facility has the advantage that medical help is readily available should a crisis arise.

The duration, intensity and frequency of exercise sessions will depend on the policy of the cardiologist and resources available. Many centres ask patients to attend two or three times weekly for three months. Exercising the patients in a group using an exercise circuit has several advantages over individually supervised exercise sessions:

1. Better utilisation of the physiotherapist's time and gymnasium space.
2. The group therapy effect of patients working together.
3. Opportunity for patients to discuss common problems with each other and with staff.

Within a class situation it will be necessary to have a system where patients' individual exercise tolerance is catered for. This can be achieved by altering:

a) speed of repetitions; b) time allowed for each exercise; c) number of repetitions to be done in the allotted time; d) resistance against which the patient is working.

The patient's natural inclination to compete and compare

performance should be discouraged. Exercises should be arranged so that the competitive element is eliminated as far as possible.

Types of Activity Suitable for Training Post-Coronary Thrombosis Patients

Endurance stimulating physical activity is preferable to strength building exercises. Activities should be enjoyable and adherence to the exercise is encouraged by variety.

Calisthenics can be used during a warm up period at the beginning of the exercise session before proceeding to heavier work. A circuit of exercises can be used, alternating arm, leg and trunk work to prevent muscle fatigue. Apparatus used in the circuit may include static bicycle, rowing machine, shoulder wheel, stools for step-ups, weighted pulleys for arm exercises, medicine balls of various weights, skipping ropes and light balls for bouncing.

EXAMPLE OF EXERCISE CLASS FOR POST-CORONARY THROMBOSIS PATIENTS

A. Warm Up Exercises
1. Arm swinging
2. Trunk side flexion
3. Alternate leg swinging
4. Trunk rotation with arm swinging
5. Knee bends

B. Circuit
1. Shoulder wheel   3 minutes
2. Rowing machine   3 minutes
3. Westminster Pulley for arm extension using weights   3 minutes
4. Step-ups on low stool   3 minutes
5. Sitting; raising and lowering 5lb medicine ball
   above head   3 minutes
6. Static bicycle   6 minutes

C. Group Activity
Volley ball

These activities are an example of an exercise class. Any similar exercises or group activity could be used to provide variety.

The resting pulse should be recorded at the beginning of the class. In order to monitor progress, the pulse can be recorded throughout the static bicycle exercise in a similar way to the recording of the exercise tolerance test. It is not necessary to record the pulse before and after every single exercise. The patient should be advised to stop exercising if he develops chest pain or severe shortness of breath and to report these symptoms to the physiotherapist immediately they occur. The patient should be rested until symptoms subside. If chest pain persists the patient should be seen and examined by the doctor.

Emergency Equipment

It would seem prudent when exercising cardiac patients to have an emergency trolley available in the physiotherapy department. The trolley should have:

a D.C. fibrillator; suction apparatus; oxygen cylinder and mask and E.C.G. leads and portable oscilloscope

The physiotherapy staff should be trained to deal with a patient in the event of a cardiac arrest. As time is of vital importance, the physiotherapist should be able to initiate external cardiac massage and artificial respiration. Medical help must be summoned immediately and most hospitals will have a cardiac arrest team to deal with such eventualities (see Chapter 3).

Home Exercises

In addition to exercising once or twice weekly in the physiotherapy department, the patients should exercise daily at home. The exercises developed by the Royal Canadian Air Force provide a very suitable progressive scheme of exercises for men and women (see references). Alternatively a list similar to that shown below could be given:

A. *Lying*
1. Raise both arms above head to touch floor behind the head
2. Alternate leg straight leg raising
3. Bend up both knees, feet resting on floor; raise pelvis and lower
4. Bend up both knees, feet resting on floor; drop both knees to one side then to the other side
5. Prone lying, back extension exercises

B. *Standing*
6. Trunk side flexion
7. Double knee bending
8. Jogging

Exercises 1–7. Start with six repeats of each exercise. Progress by adding two more repeats each week until a maximum of twenty repeats is reached.

Exercise 8: Jogging. First week – fifty jogs daily. Progress by adding ten to twenty jogs each week until about three or four hundred jogs per day are achieved.

EFFECTS OF EXERCISE

Physical activity will increase the patient's exercise capacity and general feeling of well-being. The mechanisms by which increased habitual physical activity may reduce the occurrence or severity of coronary heart disease are summarised according to Fox, Naughton and Gorman (1972).

PHYSICAL ACTIVITY MAY:

A. Increase the following
Coronary collateral vascularisation
Vessel size
Myocardial efficiency
Efficiency of peripheral blood distribution and return
Electron transport capacity
Fibrinolytic capability
Arterial oxygen content
Red blood cell mass and blood volume
Thyroid function
Growth hormone production
Tolerance to stress
Prudent living habits
Joie de vivre

B. Decrease the following
Serum lipid levels, i.e. triglycerides, cholesterol
Glucose intolerance
Obesity – adiposity
Platelet stickiness
Arterial blood pressure
Heart rate
Vulnerability to dysrhythmias
Neurohormonal overreaction
'Strain' associated with psychic 'stress'

Leisure Activities

The patients who fulfil the criteria for exercise class selection will be able to take part in numerous sporting activities. Competitive sport is usually not recommended as this introduces the stress factor. Swimming, bowls, walking, jogging, badminton, volley ball, cycling, golf, gardening, dancing and horse riding are among the long list of activities which the patients can be encouraged to participate in, depending on their preferences. Outdoor games should be avoided on cold windy days as the vasoconstriction caused by the cold puts an extra load on the circulation.

Heavy isometric work such as shovelling snow in the cold, lifting or pushing very heavy weights, e.g. pushing a car, are contra-indicated in patients with coronary heart disease.

REFERENCES

Astrand, P. O. and Rodahl, K. (1977). *Textbook of Work Physiology*, 2nd ed. McGraw-Hill Book Company.

Fox, Samuel M., Naughton, John P., and Gorman, Patrick A. (1972). 'Physical Activity and Cardiovascular Health.' *Modern Concepts of Cardiovascular Disease*, **XLI**, 4. (An official Journal of the American Heart Association.)

Royal Canadian Air Force. *Physical Fitness*. Penguin Books.

BIBLIOGRAPHY

Carson, P. et al (1973). 'Exercise Programme after Myocardial Infarction.' *British Medical Journal*, **6088**, 651.

Goble, R. E. A., Morgan, D. C. and Shaw, D. B. (1976). 'Rehabilitation in Heart Disease.' *Physiotherapy*, **62**, 11.

Lowenthal, S. L. and McAllister, R. G. (1976). 'Program for Cardiac Patients: Stress Testing and Training.' *Physical Therapy*, **56**, 10.

Morgans, Colin M. and Buston, Winifred M. (1972). 'Supervised Circuit Training after Myocardial Infarction.' *Physiotherapy*, **58**, 10.

Muldoon, D. E. (1972). 'Physiotherapy in the Rehabilitation of the Coronary Patient.' *Physiotherapy*, **58**, 10.

Nixon, P. G. F. (1972). 'Rehabilitation of the Coronary Patient.' *Physiotherapy*, **58**, 10.

Pantridge, J. F. and Adgey, A. A. (1972). 'Heart Attacks and Coronary Care.' *Physiotherapy*, **58**, 10.

Royston, G. R. (1972). 'Short-stay hospital treatment and rapid rehabilitation of cases of myocardial infarction in a district hospital.' *British Heart Journal*, **6088**, 651.

Sanne, H. (1973). 'Exercise Tolerance and Physical Training of Non-Selected Patients after Myocardial Infarction.' *Acta Medica Scandinavica*, Supplement, 551.

Thornley, P. E. and Turner, R. W. D. (1971). 'Rapid Mobilisation after Acute Myocardial Infarction.' *British Heart Journal*, **39**, 471.

McCoy, Patricia (1978). 'Rehabilitation following uncomplicated Myocardial Infarction.' *Physiotherapy*, **64**, 6.

Hampton, J. R. (1973). *The E. C. G. Made Easy*. Churchill Livingstone.
Verel, D. (1973). *Essential Cardiology: A Guide to Important Principles*. Medical and Technical Publishing Co. Ltd.

ACKNOWLEDGEMENT

The author wishes to record her thanks to all the staff of the Coronary Care Unit, the Ulster Hospital, Dundonald, Belfast. Her special thanks go to Dr. D. Boyle, M.D. and Miss S. E. Robinson, M.C.S.P., who initially stimulated her interest in Cardiac Rehabilitation. She wishes also to thank the Principal and staff of the School of Health Sciences, Faculty of Social and Health Science, Ulster College, the Northern Ireland Polytechnic, Newtownabbey, Co. Antrim BT37 OQB, Northern Ireland.

Chapter 23

A Use of Lung Function Studies

by L. H. CAPEL, M.D., F.R.C.P.

Lung function studies can help the physiotherapist assess the severity of disorders of lung function in her patients, and their response to treatment. The use of lung function studies for diagnosis is more the responsibility of medical colleagues. A discussion of the main features of lung function and the assessment of lung function in relationship to the common lung disorders may prove a useful introduction to the subject. It is also useful to an understanding of auscultation.

Lung Function and Lung Failure

The release of chemical energy within the cells of the body for the life process involves a complex series of linked chemical changes in which hydrogen ions move from one chemical system to another. At the end of the chain of reaction the hydrogen ions are mopped up by oxygen molecules in a process which forms carbon dioxide and water, which must be excreted. The function of the lungs is to exchange all the oxygen and nearly all the carbon dioxide (a small amount is excreted as bicarbonate by the kidneys) with the atmosphere. Failure of the lungs to take up oxygen or give off carbon dioxide as fast as metabolism demands leads to an accumulation of hydrogen ions in the body.

Respiratory Failure

Initially the blood becomes more acid (pH falls). The electro-positive hydrogen ions are buffered, that is, neutralised by electro-negative blood chemicals such as bicarbonate ions. The pH moves to the normal range again, but the blood bicarbonate will have risen because some of the excess hydrogen ions (positive) will have combined with bicarbonate ions (negative) in the buffering process. Evidence for the existence of respiratory failure is one or more abnormalities of the blood gases:

1. raised arterial blood carbon dioxide partial pressure
2. lowered arterial blood oxygen saturation and partial pressure
3. lowered arterial blood pH (i.e. raised blood hydrogen ion concentration; the pH notation is a simple mathematical convention which can confuse most doctors; we use it as an index)
4. increased blood bicarbonate concentration.

It is not uncommon for reduced blood oxygen saturation (and therefore partial pressure) to be the only abnormality.

THE CAUSES OF RESPIRATORY FAILURE

Respiratory failure can arise from a) disorder outside the lungs (nerves, muscle and skeleton), b) disorder of the lungs themselves, and c) disorder of the heart and blood vessels. For completion we might add that respiratory failure (with initial normal lung function) can also be caused by abnormality of the inspired air. These inspired air abnormalities are gases which are wrong in concentration or partial pressure, or toxic. Common examples are low oxygen partial pressure at altitude, toxic gases in fire, factory and home, and some complications of anaesthesia. Haemoglobin poisons, such as carbon monoxide and severe anaemia, interfere with oxygen transport to the cells. Cell poisons such as cyanide prevent the use of oxygen transported to the cells. Each of the above causes respiratory failure.

DISORDER OUTSIDE THE LUNGS

Neuromuscular Damage

Impairment of consciousness by head injury, drug overdose or anaesthetic may be as dangerous for the depression of lung ventilation which results, as from any damage elsewhere. Nerve damage without impairment of consciousness, for example in poliomyelitis and acute polyneuritis, impairs lung ventilation by preventing normal function of the intercostal muscles. The diaphragm may be paralysed on one side by a neoplasm involving the phrenic nerve.

Thorax: Fractured or Distorted

Fractured thorax is common after steering wheel injury (no seat belt!) on the roads and industrial and other crush accidents.

The danger is flail chest wall, that is, the chest wall falls in on inspiration preventing lung expansion and inhalation of air. (First aid, incidentally, is to strap the chest).

The distorted thorax of kyphoscoliosis causes lung failure only when severe, and in later years. The damage to lung function arises from uneven ventilation of the lungs which causes arterial blood oxygen unsaturation. Interestingly enough, in kyphosis without scoliosis, as in ankylosing spondylitis, impairment of lung ventilation is symmetrical, and so there is no uneven ventilation of the lungs and hence no arterial blood unsaturation. We shall see how uneven ventilation of the lungs can result in unsaturation.

Pleural Disorder

Pneumothorax, pleural effusion, hydropneumothorax and thickening of the pleura reduce the volume of the lung and also impair ventilation.

LUNG DISORDER

Lung function may be impaired by a) airway narrowing, b) by alveolar damage or loss and c) by bloodway narrowing or block (pulmonary arteries, alveolar capillaries and pulmonary veins). The airway, alveoli and bloodway all may be involved in any particular illness, but commonly we discuss the illness as if disorder of one system predominates. Because airway narrowing is the commonest feature of lung disorder and because there are simple and precise ways of detecting and assessing it, it is customary to distinguish two main groups of lung disorder: lung disorder with airway narrowing, i.e. obstructive lung disorder and lung disorder without airway narrowing, i.e. non-obstructive lung disorder. Non-obstructive lung disorder is commonly called restrictive lung disorder. Most people find the term restrictive convenient; I dislike it as it means no more than non-obstructive and may obscure the great uncertainty which may exist about the description of the lung disorder in question. These disorders may be unevenly distributed about the lung. This unevenness of distribution is important.

Airway Narrowing With and Without Alveolar Disorder

Local airway narrowing is commonly caused by neoplasm or foreign body.

General airway narrowing is caused by a) excess secretion in the

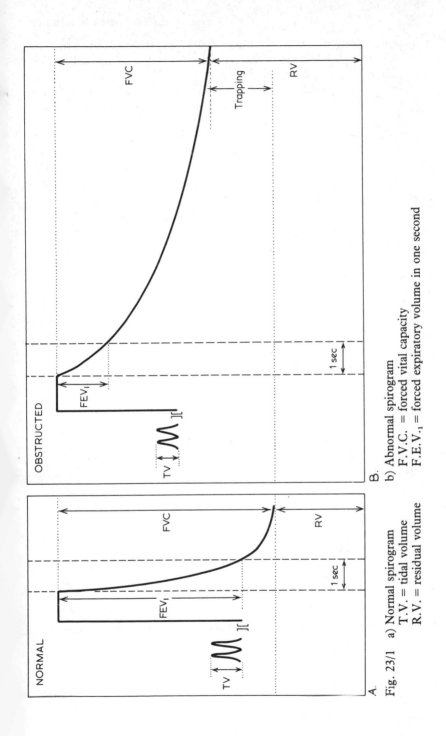

Fig. 23/1 a) Normal spirogram
T.V. = tidal volume
R.V. = residual volume

b) Abnormal spirogram
F.V.C. = forced vital capacity
F.E.V.₁ = forced expiratory volume in one second

airway, b) congestion of the mucous membrane lining the airway, c) spasm of smooth muscle in the wall of the airway and d) pressure on the airway by the air trapping mechanism. Air trapping is a consequence of loss of alveolar elasticity. In quiet breathing expiration is mainly passive: the thorax and diaphragm relax, and the lung expires air by elastic retraction of alveoli stretched during the previous inspiration. If this elasticity is lost, then expiration must be by outside pressure on the alveoli from thorax and diaphragm. This pressure falls also on the airway, narrowing it and in places closing it, so making expiration difficult and trapping air in the lungs (see Fig. 23/1b). Because of trapping, total lung volume increases. Residual lung volume (see Fig. 23/1a and 1b) i.e. the volume of air left in the lungs at the end of a complete expiration, also increases. This is another way of saying that the patient is breathing with the lungs in a more inflated position than in health. In some patients with long standing airway narrowing the inflated chest posture and tense neck muscles are all too obvious. If we look at the spirogram of a patient in health (see Fig. 23/1a) or with airway narrowing (see Fig. 23/1b) we see that the slope becomes steeper towards the position of full inspiration. The steeper the slope on the trace the faster the airflow making it: it follows that the more inflated the lung, the faster it can blow. In addition to the high shoulders and the inflated chest, the patient with very severe airway narrowing (usually due to emphysema) may breathe out through pursed lips. It is as if there is an attempt to pull on the connective tissue airway supports by inflating the chest, and to exert back pressure from the lips on their inside by pursed lip expiration so opposing the tendency to airway closure by trapping.

A simultaneous recording of inspired and expired airflow velocity and of the moment-to-moment lung volume at which the flow volume occurs shows this dramatically. Figure 23/2a is from a healthy individual. It shows tidal breathing at rest and the recording made during forced inspiration and forced expiration. The forced inspiratory flow rate increases and decreases smoothly as the lungs fill from the fully expired to fully inspired position. The forced expiratory flow rate, on the other hand, rises sharply and then falls rapidly because of the expiratory airway narrowing which occurs even in health. In airway narrowing (due to emphysema) the pattern of tidal breathing at rest more or less resembles that in health (see Fig. 23/2b and 3a). On forced inspiration in emphysema there is a smooth change as in health, only with lower peak flow rate at the mid-inspiratory maximum (see Fig. 23/2b and 3a). On forced expiration, however, the rapid increase in flow rate is soon slowed, and maximum forced expiration, because of trapping, results in a flow rate no greater than that achieved during

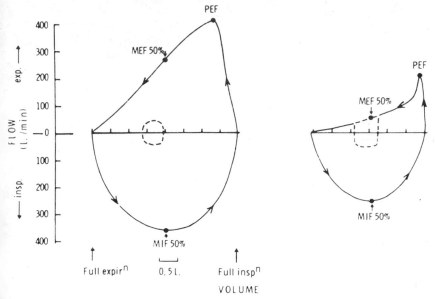

Fig. 23/2   a) Normal flow volume curve. b) Flow volume curve in a patient with airways obstruction. M.E.F. = mid-expiratory flow M.I.F. = mid-inspiratory flow P.E.F. = peak expiratory flow

quiet breathing (see Fig. 23/2b and 3a). This is the burden of severe emphysema: the harder the patient tries to breathe out, the more difficult it is for him.

Figure 23/3b shows an experiment in which an expiratory obstruction (a 4mm hole) mimics pursed lip breathing. The arrow points to a slight increase in expired flow velocity in this case. This form of recording forced expiration and inspiration, the flow volume curve, is informative, but the instruments are more complicated and costly than those used for conventional spirometry. Mathematically the flow/volume curve shown here is identical with the volume/time curve of conventional spirometry, and for clinical management spirometry is much more practical.

Airway narrowing reduces the vital capacity (V.C.) of the lungs (see Fig. 23/1a and 1b), that is, the largest volume of air which can be slowly expired after a full inspiration. In lung disorder with airway narrowing we have seen that both the total lung capacity and the residual lung volume are increased. Further, residual lung volume is increased proportionately more than total lung capacity. Since the vital capacity is the largest breath and vital capacity plus residual

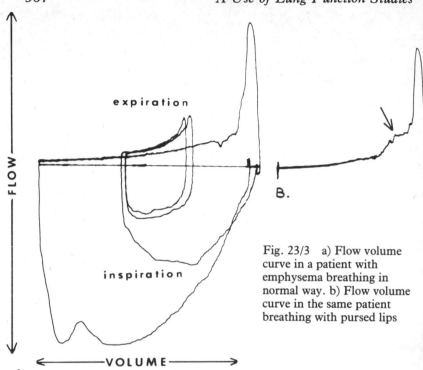

Fig. 23/3   a) Flow volume curve in a patient with emphysema breathing in normal way. b) Flow volume curve in the same patient breathing with pursed lips

volume equals total lung capacity, it follows that vital capacity in airway narrowing will be reduced – squeezed out as it were, by the increase in the residual volume.

There is another way of looking at this reduction in vital capacity. At the end of a full expiration in both healthy persons and in those with lung disorders the vital capacity is limited by closure of the airways. In airway narrowing the trapping mechanism closes the airways sooner than would have occurred in the healthy lung.

In patients with airway narrowing the vital capacity is not only smaller in volume than expected for an individual of the patient's age, sex and stature, it is also more slowly expired. This is seen from the shallow slope of the Forced Expiratory Spirogram (see Fig. 23/1b). The spirogram trace is shallow because the recording paper moves a long way horizontally as the pen travels slowly down. If you visit the lung function testing department of your hospital, or use a recording spirometer yourself, this will usually be seen dramatically during the most routine testing sessions. As an index of the speed at which the vital capacity can be expired we record the maximum volume of air which can be forcibly expired in one second during a complete expiration after a full inspiration, the F.E.V.$_1$ (see Fig. 23/1a and 1b). The trace also gives us the Forced Vital Capacity, the F.V.C., which is smaller than the slow or relaxed vital capacity because forcible expiration traps air more effectively than slow expiration. The F.E.V.$_1$ is an important index of airway narrowing; its magnitude depends not only on the severity of airway narrowing but also, because it is related to the vital capacity, on the age, sex, and stature of the subject. We can greatly reduce the influence of age, sex and stature and greatly increase the usefulness of the F.E.V.$_1$ as an index of the severity of airway narrowing by expressing it as a percentage of the V.C. or F.V.C. (F.E.V.$_1$ %V.C. or F.E.V.$_1$ %F.V.C.). We can say that if the F.E.V.$_1$ %V.C. is less than 75 then some airway narrowing is probable, and if it is less than 70 then airway narrowing is almost certain; the smaller the percentage the more severe the airway narrowing. A patient with severe airway narrowing may have an F.E.V.$_1$ %V.C. in the region of 30 to 40, for example. All these figures are, of course, suggestions. The normal value for F.E.V.$_1$ % is commonly given as 80, presumably for healthy non-smokers. It is of interest that in a group of apparently healthy ambulance drivers I found the average F.E.V.$_1$ %V.C. to be 75, presumably because most were smokers.

Spirometry and other simple methods may be used to assess the presence and severity of airway narrowing and any change in its severity with the progress of the disorder or in response to treatment. This is perhaps the most important practical use of lung function testing for the physiotherapist.

Clinical Patterns of Airway Narrowing

Airway narrowing is the functional feature common to bronchitis, asthma and emphysema. Bronchitis is recognised by cough and expectoration – a clinical definition, asthma by variable airway narrowing – a functional definition, and emphysema by inflation of alveoli and breakdown of alveolar walls – a histological definition. These conditions are not uncommonly found together in older persons.

Asthma is common in younger people, and cough and expectoration (bronchitis) may be a feature of it as well as wheeze. In some asthmatics the only evidence may be the symptom of wheeze at night or wheeze on exercise, with normal spirometry when tested at rest during the day. In most asthmatics, however, spirometry will show the characteristic variability: an increase in values of 15–20% after isoprenaline inhalation.

Bronchitis becomes commoner after middle age. Most bronchitics suffering disability from it are smokers. If cough and expectoration is present for as much as three months of the year for as long as two years, it is chronic. Spirometry shows airway narrowing and some degree of reversibility in the typical chronic bronchitic. It would be reasonable to say that the condition is bronchitis with asthma according to our definition, but some variability of airway narrowing in chronic bronchitis is taken for granted. Troublesome cough and expectoration without important airway narrowing by spirometry can be a feature of bronchiectasis: this is fortunately now a rare condition but not uncommonly seen by the physiotherapist since physiotherapy is so important in its management. Bronchitis, asthma and bronchiectasis have this in common, that to a greater or lesser extent in each case they respond to management.

Emphysema is irreversible: spirometry typically shows severe slightly variable (say about 10%) airway narrowing. The chest radiograph shows the inflated transradiant lung fields consequent on loss of lung tissue and loss of lung retractility. Management is by attempts to control the bronchitis and small degree of reversible airway narrowing which go with it, and by breathing exercises which attempt to help the patient breathe just a little more efficiently, that is, slightly to reduce the trapping effect. Unfortunately the physiotherapist will rarely be rewarded for her pains by an improvement in spirometry or other lung function tests. This may be because the tests are too crude, and, of course, tests of forced breathing would not show the results of relaxed breathing.

Alveolar Damage Without Airway Narrowing (Non-obstructive or restrictive disorders)

Alveoli may be involved in inflammation due to virus and bacteria infection, industrial toxins and the auto-immune processes. These are all forms of pneumonia. The process may be generalised or localised. It may be transient or it may proceed to fibrosis. Fibrosis leaves a smaller number of functioning alveoli, a smaller lung and a stiffer lung. The total lung capacity is reduced and this reduces the vital capacity. Since there is no air trapping the residual volume of the lung is not increased, and, indeed, it is reduced. Since the Vital Capacity (V.C.) is reduced the $F.E.V._1$ is reduced. Most important, however, the $F.E.V._1$ %V.C. is not reduced: it will remain over 70. Since the lung is stiff the airways will be well held against the trapping tendency, and in patients with severe pulmonary fibrosis we may even see the $F.E.V._1$ %V.C. higher than the normal value – say over 80.

SPIROMETRY AND DISORDERS WITH AND WITHOUT AIRWAY
NARROWING

Thus the F.E.V.$_1$ %V.C. ratio is used to distinguish lung disorders
with and without airway narrowing. We might go further and say that
reduction in the V.C. is an index of the presence of lung disorder of
any sort, and the F.E.V.$_1$ %V.C. may be used to distinguish obstructive from non-obstructive disorder. Unfortunately there is a snag: we
cannot know what the patient's vital capacity would be if well, and so
must rely on Tables of predicted values. It is only when the patients
are more than, say, 20% below predicted that we can say that they are
abnormal. This is very crude, and there are many patients with lung
disorder whose V.C. is in the normal range. The F.E.V.$_1$ %V.C. is,
however, a reliable index of the presence or absence of airway narrowing which can be severe enough to cause symptoms.

Pulmonary embolism causes bloodway narrowing by obstruction.
Diagnosis of this condition is not straightforward. It is more likely to
affect the blood gases than to affect spirometry.

Patients with *emotional hyperventilation* may come the physiotherapist's way. This may occur in patients with healthy lungs (sor-
row, worry and frustration bring on the trouble), and in patients with
lung disorder (especially asthma).

This emotional hyperventilation may be diagnosed by noticing the
occasional deep inspiration with sighing, and often confirmed by
showing that blood carbon dioxide is low. Occasionally there will be
plain hysteria or malingering, recognised by a very irregular spirogram: it begins well and becomes uneven, or begins uneven and ends
reasonably well. It is difficult to fake the spirogram.

USE OF LUNG FUNCTION TESTS

Lung function tests may be used to help in the management of
patients and academically to help in the study of lung disease. The
tests of practical use to the physiotherapist are the simple tests of
ventilatory capacity for patients with airway narrowing, and blood gas
analysis for patients with severe acute illness. Tests of ventilatory
capacity give some information about the nature of the lung disorder.
Careful assessment of effort intolerance grading and blood gas analysis
give some information on the consequence of the disorder, and sometimes something of the nature of the disorder may be inferred as well.
How can these tests be useful to the physiotherapist?

Tests of Ventilatory Capacity

Tests of ventilatory capacity are made with a spirometer which may be wet or dry. These spirometers will give recordings of the V.C. The F.V.C. and the F.E.V.$_1$ %V.C. can be derived for the diagnosis of airway narrowing and as an index of its severity, as we have seen. If the diagnosis of airway narrowing has been made then measurement of the Peak Expiratory Flow Rate (P.E.F.R.) is a convenient instrument (indeed, the most convenient), to give an index of its severity. The P.E.F.R. is recorded using a Peak Flow Meter or a Peak Flow Gauge. Recording of the Forced Expiratory Time (F.E.T.), (the time required to complete a forced expiration after a full inspiration), may be carried out using only a watch: over six seconds suggests airway narrowing.

Airway narrowing is present if the F.E.V.$_1$ %V.C., the P.E.F.R. or the F.E.T. are reduced. The chest radiograph may be normal, or show inflated lung fields. Variability of the airway narrowing is shown by an increase in the V.C., the F.V.C., the F.E.V.$_1$ or P.E.F.R. about five minutes after isoprenaline inhalation (isoprenaline is potent and quick acting). An increase of 15% is a common arbitrary choice. The F.E.V.$_1$ %V.C. is not a useful index of variability since both F.E.V.$_1$ and V.C. tend to change in the same direction, and so the change in the ratio may be small. Whether this variability is called asthma is a matter of definition. In patients with airway narrowing ventilatory capacity can vary considerably during the day, and this must be taken into account in assessing response to management. Ventilatory capacity is nearly always at its lowest ebb on rising from sleep. Some asthmatics are especially bad at this time. These patients have been called morning dippers because their Peak Flow can be low (very occasionally dangerously low) at this time.

Diffuse lung disorder without airway narrowing is present if there is diffuse radiological change, commonly indicating pulmonary fibrosis, with or without reduction in vital capacity and with the F.E.V.$_1$ %V.C. and P.E.F.R. in the normal range. Of course pulmonary fibrosis and airway narrowing will often be found together. The efficient management of the airway narrowing is then specially important.

Blood Gas Analysis and pH

Attention to blood gas analysis is important to the physiotherapist mainly in the management of the acutely ill patient. Here the main dangers are arterial blood oxygen unsaturation and the fall in arterial blood pH which may go with it.

What can cause arterial blood oxygen unsaturation? Alveolar damage and alveolar loss, especially in lungs already damaged, are obvious causes. Less obvious but more important is uneven matching of ventilation and circulation in different parts of the lungs. Ventilation/perfusion imbalance is a commonly used term for this. In a healthy person at rest something like five litres of air and five litres of blood per minute meet in the three hundred million alveoli of the lung, where they are separated by alveolar tissue thinner than the finest paper. A red blood cell flicks through an alveolar capillary in less than one second. During this time, in health and disease, it reaches the same oxygen and carbon dioxide partial pressure as the air in the alveolus. Partial pressure is not an easy concept. Air contains about 21% oxygen. At sea level where the barometric pressure is about 760 millimetres of mercury (mm Hg) this pressure is made up mainly by the pressure exerted by oxygen, nitrogen and water vapour. The pressure of water vapour is about 50mm Hg, leaving 710mm Hg for oxygen and nitrogen; 21% of 710mm Hg is about 150mm Hg, which is the partial pressure of oxygen in the lungs. Up a high mountain the air is rarefied and though it still contains 21% oxygen, the partial pressure of oxygen will be much less.

We must now relate partial pressure of oxygen in the blood to oxygen saturation. A remarkable feature of haemoglobin is the disproportionate relationship between its oxygen saturation and oxygen partial pressure. Oxygen saturation of haemoglobin is the ratio of the oxygen content of the haemoglobin to the capacity of the haemoglobin to hold oxygen when fully saturated: it is the ratio of the oxygen it actually does hold, to its maximum capacity to hold oxygen. The relationship between oxygen partial pressure and oxygen saturation in the blood is such that it facilitates oxygen uptake in the lungs and delivery by the blood to the tissues in the body.

Now to the question again: how does ventilation/perfusion imbalance cause saturation? Let us assume that half the alveoli in the lungs are working normally and half abnormally in that they are receiving too little ventilation for their circulation. The blood leaving the underventilated alveoli will be unsaturated. Blood leaving the well-ventilated alveoli will be normally saturated. The mixture of saturated and unsaturated blood gives unsaturation. Can an increase in the ventilation of the good alveoli take up more oxygen and so make up for the poorly ventilated alveoli? NO: because the blood leaving the well-ventilated alveoli is already 100% saturated, and blood cannot be more than 100% saturated. So unevenness of ventilation and perfusion must lead to arterial blood oxygen unsaturation and the dire consequences of this.

Let us now examine some typical findings for the blood gas analysis in some common conditions.

1. *In mild chronic asthma* the blood gases are normal. With a slight increase in severity the arterial blood carbon dioxide pressure (P_{CO_2}) tends to fall while the oxygen partial pressure (P_{O_2}) remains normal. We may say that the patient is 'overventilating'. If the condition worsens then the P_{O_2} can begin to fall, a worrying event. If the arterial blood P_{CO_2} then rises, and the arterial blood P_{O_2} falls the situation is dangerous. Incidentally, an increasing pulse rate will be a simple indication of this bad turn of events. For the asthmatic in respiratory disorders we give oxygen in high concentration (35–40%) to help the unsaturation and the high oxygen cost of the laboured breathing.

2. *As bronchitis with emphysema* becomes more severe so that the arterial blood P_{O_2} tends to fall and the arterial blood P_{CO_2} to rise. The pH is likely to remain in the normal range except in dangerous acute exacerbations with low P_{O_2} and high P_{CO_2}. In severe exacerbations oxygen is given in low enrichment concentration at first (say 24%) because it may cause drowsiness and decrease ventilation so increasing the arterial blood P_{CO_2} and reducing the pH (contrast this with the alert frightened hard breathing asthmatic). The pH falls because hydrogen ions are accumulating and CO_2 is remaining as carbonic acid.

3. *In pure emphysema* the blood gases may be normal at rest even though the patient is housebound. This is because the damage to ventilation and circulation are each evenly distributed about the lung with respect to each other: alveolar damage affects alveolar ventilation and alveolar capillary circulation more or less equally. With exertion in emphysema the P_{O_2} falls and the P_{CO_2} rises.

Note that a patient with chronic bronchitis and emphysema with reduced P_{O_2} and raised P_{CO_2} can go shopping, while the same blood gas findings in a patient with asthma or emphysema could mean dangerous acute illness. It will have been guessed by now that there is no necessarily close relationship between ventilatory capacity and the blood gases.

4. *In pulmonary fibrosis* without obstruction the P_{O_2} may be at the lower limit of normal with the P_{CO_2} also at the lower limit of normal. The patient can and does increase breathing. This reduces the P_{CO_2}, the level of which tends to follow the ventilation volume, but ventilation perfusion imbalance keeps the P_{O_2} low.

5. *In pulmonary embolism* the findings are the same. Here there will be alveoli ventilated but not circulated. There will be a loss of effective alveolar surface area and slight fall in arterial blood P_{O_2}. There will be

a fall in P_{CO_2} because the patient tends to increase the volume of ventilation.

6. *In kyphoscoliosis* of any severity ventilation of the lungs is uneven, and some regions of the lungs underventilated. Towards the end of life this may cause arterial blood oxygen unsaturation and the complications which follow.

7. *Cor pulmonale* or, as I prefer to call it, *hypoxaemic heart failure* arises from chronic hypoxaemia, that is, prolonged reduction in arterial blood P_{O_2}. This increases pulmonary artery resistance and hence pulmonary artery pressure, which in turn adds an extra burden to the right ventricle. The overburdened right ventricle enlarges – its volume increases and its wall thickens. The neck veins become engorged and the ankles swell. Less obvious will be the brain damage (a very irritable patient often) and damage to liver and kidneys. Hypoxaemia both slows the machinery and damages the works. In addition to the heart failure there will, of course, be the burden of the chronic lung disease which caused the hypoxaemia: this may be obstruction when the F.E.V.$_1$ %V.C. will be low and the P_{CO_2} high, as in severe bronchitis with emphysema, or non-obstructive, when the F.E.V.$_1$ %V.C. will be normal and the P_{CO_2} normal or reduced. Diuretics are important in management as they remove water via the kidneys from all tissues, including the lungs. This enables the lungs to ventilate better.

Effort Tolerance Grading

Whatever the patient's condition, and whether due to lung or other disorder, a careful note of the severity of the patient's effort intolerance will help in recording the severity of their condition and change in outpatients, and in assessing the other tests used. The following grading (it closely resembles the Medical Research Council Grading) is recommended:

EFFORT INTOLERANCE GRADES	
0. Can hurry up hill 1. Unable to hurry up hill 2. Unable to hurry on level	Mild
3. Unable to maintain normal walking pace on level 4. Unable to walk $\frac{1}{4}$ hour ($\frac{1}{4}$ mile approx.) without stopping	Moderate
5. Unable to walk 3 mins. (100 yards) without stopping	Severe

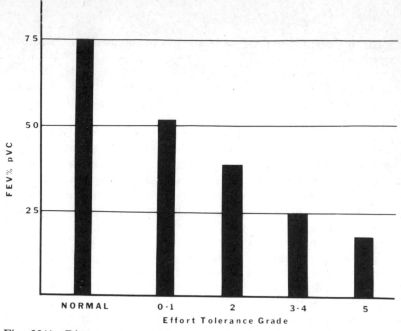

Fig. 23/4 Diagram showing the relationship between the effort tolerance grading and the F.E.V. % pV.C. (predicted vital capacity)

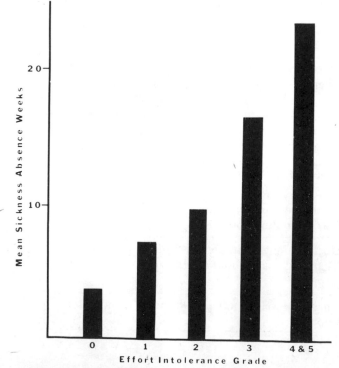

Fig. 23/5 Diagram, showing the relationship between the effort tolerance grading and the mean sickness absence

In two large series of patients with airway narrowing seen at the London Chest Hospital it was found that this grading of effort into-lerance was fairly closely related to the F.E.V.₁ percentage of pre-dicted Vital Capacity (see Fig. 23/4) and sickness absence during the preceding three years (see Fig. 23/5).

Auscultation

Auscultation in conjunction with the chest radiograph will help in the assessment of the severity of airway narrowing and in the detection of lung congestion, lung fibrosis, bronchiectasis and emphysema.

Clearing the Airway

The physiotherapist's help in the management of patients with acute lung disorder with retention of secretions and in the management and training of patients with asthma, bronchitis, bronchiectasis and cystic fibrosis can be the key to their improvement. Lung function tests can help in assessing progress and their study can help towards a better understanding of patients suffering the burden of lung disorder.

BIBLIOGRAPHY

Comroe, J. H. (1974) *The Lung: Clinical Physiology and Pulmonary Function Tests*, 2nd ed. Year Book Medical Publishers. Chicago, U.S.A.

ACKNOWLEDGEMENT

The author thanks Mr. D. Connolly, A.R.P.S., the Principal Photographer of the Institute of Laryngology, London, for his help with the illustrations and Mrs. Carol Hodder and Mrs. Jane Jones for preparing the material for them.

List of Useful Organisations

Action on Smoking and Health (ASH)
27/35 Mortimer Street
London W1N 7RJ   01–637 9843

Asthma Research Council
12 Pembridge Square
London W2 4EH   01–229 1149

The British Heart Foundation
57 Gloucester Place
London W1H 4DH   01–935 0185

The British Thoracic and Tuberculosis Association
30 Britten Street
London SW3 6NN   01–352 2194

The Chest, Heart and Stroke Association
Tavistock House North, Tavistock Square
London WC1H 9JE   01–387 3012

The Chest, Heart and Stroke Association (Scotland)
65 North Castle Street
Edinburgh EH2 3LT   031–225 6527

The Cystic Fibrosis Research Trust
5 Blyth Road, Bromley
Kent BR1 3RS   01–464 7211

Index